Comprehensive Virology 15

Comprehensive Virology

Edited by Heinz Fraenkel-Conrat
University of California at Berkeley

and Robert R. Wagner
University of Virginia

Editorial Board

Comprehensive

Edited by

Heinz Fraenkel-Conrat

Department of Molecular Biology and Virus Laboratory
University of California, Berkeley, California

and

Robert R. Wagner

Department of Microbiology
University of Virginia, Charlottesville, Virginia

Virology

15

Virus-Host Interactions

Immunity to Viruses

PLENUM PRESS · NEW YORK AND LONDON

Library of Congress Cataloging in Publication Data

Fraenkel-Conrat, Heinz, 1910-
  Virus-host interactions.

  (Their Comprehensive virology; v. 15)
  Includes index.
  1. Host-virus relationships. 2. Virus diseases—Immunological aspects. I. Wagner,
Robert R., 1923-   joint author. II. Title. III. Series. [DNLM: I. Viruses—Im-
munology. II. Immunity. QW160 C737 v. 15]
QR357-.F72 vol. 15 [QR492]   576'.64'08s [616.9'2]   79-26533
ISBN 0-306-40262-9

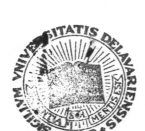
© 1979 Plenum Press, New York
A Division of Plenum Publishing Corporation
227 West 17th Street, New York, N.Y. 10011

Printed in the United States of America

Foreword

The time seems ripe for a critical compendium of that segment of the biological universe we call viruses. Virology, as a science, having passed only recently through its descriptive phase of naming and numbering, has probably reached that stage at which relatively few new—truly new—viruses will be discovered. Triggered by the intellectual probes and techniques of molecular biology, genetics, biochemical cytology, and high resolution microscopy and spectroscopy, the field has experienced a genuine information explosion.

Few serious attempts have been made to chronicle these events. This comprehensive series, which will comprise some 6000 pages in a total of about 18 volumes, represents a commitment by a large group of active investigators to analyze, digest, and expostulate on the great mass of data relating to viruses, much of which is now amorphous and disjointed, and scattered throughout a wide literature. In this way, we hope to place the entire field in perspective, and to develop an invaluable reference and sourcebook for researchers and students at all levels.

This series is designed as a continuum that can be entered anywhere, but which also provides a logical progression of developing facts and integrated concepts.

Volume 1 contains an alphabetical catalogue of almost all viruses of vertebrates, insects, plants, and protists, describing them in general terms. Volumes 2–4 deal primarily, but not exclusively, with the processes of infection and reproduction of the major groups of viruses in their hosts. Volume 2 deals with the simple RNA viruses of bacteria, plants, and animals; the togaviruses (formerly called arboviruses), which share with these only the feature that the virion's RNA is able to act as messenger RNA in the host cell; and the reoviruses of animals and plants, which all share several structurally singular features, the most important being the double-strandedness of their multiple RNA molecules.

Volume 3 addresses itself to the reproduction of all DNA-containing viruses of vertebrates, encompassing the smallest and the largest viruses known. The reproduction of the larger and more complex RNA viruses is the subject matter of Volume 4. These viruses share the property of being enclosed in lipoprotein membranes, as do the togaviruses included in Volume 2. They share as a group, along with the reoviruses, the presence of polymerase enzymes in their virions to satisfy the need for their RNA to become transcribed before it can serve messenger functions.

Volumes 5 and 6 represent the first in a series that focuses primarily on the structure and assembly of virus particles. Volume 5 is devoted to general structural principles involving the relationship and specificity of interaction of viral capsid proteins and their nucleic acids, or host nucleic acids. It deals primarily with helical and the simpler isometric viruses, as well as with the relationship of nucleic acid to protein shell in the T-even phages. Volume 6 is concerned with the structure of the picornaviruses, and with the reconstitution of plant and bacterial RNA viruses.

Volumes 7 and 8 deal with the DNA bacteriophages. Volume 7 concludes the series of volumes on the reproduction of viruses (Volumes 2–4 and Volume 7) and deals particularly with the single- and double-stranded virulent bacteriophages.

Volume 8, the first of the series on regulation and genetics of viruses, covers the biological properties of the lysogenic and defective phages, the phage-satellite system P 2–P 4, and in-depth discussion of the regulatory principles governing the development of selected lytic phages.

Volume 9 provides a truly comprehensive analysis of the genetics of all animal viruses that have been studied to date. These chapters cover the principles and methodology of mutant selection, complementation analysis, gene mapping with restriction endonucleases, etc. Volume 10 also deals with animal cells, covering transcriptional and translational regulation of viral gene expression, defective virions, and integration of tumor virus genomes into host chromosomes.

Volume 11 covers the considerable advances in the molecular understanding of new aspects of virology which have been revealed in recent years through the study of plant viruses. It covers particularly the mode of replication and translation of the multicomponent viruses and others that carry or utilize subdivided genomes; the use of protoplasts in such studies is authoritatively reviewed, as well as the nature of viroids, the smallest replicatable pathogens. Volume 12 deals with special groups of viruses of protists and invertebrates which show properties that set them apart from the main virus families. These are the lipid-containing phages and the viruses of algae, fungi, and invertebrates.

Volume 13 contains chapters on various topics related to the structure and assembly of viruses, dealing in detail with nucleotide and amino acid sequences, as well as with particle morphology and assembly, and the structure of virus membranes and hybrid viruses. The first complete sequence of a viral RNA is represented as a multicolored foldout.

Volume 14 contains chapters on special and/or newly characterized vertebrate virus groups: bunya-, arena-, corona-, calici-, and orbiviruses, icosahedral cytoplasmic deoxyriboviruses, fish viruses, and hepatitis viruses.

This volume deals with immunological reactions to viruses. Several subsequent volumes will deal with virus–host relationships and with methodological aspects of virus research.

Contents

Chapter 2

Interaction of Viruses with Neutralizing Antibodies

Benjamin Mandel

Chapter 3

Humoral Immunity to Viruses

Neil R. Cooper

Chapter 4

Cellular Immune Response to Viruses and the Biological Role of Polymorphic Major Transplantation Antigens

R. M. Zinkernagel

Chapter 5

Interferons

E. De Maeyer and J. De Maeyer-Guignard

Immune Responses, Immune Tolerance, and Viruses

Michael B. A. Oldstone

Department of Immunopathology
Scripps Clinic and Research Foundation
La Jolla, California 92037

1. INTRODUCTION

Exactly how viruses or other microbes can persist in the host they invade is one of the most challenging problems in animal virology and an intellectual puzzle in biology. Because the immune system is responsible for purging these agents from the host, their continued presence has long been equated with partial or total malfunction of the appropriate immune response.

Reflecting on the early observations of Eric Traub (1936*a,b*) concerning natural infections of mice with lymphocytic choriomeningitis virus (LCMV) as well as examination of chimeric cattle by Ray Owen (1945), Burnett and Fenner postulated (1949, 1959) nearly three decades ago that clonal elimination of immunocompetent cells is the basis for immunological tolerance to viruses and self antigens, respectively. Immunological tolerance is defined as the state of specific refractoriness in responding to an antigen (virus) following a prior exposure to that antigen (virus). The concept that individuals can become immunologically tolerant to viruses, especially LCMV and retroviruses, was championed by many investigators during the 1950s and 1960s (Burnett and Fenner, 1949; Hotchin and Cinits, 1958; Volkert and Larsen, 1965; Traub, 1960; Gross, 1961). This conclusion followed observations that, after exposure to virus *in utero* or at birth, adult animals retained infectious virus throughout life, but free antibody(ies) to that virus was not detected in their circulations.

Reappraisal of this conclusion has paralleled the outburst of recent knowledge defining the subcomponent cell populations of the immune system and their interactions in generating immune responses, coupled with new technology for measuring immune response products, especially in the presence of virus. Although several unanswered questions remain, the overwhelming evidence indicates that immune responses accompany most, if not all, viral infections, and that classical immunological tolerance does not occur.

This chapter will present the evidence that has accumulated regarding the generation of antiviral immune responses during virus persistence. Toward understanding such responses to viruses, we will first describe immune responses to antigens other than virus as presently understood; then we will dissect immune responses and discuss ways of investigating immune tolerance.

2. IMMUNE SYSTEM

2.1. Organization, Interaction, and Genetic Control

Conceptually, over the last decade a revolution has occurred in our understanding of the biology and function of the immune system. It is now abundantly clear (1) that both the making of antibody and the mediation of immune responses by cells are end products of cellular collaboration, which is (2) associated with unique subsets of both thymus-derived (T) and bone-marrow-derived (B) lymphocytes, and (3) that regulation is under genetic control. The end result is measured as a specific immune response initiated by a specific antigen and associated with unique interactions among macrophages, T-cell subsets, and B cells. The immune product results from a series of minute regulations from a network of unique cells (Jerne, 1974) involving such events as cell–cell interactions and release of mediators that can enhance or suppress the immune response. Alterations in expected immune responses following exposure to antigens may occur at any one of several stages. Studies in which replicating agents are the antigens may lead to information concerning generation and control of immune responses. Further, viruses themselves, when they infect immunocompetent cells, may be used as probes toward understanding each step in lymphocyte differentiation and function.

Cell subsets of the immune system are often distinguished from one another in terms of their functions or the unique cell-surface determinants they carry (Raff, 1977; Mitchell, 1977; Gershon, 1974; Katz, 1977; Greaves *et al.*, 1974). On the basis of several properties, particularly their content of unique cell-surface determinants that bind specific reagents, reasonably homogeneous subsets can be segregated from the total populations of immune cells so that their functions and interactions can be analyzed. Evidence for cellular collaboration has been documented for T-cell–B-cell, T-cell–T-cell, T-cell–macrophage, and B-cell–macrophage interreactions. Cellular collaboration is exemplified as follows: antigen-specific helper factors are released from T lymphocytes bearing Ly1 antigens on their surfaces (helper T cells). These factors, under genetic restraints, bind to macrophages. In turn, macrophages induce a unique clone of B cells, again under genetic restriction, to proliferate and differentiate into plasma cells, which release specific antibody. Modulating effects between T-helper lymphocytes and T-suppressor lymphocytes are important in regulating such responses (reviewed in Katz, 1977).

The genetic control over antibody synthesis (McDevitt and Landy, 1972) has been noted at the level of B cells (Benacerraf and McDevitt, 1972; Taussig *et al.*, 1974), T cells (Benacerraf and McDevitt, 1972), and macrophages (Weiner and Bandieri, 1974). In addition, several cytotoxic T-cell responses to virus infections (Cole *et al.*, 1972; Doherty and Zinkernagel, 1974; Zinkernagel and Doherty, 1973) and to products of tissue- and adjuvant-induced autoimmune diseases, i.e., allergic encephalomyelitis (reviewed by Paterson, 1977; Gonatas and Howard, 1974; Williams and Moore, 1973), are under genetic restriction and regulation. Thus the control of immune responses is manifested in a number of different ways during virus infections and autoimmune responses.

2.2.   Measurement of Immune Responsiveness: Antigen-Binding Cells

Evaluating experiments on alterations of immune function (enhancement or suppression) requires knowledge of the strengths and limitations of techniques used to measure them. Total populations and subpopulations of immunocompetent cells can be measured on the basis of functional assays and unique cell-surface markers (Katz, 1977). However, some of these markers may change during differentiation. Hence detection and description of cell surface markers on lymphocytes are, in part, relative to the conditions of the assay. Despite the limitations, a vast and informative body of data now exists (Greaves *et al.*, 1974; Katz, 1977) and T-cell-specific helper cells, suppressor cells, and cytotoxic cells can be marked, segregated, and isolated. Antigen-specific immunocompetent cells can be detected by using radiolabeled antigens (Nossal and Ada, 1971) that react with specific receptors on T and/or B cells or their subpopulations. Hence antigen-specific T and/or B cells can be identified within a population and quantitated. In an extension of this technique, one uses antigen radiolabeled at a high specific activity so that cells binding this antigen can be eliminated on the basis of radioactive injury. Thereafter, the function usually performed by these cells is no longer present. The use of such an assay to cause suicide of antigen-specific cells in combination with reconstitution experiments has been helpful in charting specific immune response interactions.

2.3. Measurement of Immune Responsiveness: B-Cell Products (Antibodies)

When antibodies form and circulate free of antigen, they are easily detected by any of a wide variety of techniques (Lennette and Schmidt, 1979; Bloom and David, 1976). These consist of both primary (radiobinding assays, fluorescent binding assays) and secondary (complement fixation, hemagglutination inhibition, lysis of infected cells in the presence of complement or lymphocytes bearing Fc receptors) binding assays. In contrast, when antibodies and antigen are both present, antibody may not be detectable by such assays; instead one must measure antigen–antibody complexes (Oldstone and Perrin, 1979; Theofilopoulos and Dixon, 1976; Zubler and Lambert, 1976). When antibodies complex with antigen, their quantitation is difficult unless antibody is measured before it reaches the antigen. This is best done by quantitating the numbers of antibody-secreting cells in a Jerne plaque assay (Jerne and Nordin, 1963).

2.4. Measurement of Immune Responsiveness: T-Cell Activities

T-suppressor- and T-helper-specific functions are measured in biological systems in which enhanced or suppressed immunological activity is quantitated. For example, some *in vitro* assays use pokeweed mitogen to stimulate B cells in the presence of added T-helper or T-suppressor cells. The amount of immunoglobulin made and released in the fluid phase or the number of plasma cells generated in culture is quantitated (Moretta *et al.*, 1977; Oldstone *et al.*, 1977). The activity of cytotoxic T cells can be quantitated by the use of a ^{51}Cr release assay (Brunner *et al.*, 1976). Target cells tested are radiolabeled with ^{51}Cr and reacted with different amounts of primed cytotoxic T cells. The number of cytotoxic T cells present in the reaction correlates directly with the degree to which the lysed cells release ^{51}Cr.

3. IMMUNE RESPONSES IN NONVIRAL SYSTEMS

3.1. Immune Regulation

The tuning of the immune system is the result of a balance between factors that enhance and suppress the immune system. Lack of control leading to overbearing immune enhancement occurs, for example, with polyclonal activation of immune cells, which can lead to autoallergic reactions and resultant disease. This is not the subject of this chapter. The opposite extreme, immunological tolerance, will be considered in detail.

By definition, immune tolerance refers to the lack of response to an antigen previously contacted. Conceptually immune tolerance can occur via divergent mechanisms which may have their effects on B cells, T cells, and/or macrophages. Although the end stage is unresponsiveness, the routes to that end differ. Immune tolerance results from either central unresponsiveness or peripheral unresponsiveness.

3.2. Central Tolerance

Central tolerance or unresponsiveness refers to the irreversible loss of competent lymphocytes and can occur by clonal elimination or clonal dysfunction. Burnett originally postulated that a mechanism of clonal elimination could provide a biological basis for cell tolerance (1959). The scheme indicates that during T-cell, B-cell, or macrophage maturation, interaction with specific antigen may occur. The antigen binds with specific antigenic receptors on the cell surface, leading to the inactivation and clonal elimination of these potentially immune functioning cells. Thus far the most meaningful experiments in this vein involve B-cell tolerance, perhaps owing to the ease in measuring the final product, i.e., antibodies. Experimental evidence for central unresponsiveness has been provided in several laboratories (Chiller and Weigle, 1975; Katz and Benacerraf, 1974) by showing the deletion of specific antigen-binding cells. Although no antigen-binding cells should be detected during central tolerance (clonal deletion), they may similarly fail to form during peripheral unresponsiveness because of ligand interaction (see below). Before tolerance can be broken and immune responsiveness restored, new cells must regenerate from precursor stem-cell pools. Clonal deletion implies three major points. First, specific antigen-binding B or T lymphocytes must be absent. Second, in most systems studied, immunity is lacking during the induction period of tolerance. Third, maintenance of tolerance is dependent directly on the continued presence of antigen rather than indirectly on antigen-induced regulation factors such as suppressor cells or antigen–antibody complexes.

Clonal dysfunction indicates that the clones are not eliminated but rather lack normal activity that would produce immune responsiveness. Viruses are permissive for and can persist in cells of the immune system (Notkins *et al.*, 1970; Doyle and Oldstone, 1978; Popescu *et al.*, 1977). Could viruses alter lymphocyte function(s)? Although it is not known whether such lymphocyte dysfunction occurs, it is clear that viruses can persist in some differentiated cells (neuroblastomas) and alter their luxury (differentiation) function without altering their vital function (growth, cloning efficiency, survival). Differentiated functions of neuroblastoma cells (making the transferase and/or esterase needed to synthesize or degrade acetylcholine) can be uniquely impaired during persistent LCMV infection, both *in vitro* and *in vivo* without altering the vital functions of cultured cells or those in an intact animal (Oldstone *et al.*, 1977a). However, despite the many clinical observations of impaired immune responses during virus infections (von Pirquet, 1908; Notkins *et al.*, 1970), there is no direct evidence yet that viruses infecting lymphocytes or macrophages can cause their dysfunction without their death.

3.3. Peripheral Tolerance

Peripheral unresponsiveness indicates that cells competent for immune responses are present but cannot be induced to respond. Any of several mechanisms could produce peripheral tolerance. For example, ligands may induce inactivation of immunocompetent lymphocytes by receptor blockade, and not by their deletion. Antibodies generated to idiotypic or allotypic determinants of cell-surface receptors can bind and complex with receptors on the cell surface. The resultant antigen–antibody complex is internalized by the cell, and the receptor is cleared from its surface (reviewed by Schreiner and Unanue, 1976). Recent observations indicate that antibody-induced capping and modulation of immunoglobulin receptors on the surfaces of lymphocytes obtained from young (less than 2-week-old) mice lead to a marked delay in the reexpression of cell-surface antigens as compared to capping and modulation of lymphocytes taken from adult animals (Sidman and Unanue, 1975; Raff *et al.*, 1975). Hence the age and presumably state of differentiation of the immunocompetent cell at the time of ligand-induced inactivation can determine whether immune unresponsiveness occurs for a short time (less than 18 hr) or a long time (5–7 days, the length of time that murine lymphocytes were cultured). When ligand-induced inactivation occurs, previously immunocompetent cells thereafter lack the capacity to bind specific antigens; thus functionally no antigen-binding cells are present. The absence of antigen-binding cells, *per se*, does not differentiate central (deletion of cells) from peripheral (nondeletion) unresponsiveness.

Antibody-mediated suppression of specific immune responses occurs and can be accomplished experimentally with a wide variety of both soluble and particulate antigens. The mechanisms involved can be multiple. This includes the competition between antibody and antigen for recognition sites on immunocompetent cells and the formation of antigen–antibody complexes which in appropriate ratios may inhibit helper function and primed T cells or act at the macrophage level (reviewed in Katz, 1977). Further, antigen–antibody complexes at appropriate valences may be tolerogenic.

In addition to antibody-induced suppression resulting in immune unresponsiveness, suppressor cells actively inhibit various stages of immune responsiveness in many systems with the same end result (reviewed by Gershon, 1974; Gershon *et al.*, 1972; Ha *et al.*, 1974). Mice make suppressor cells in response to a variety of soluble and particulate nonviral antigens and may do so during virus infection (Rollinghoff *et al.*, 1977). Suppressor cells are believed to act via the secretion of a soluble product and have been defined in mice on the basis of expression both θ and Ly23 surface antigens. Suppressor T cells have also been demonstrated in humans (Moretta *et al.*, 1977; Oldstone *et al.*, 1977*b*; Waldman *et al.*, 1974). Of interest are the findings of Moretta *et al.* (1977) that T-suppressor cells, which have Fc receptors for human IgG (T.G), ordinarily remain inactive in the peripheral blood until activated by immune complexes. In contrast, such T-suppressor cells found in cord blood lymphocytes from human newborns are functionally active (Oldstone *et al.*, 1977*b*). Whether suppressor cells form in humans during virus infection and influence their immune reactions is unknown at present. Huddlestone *et al.* (1979) recently observed replication of measles virus in T.G and T.M (T lymphocytes having Fc receptors for IgM and acting as T-helper cells) cells (Fig. 1). Measles virus infects human lymphoid cells (Joseph *et al.*, 1975; Katz and Enders, 1965; White and Boyd, 1973; Gresser and Chany, 1963), after which these cells' responses to several antigens become suppressed, i.e., loss of tuberculin reactivity (von Pirquet, 1908; reviewed Finkel and Dent, 1973*a,b*; Fireman *et al.*, 1969; Smithwick and Berkovich, 1966; Zweiman *et al.*, 1971). Hence Huddlestone's findings may be relevant in understanding these virus-induced alterations in immune responses.

Several experimental systems have characterized peripheral unresponsiveness according to the following criteria: First, antigen persists for long periods of time during peripheral unresponsiveness. Second, although spleen cells do not respond to these antigens in the tolerized host, they do respond following adoptive transfer. Third, specific antigen-binding lymphocytes are present. Fourth, antibody is produced transiently during the period of tolerance induction.

3.4. Divergence in B- and T-Cell Tolerance

Several elegant experiments have defined B- and T-cell participation in immunological tolerance of mice to human γ-globulin (Chiller and Weigle, 1973; Chiller and Weigle, 1975) and may offer important leads for understanding unresponsiveness associated with some virus infections. In these experiments, heterologous human γ-globulin is immunogenic in adult mice unless deaggregated and rendered monomeric, in which case it induces tolerance. Hence the injection of monomeric human γ-globulin followed by a challenge with aggregated human γ-globulin fails to yield an immune response. In contrast, injection of a non-cross-reacting antigen, such as turkey γ-globulin, incites the expected response, indicating the specificity of tolerance induction. This specificity is also seen in models of virus infection, as is discussed later (see Fig. 4).

γ-Globulin can induce tolerance via both specific B and/or specific T cells (Chiller and Weigle, 1975; Chiller *et al.*, 1970), indicating that both cell types can be rendered unresponsive to the same antigen. Specific T- and B-cell populations each display distinctive temporal kinetic patterns of tolerance induction, maintenance, and spontaneous

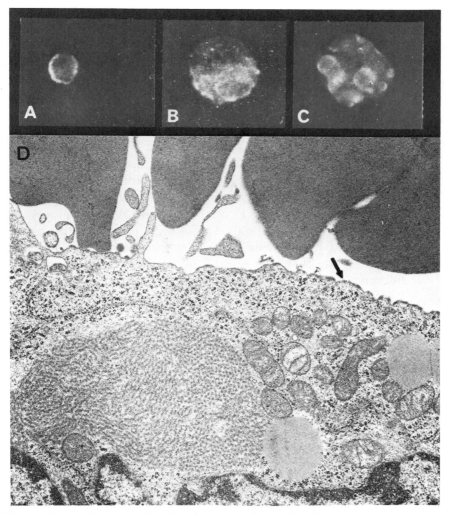

Fig. 1. Replication of measles virus in thymus-derived lymphocytes (T.G) known ordinarily to have immune suppressor activity. T-suppressor-cell function had been
recorded in *in vitro* experiments using B-cell activation by pokeweed mitogen (Moretta
et al., 1977; Oldstone *et al.*, 1977*b*). Such T cells have Fc surface receptors for IgG.
A,B,C: Presence of measles virus antigens on the surfaces of T.G cells using a direct
immunofluorescence assay. Six days after infection with Edmonston strain measles
virus, unfixed T.G cells were stained with a fluorescein-conjugated monospecific antibody to measles virus. D: Electron micrograph of a similarly infected cell, fixed with
2% gluteraldehyde. Measles-virus-induced alteration of the plasma membrane is
designated by the arrow. Nucleocapsids are seen in the cytoplasm of the T.G cell.
15,000×. From Huddlestone *et al.* (1979).

termination. T cells obtained from thymuses or spleens are rendered unresponsive in short periods of time, usually less than 24 hr, but B cells do not become unresponsive for 2–4 days and those in bone marrow not until 8–15 days after introduction of a specific tolerizing antigen. The maintenance of tolerance also varies in time. T cells derived from the thymus remain tolerant for 120–130 days, whereas T cells derived from spleens are tolerant for 100–150 days after the injection of tolerizing antigen. In contrast, B cells from the spleen maintain tolerance for 50–60 days and those from the bone marrow last 40–50 days after being tolerized by antigen. Hence tolerance is initiating earliest and remains longest in the T-cell population. The unresponsiveness in B cells takes longer to begin and is quicker to end. The T cells described here are helper cells; at this point neither T-suppressor cells nor T-cytotoxic cells have been rendered tolerant. Another observation of particular interest is that the onset and maintenance of tolerance in the animals tested experimentally parallel the time interval of T-cell tolerance rather than that of B cells (Table 1). Further, the induction of B-cell tolerance requires higher concentrations of tolerogen than the induction of T-cell tolerance. Thus it is possible experimentally to demonstrate that T cells become unresponsive in the presence of B-cell competence, especially when small doses of tolerogen are used. With a large tolerizing dose both T cells and B cells become unresponsive. B-cell tolerance can occur in the presence of large amounts of specific antigen and may be associated with antigen blockade of B-cell receptors.

TABLE 1

Kinetic Pattern of Immunological Tolerance in Lymphocyte Populations[a]

Populations of lymphocytes	State of tolerance (days)	
	For induction	For maintenance
Thymus	<1	120–135
Bone marrow	8–15	40–50
Spleen		
T cells	<1	100–150
B cells	2–4	50–60
Whole animal	<1	130–150

[a] Note the different kinetic patterns in the induction and maintenance of tolerance for T lymphocytes and for B lymphocytes. A/J mice were injected with 2.5 mg of deaggregated human γ-globulin on day 0. Data obtained from Chiller and Weigle (1975).

Macrophages may also play a role in the establishment of unresponsiveness. In the systems thus far studied, the participation of macrophages is antigen nonspecific and is under genetic control (Lukic et al., 1975a,b; Fujiwara and Cinader, 1974). It is presumed that the immunological defect related to macrophages lies in their handling of antigen.

3.5. Breaking of Immune Tolerance

The tolerance induced with a T-cell-dependent antigen can be terminated by several specialized maneuvers. With unresponsiveness in T cells but competency in B cells, the lack of T-helper-cell function can be bypassed either by triggering B cells with nonspecifically activated T cells, for example, by superimposing an allogeneic effect (Katz et al., 1971), or by the use of a polyclonal B-cell activator, such as lipopolysaccharide (Chiller and Weigle, 1973; Coutinho and Moller, 1975). Lipopolysaccharide substitutes for the T-helper cell and actually circumvents the need for T cells in T-cell–B-cell collaboration. T-helper-cell tolerance is broken only when specific B cells are in a state of responsiveness. Hence even using both the allogeneic effect and B-cell polyclonal activators in mice whose T and B cells are unresponsive does not generate an immune response.

Although the induction of specific cytotoxic T cells may depend on antigen–macrophage–T-cell interaction (Zinkernagel et al., 1978), the recognition and destruction of targets by cytotoxic T cells occur in the absence of macrophage and B-cell interactions (reviewed by Doherty et al., 1974). Rollinghoff et al. (1977; Pfizenmaier et al., 1977) have suggested that suppressor cells inhibited cytotoxic T cells of mice infected with herpes simplex type 1 virus infection from lysing herpesvirus-infected targets. Presumed deletion of these suppressor cells was needed to see the virus specific cytotoxic T-cell activity. This was achieved either by prolonged culture in vitro or by use of cycloheximide in vivo.

4. IMMUNE RESPONSES IN VIRAL SYSTEMS

Many reports describe immune reponses of hosts to infectious viruses as well as the effects of virus infection on the host's ability to generate immune responses. Viruses can replicate in those cells which form the constituent parts of the immune system (reviewed Notkins et al., 1970; Wheelock and Toy, 1973) and can also alter the normal route of travel and localization of immunocompetent cells (Woodruff and

Woodruff, 1975). In addition, viral antigens *per se* actively compete with nonviral antigens in stimulating immune responses (Oldstone, *et al.*, 1973). Therefore, the effects of viruses on the already complex immune system present an additional dimension of subtlety.

4.1. Responses to Nonviral Antigens

Mice acutely or persistently infected with any of a variety of DNA and RNA viruses may respond aberrantly to other antigens when compared to uninfected matched controls, as measured by antibody production, immunoglobulin levels, induction of immunological tolerance, graft rejection, graft-vs.-host reaction, delayed-type skin reaction, lymphocyte transformation, and phagocytosis (reviewed by Notkins *et al.*, 1970). The responses observed depend on the state and dose of antigen given and virus infection under study (Oldstone *et al.*, 1974). It is important to recognize that abnormalities in the immune responsiveness of infected mice against one antigen do not necessarily indicate overall immunlogical incapacity. For example, mice persistently infected with LCMV made significantly lower responses than uninfected control mice against mammalian and avian immunoglobulins. This depression in immune responses was not associated with differences in antibody avidity or antigen handling by macrophages but correlated directly with decreased numbers of antibody-forming cells. In contrast to the hyporesponsiveness to immunoglobulin antigens by mice infected with LCMV, their immune responses to antigens like sheep red blood cells and keyhole limpet hemocyanin were normal over wide dose ranges, compared to responses of uninfected controls (Oldstone *et al.*, 1973).

Other virus may similarly depress or even enhance immune responses to some antigens. Von Pirquet (1908) noted that positive tuberculin reaction in children with tuberculosis became negative during infection with measles virus, and later workers confirmed these findings (reviewed Finkel and Dent, 1973*a,b*). Depressed responses to a variety of antigens occurred in rodents infected with leukemogenic viruses, and lactic dehydrogenase virus enhanced the capacity of mice to make antibodies to human IgG. Recent studies with murine hepatitis virus correlated continuous production of interferon during persistent viral infection and alterations of the immune response with the strain of mice infected (Virelizier *et al.*, 1976). Interferon is known to alter a variety of immune responses (de Maeyer *et al.*, 1975; de Maeyer-Guignard *et al.*, 1975) as well as modulate histocompatibility antigens

(Lindahl *et al.*, 1973, 1974, 1976). Thus many factors may play a role in the regulation of immune responses during virus infection.

Although relatively few viruses have been studied sufficiently in relation to the generation of immune responses to numerous nonviral antigens over wide range of doses, nevertheless it is clear that virus infections can profoundly alter the performance of the immune system. However, more detailed and controlled information is needed and is best obtained by systematically studying immune functions after animals or cells are infected with different viruses. By influencing immune functions, viruses may produce important secondary biological effects. Viruses that depress humoral or cellular immunity may render the host more susceptible to other infectious agents or less in control of transformed and malignant cells. Conversely, the ability of viruses to enhance humoral or cellular immunity may be an important factor in the etiology of autoimmune diseases.

4.2. Responses to Viral Antigens

Although there is a vast amount of information about the immune response to infectious virus, little designates whether viral antigens are thymic dependent or independent. The repeating antigenic determinants of viral antigens, if associated with appropriate spatial relationships, might effectively interact with and trigger B cells without the need of T-cell collaboration. Clarification of this and related issues rests on the availability of purified viral antigens for use in measuring the generation of humoral and cell-mediated immune responses. Additional research with mice that are genetically or experimentally rendered thymusless should allow the determination of T-cell dependency of viral antigens.

Most of our knowledge as to the T dependency of viral antigens comes from experiments in which a battery of RNA and DNA viruses were inoculated into genetically athymic mice (nude) or their thymically normal littermates (Burns *et al.*, 1975). Only limited interpretations of these experiments are available as the viral antigens used were not purified and did not cover a wide range of doses, and the antibodies were measured by several indirect secondary techniques so that the results were not truly comparable. Nevertheless, this is the best available information and the data indicated that athymic mice made antibody responses after infection with Coxsackie B1 virus, endomyocarditis virus, vesicular stomatitis virus, and Sindbis virus, just as their thymically normal littermates did. In contrast, athymic mice failed to respond to influenza PR8, simian virus 5, Sendai virus, mumps virus, minute virus of mice, mouse adenovirus, herpes simplex type 1 virus, and simian virus 40, while the same controls did make humoral responses. These results suggest strongly that immune responses generated against picornaviruses, rhabdoviruses, and togaviruses are T-cell independent, whereas responses against orthomyxovirus, paramyxoviruses, parvoviruses, adenoviruses, herpesviruses, and papoviruses tested are T-cell dependent.

4.3. Interactions between Viruses and Leukocytes

Viruses or viruslike particles have been found in the thymus, lymph node, spleen, bone marrow, stem cell, plasma cell, lymphocyte, macrophage, monocyte, polymorphonuclear leukocyte, and Kupffer cell (reviewed by Notkins *et al.*, 1970; Wheelock and Toy, 1973), indicating the permissivity of such cells for viruses. In addition to these observations *in vivo*, the interaction of viruses with lymphocytes and macrophages has been studied carefully *in vitro*. The following discussion covers a few of the most interesting recent observations related to vesicular stomatitis virus (VSV), measles virus, influenza virus, Dengue hemorrhagic fever virus, Epstein–Barr virus (EBV), cytomegalovirus and LCMV.

Replication of VSV by lymphocytes appears to be controlled by several restrictions (reviewed by Bloom *et al.*, 1977). While it is clear that resting lymphocytes can be infected by VSV, replication and release of virus from lymphocytes require their activation. The requirement for lymphocyte activation is not unique to VSV but is in force for cytomegalovirus, Newcastle disease virus, and poliomyelitis virus. Studies with murine and human lymphocyte populations indicate that infectious VSV is produced selectively in activated T cells but little, if any, virus replicates in B cells. This replication of infectious VSV can be generated *in vitro* with mitogens or in mixed leukocyte reactions or *in vivo* during allogeneic cell transfer.

In contrast to the reported T cell's specificity for VSV, measles virus infects B cells and macrophages as well as T cells (Joseph *et al.*, 1975; Sullivan *et al.*, 1975; Lucas *et al.*, 1978). Of interest is the observation that, following measles virus exposure, resting lymphocytes express little, if any, viral antigen, but after mitogenic stimulation the vast majority of lymphocytes express viral antigens (Lucas *et al.*, 1978; Huddlestone *et al.*, 1979).

Two unexpected findings mark research on the interaction between influenza virus or dengue hemorrhagic fever virus and leukocytes. The surfaces of peripheral blood lymphocytes removed from patients during the peak reaction to infection by influenza virus contained viral antigens (Wilson *et al.*, 1976). Influenza viruses are traditionally believed to replicate only in the respiratory tract epithelium and not to produce viremia. Wilson's findings may provide important leads in understanding that the pathogenesis of influenza virus infection may result from a more general dispersion of viral antigens or virus and bear similarities to other virus–lymphocyte interactions. Marchette *et al.* (1976) infected cultures of peripheral blood leukocytes with dengue virus and noted an immunological dependence for viral replication. Dengue viruses of types 1, 2, and 4 replicated in cultures of peripheral blood leukocytes from Dengue-immunized rhesus monkeys. In contrast, Dengue virus failed to multiply in peripheral blood leukocytes from nonimmune monkeys. These findings may offer leads in explaining the Dengue shock syndrome that occurs in immune and not in nonimmune individuals.

Several studies have demonstrated an association between the receptor for EBV and the third component (C3) of complement on human lymphoid cells (Jondal *et al.*, 1976; Yefenof *et al.*, 1976). In studies of over 50 cultured lines, the expression of these two receptors correlated. The vast majority of cells expressing EBV receptors also expressed C3 receptors and, conversely, cells lacking C3 receptors usually did not contain EBV receptors. In blocking experiments, covering of C3 receptor binding with purified C3 prevented EBV from attaching and, conversely, the blocking of the EBV receptor with EBV kept C3 from binding to the cell's surface. The relative positions of C3 and EBV receptors on the plasma membrane were demonstrated by using isofluorescein- or rhodamine-conjugated antibodies and cocapping techniques. After this two-color staining for EBV receptors and C3 receptors, the cells' plasma membranes displayed complete overlapping of green and red fluorescence from both stains. Capping of EBV receptors induced cocapping of C3 receptors and *vice versa* on human B lymphocytes, again indicating the close association between the EBV and C3 receptors.

Cytomegalovirus can invade murine B cells and resides there in a latent state (Olding *et al.*, 1975, 1976). In spleen cells harvested from several strains of mice latently infected with murine cytomegalovirus (MCMV), infectious virus was activated by cocultivation with allogeneic permissive feeder cells. In contrast, infectious virus was not released following cocultivation on syngeneic permissive mouse embryo cells. MCMV was found in the B-cell population and not in T cells when depletion and reconstitution techniques were used. In other studies (Brautigam *et al.*, 1979), more than 82% of peritoneal macrophages harvested from latently infected mice following stimulation with thioglycollate (activated macrophages) contained viral DNA as detected by *in situ* hybridization. Infectious virus was recovered with ease from over 90% of these macrophages following cocultivation with syngeneic or allogeneic permissive mouse embryo cells. Although more than 82% of peritoneal macrophages that were not stimulated with thioglycollate (resident macrophages) also contained viral DNA, less than 10% of these released infectious virus. It is not clear whether the fact that activated macrophages yielded infectious virus but resident macrophages did not was caused by a unique population of macrophages recruited to the peritoneal cavity after stimulation, the initiation of DNA synthesis in activated macrophages needed for CMV synthesis, or the release of several protease, collagenase-, and plasminogen-activating enzymes by activated macrophages. Like CMV, a variety of other viruses persist in peritoneal macrophages (Mims and Subrahmanyan, 1966; Notkins *et al.*, 1970).

Recently two groups (Doyle and Oldstone, 1978; Popescu, 1978) independently found replicating LCMV in subpopulations of circulating blood mononuclear cells harvested from mice persistently infected with LCMV. Popescu *et al.* (1977) inoculated the WE3 strain of LCMV into NMRI mice within the first 24 hr of life. The mice became persistent carriers of LCMV throughout their lives, and approximately 3% of their peripheral blood leukocytes contained viral antigen and produced infectious virus. The same authors examined an adult house mouse with naturally acquired persistent LCMV infection and found resident virus in the circulating blood leukocytes. Limited morphological studies indicated that the infected cells were neither lymphoblasts nor mononuclear phagocytes but rather were lymphocytes. Doyle and Oldstone (1978), using several strains of mice infected congenitally *in utero* or neonatally at birth with Armstrong strain LCMV, similarly detected LCMV in mononuclear cells harvested from the circulating blood of adult mice. These cells contained infectious virus according to an infectious center assay, and lymphoid cells harvested from the animals' peripheral blood, spleens, thymuses, and bone marrow released LCMV. However, virus was not present in a fully infectious form either within the cells or on their surfaces. After depletion and reconstitution experiments with specific cell types, the mononuclear cells replicating LCMV were classed as B cells, T cells, and phagocytic monocytes. In addition to these results with persistently infected mice, adult mice acutely infected with LCMV had infectious centers in peripheral blood and splenic mononuclear cells. Three to four days after viral inoculation infective centers peaked, then decreased to below detectable levels by the eighth day. In contrast, in persistently infected mice, infectious centers were demonstrable throughout the animals' life. At present it is not known whether virus replicates preferentially in particular subpopulations of T cells (suppressor, helper, or cytotoxic) or whether cells harboring virus fail in their differentiated immune function(s).

B and T lymphocytes and their products and mononuclear phagocytes represent important factors in limiting the spread and continuity of virus infection. It is of interest, then, that viruses may directly or indirectly affect the function of such immunocompetent cells via replication or by alteration of cell-surface determinants. Further, the accompanying release of lymphokines such as interferon may affect immune responses. These interactions between viruses and cells of the immune system have been analyzed predominantly *in vitro* and rarely *in vivo*. Most studies show that resting lymphocytes and macrophages or particular subpopulations of lymphocytes in cultures can be infected with various DNA and RNA viruses and that, on activation, the permissive lymphocytes express viral antigens and replicate infectious virus. Adding biological significance to these *in vitro* observations is the increasing number of reports that viruses can replicate for long periods in lymphocytes and macrophages of infected, intact animals.

5. IMMUNE TOLERANCE IN VIRAL SYSTEMS

5.1. LCMV Infection

LCMV infection of mice is an extremely informative model in which the parameters for pathogenesis of both acute and persistent infections have been studied (Rowe, 1954; Hotchin and Cintes, 1958; Oldstone and Dixon, 1969, 1972; Zinkernagel and Doherty, 1973). This model provides the framework in which virus-induced immune complex disease has been recognized and evaluated (Oldstone and Dixon, 1967, 1969; Oldstone, 1975; Buchmeier and Oldstone, 1978). The recent concept that viruses can curtail the physiological (luxury) functions of differentiated (neuroblastoma) cells but leave their vital functions intact derives from the LCMV-murine model of infection (Oldstone *et al.*,

1977*a*). In addition, LCMV infection provided the first evidence for the arousal of T-cytotoxic killer cells in virus infection (Cole *et al.*, 1973; Marker and Volkert, 1973) and the observation that cytotoxic T cells recognize and kill virus-infected targets only when specific viral antigens and the D and/or K components of the major murine *H-2* gene complex both participate appropriately (Zinkernagel and Doherty, 1973).

The concept of virus-induced immune tolerance evolved from the observations that mice infected *in utero* or at birth with LCMV carry infectious virus in their tissues throughout life in the absence of detectable complement-fixing or neutralizing antibody(s) (Traub, 1936*a*; Volkert and Larsen, 1965). This was also based on the observations of the two different courses in acute and chronic infection in mice with LCMV. In the first instance, infection of weanling or adult mice, depending on the virus dose and site of inoculation, led either to death or to recovery and immunity. The tissue injury found in mice with acute virus infections is immunopathological in nature (Rowe, 1954) as shown by experiments in which immune function is terminated (by irradiation, thymectomy, antimetabolic agent treatment, antilymphocytic treatment or complement depletion) and later reconstituted by adoptive transfer of specific sensitized spleen cells. In the contrasting second instance, mice are infected *in utero* or shortly after birth and carry high titers of virus throughout life (persistent infection) without complement-fixing antibodies. Why does the host's immune system fail to clear this virus? With the recent definition of the protein structure of LCMV and the identification of viral structural and cell-associated polypeptides, assays for B-cell and T-cell anti-LCMV immune responses can now be performed to answer this question.

LCMV contains three major structural polypeptides (Buchmeier and Oldstone, 1978; Buchmeier *et al.*, 1978) (Fig. 2). The largest of these is a nonglycosylated nuclear protein of approximately 63,000 daltons found inside the virion and associated with a dense ribonucleoprotein complex. Two glycopeptides, termed gp1 and gp2, of approximately 54,000 and 35,000 daltons, respectively, are localized on the virion surface as shown by proteolytic digestion of intact viruses (Buchmeier *et al.*, 1978). Peptide maps of gp1 and gp2 indicate that they are independent polypeptides and that gp2 is not a cleavage product of gp1. BHK21 and L929 cells infected with LCMV and then labeled with $[^{35}S]$methionine or $[^{14}C]$glucosamine synthesize nuclear capsids, gp1, and gp2 as well as an apparently nonstructural glycopeptide designated gpc, whose size is 74,000–75,000 daltons. The relationship of this cell-associated gpc to gp1 and gp2 is not completely

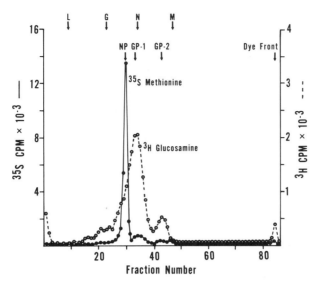

Fig. 2. Polypeptide profile of purified LCMV by SDS-PAGE. Purified LCMV, radiolabeled with [³⁵S]methionine (●———●) and [³H]glucosamine (O---O) was electrophoresed on a 12.5% acrylamide gel. The gel was sliced into 1-mm fractions, and the amount of radiolabel in each fraction was determined by liquid scintillation counting. The migration positions of the polypeptides of VSV (Indiana strain), L (molecular weight ~ 160,000), G (molecular weight 68,000), N (molecular weight 54,000), and M (molecular weight 27,000) were determined on a parallel gel and are indicated at the upper part of the figure. See Buchmeier and Oldstone (1978) for experimental details.

clear, although gpc is a precursor of gp1. Gp1 is likely the only one of the three glycopeptides that is expressed on the surfaces of infected cells.

5.2. B-Cell Responses to LCMV

After mice are infected *in utero* or at birth with LCMV, their circulating blood contains LCMV antigens and antibody in immune complexes as detected by the significant reduction of the virus's infectious titer following removal of immunoglobulin (presumably anti-LCMV antibody) with a rabbit antibody to mouse immunoglobulin or the removal of complement with a rabbit antibody to mouse C3 (Oldstone and Dixon, 1969, 1972). In contrast, removing albumin from the sera or plasma of mice persistently infected with LCMV does not lower the titer of infectious virus, ruling out the possibility of nonspecific trapping. Other assays are similarly positive for virus–antibody complexes;

for example, sera or plasma from mice persistently infected with LCMV contain circulating complexes as shown by the C1q precipitin test and the Raji-cell immune precipitation test (Oldstone, 1978), both of which detect complement-bound circulating immune complexes, and by analytical ultracentrifugation (Oldstone *et al.*, 1975). One characterizes the specific antibodies in these circulating complexes by treating the euglobulin fraction with 0.02 M glycine HC1, pH 2.8, to dissociate the antigen–antibody complex(es). The recovered immuno-globulin is incubated with [^{35}S]methionine-labeled LCMV polypeptides and [^{3}H]glucosamine-labeled LCMV polypeptides, after which the resultant immune precipitates are analyzed for all the viral polypeptides of LCMV. Results indicate that antibodies to all LCMV polypeptides are in the circulation. In contrast, immunoglobulins found in sera of uninfected mice and of mice with immune complex diseases unrelated to LCMV do not react against LCMV antigens.

Immune complexes formed during persistent virus infections frequently deposit in tissue with limiting basement membranes like glomeruli of the kidney and choroid plexi of the brain and arteries (Oldstone, 1975). In several model systems it has been possible to elute the immunoglobulins complexed in the glomeruli, free the immuno-globulin from the bound antigen, and determine its specificity against viral antigens. Immunoglobulin eluted from immune complex deposits in glomeruli of adult mice persistently infected with LCMV precipitated specifically with all of the major viral polypeptides of LCMV (Buch-meier and Oldstone, 1978) (Fig. 3). As controls, immunoglobulin eluted from the sera of uninfected mice or from tissue deposited immune com-plexes unrelated to LCMV does not contain LCMV antigens, and the eluates from mice persistently infected with LCMV do not immuno-precipitate with unrelated viruses (Table 2).

The above results embody the characteristic activity of the B-cell immune response and clearly demonstrate that mice persistently infected with LCMV are responsive to all of the LCMV polypeptides at the B-cell level, and their inability to clear virus does not result from the failure to produce antiviral antibody(ies). Previous difficulties in demonstrating antibodies in this model arose primarily because the assays used could not measure antibodies bound to antigens (immune complexes). At present it is not known whether the various polypeptides of LCMV constitute T-cell-dependent or -independent antigens. If it is determined that the antibody responses to LCMV polypeptides require T-helper-cell function, then the data at hand indicate no unresponsive-ness during persistent LCMV infection at the T-helper-cell level.

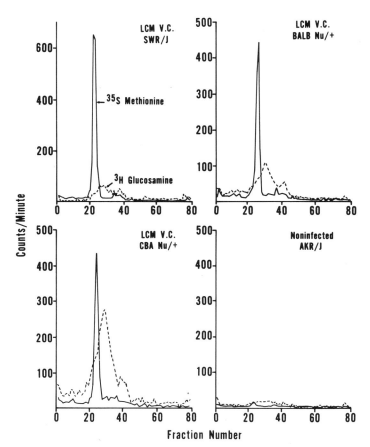

Fig. 3. Immune precipitation of the polypeptides of LCMV by Ig eluted from the renal glomeruli of adult mice which had been persistently infected with LCMV since birth (V.C.). The quantities of eluted immunoglobulin indicated below were mixed with radiolabeled viral antigen: SWR/J, 6.5 μg; CBA *Nu*/+, 2.8 μg, BALB *Nu*/+, 4.2 μg; AKR/J, 3.2 μg. The resultant immune precipitates were analyzed on 12.5% gels as described in Fig. 2. AKR/J mice have retrovirus antigen–antibody immune complexes (see Fig. 5) and were not infected with LCMV. See Buchmeier and Oldstone (1978) for experimental details. Data extend the findings in Table II and clearly demonstrate that mice persistently infected with LCMV are not tolerant on the B-lymphocyte level. Antibody responses to all the LCMV structural polypeptides are made.

5.3. T-Cell Responses to LCMV

Clearance of LCMV *in vivo* and destruction of LCMV-infected target cells *in vitro* during acute infection require in large part the participation of cytotoxic T lymphocytes (Zinkernagel and Doherty, 1973;

TABLE 2

Immune Precipitation of LCMV and Pichinde Virus Proteins by Ig Eluted from the Glomeruli of Mice Persistently Infected (VC) with LCMV or Other Viruses[a]

Ig eluted from glomeruli of	μg Ig per reaction	Viral antigen	% of offered cpm precipitated[b]	
			[³H]-Glucosamine	[³⁵S]-Methionine
SWR/J (LCM VC) Expt. 1	15	LCMV	ND[c]	29.2
		PV	ND	4.1
SWR/J (LCM VC) Expt. 2	13	LCMV	13.7	57.4
		PV	3.3	4.3
SWR/J (LCM VC) Expt. 3	6.5	LCMV	14.2	48.3
		PV	3.0	4.9
CBA/WEHI *Nu/+* (LCM VC)	2.8	LCMV	30.5	34.2
		PV	4.1	6.4
BALB/WEHI *Nu/+* (LCM VC)	4.2	LCMV	16.1	31.0
		PV	4.1	4.9
AKR [MuLV (AKR) VC][d]	3.2	LCMV	4.8	4.9
		PV	5.3	7.2
NZB (polyoma VC)[e]	2.2	LCMV	6.7	7.4
		PV	ND	ND
GP anti-LCMV[f]	ND	LCMV	19.2	73.9
	ND	PV	2.6	7.2
GP anti-PV[g]	ND	LCMV	3.0	4.5
	ND	PV	27.0	73.1
Nonimmune GP serum	ND	LCMV	ND	6.4
	ND	PV	ND	3.8

[a] Note the specificity of the immunoglobulin eluted from the glomeruli of mice persistently infected with LCMV for LCMV antigens. Data indicate that mice are not tolerant but make antibody responses to LCMV.

[b] Mean offered cpm: LCMV, ³H 17,000; ³⁵S 9600; Pichinde virus (PV), ³H 17,000; ³⁵S 8300 (see Buchmeier and Oldstone, 1978, for experimental details).

[c] ND, Not done.

[d] Retrovirus–antiretrovirus immune complexes.

[e] DNA–anti-DNA, nuclear antigen–antinuclear antigen, polyoma–antipolyoma virus, and retrovirus–antiretrovirus immune complexes form and then deposit in the glomeri of New Zealand black mice persistently infected with polyoma virus (Dixon *et al.*, 1971).

[f] Guinea pig antibody to LCMV.

[g] Guinea pig antibody to PV.

Zinkernagel and Welsh, 1976). LCMV continuously exists in the mice it persistently infects and mice persistently infected with LCMV are not tolerant at the B-cell level. Tolerance can exist at the T-cell level while B-cell responses are functional (see Section 3). This sequence of evidence has led to the evaluation of cytotoxic T-cell responses in persistently infected mice. Several investigators have consistently been unable to demonstrate the presence of virus-specific cytotoxic T cells in the spleens of mice persistently infected with LCMV (Zinkernagel and Doherty, 1974; Cole *et al.*, 1973; Marker and Volkert, 1973; Cihak and Lehmann-Grube, 1978). Others have found low levels of cytotoxic T cells occurring transiently in such mice (Oldstone and Dixon, 1971, 1973; Lundstedt, 1969). This difficulty in detecting virus-specific cytotoxic T cells may rest on either a central or a peripheral blockage of the immune response. As mentioned in Section 4.3, LCMV is harbored in both circulating and splenic T cells of the infected mice. However, there is no evidence yet that the T cells carrying virus are in fact cytotoxic T cells. The use of anti-Ly23 sera to delete cytotoxic T cells while scoring infectious centers as well as enriching the cytotoxic T-cell population by using a fluorescence-activated cell sorter in parallel with LCMV antigen-binding studies of immunocompetent cells should settle this issue. Figure 4 shows the ability of mice persistently infected with LCMV to generate immune-specific cytotoxic T cells to Pichinde-virus-infected targets while not generating cytotoxic T cells to LCMV-infected targets (Buchmeier *et al.*, unpublished data). Pichinde virus is a member of the arenavirus group, as is LCMV.

Recent evidence suggesting a peripheral mechanism for immune unresponsiveness of cytotoxic T cells comes from several different sources. Zinkernagel and Doherty (1974) injected allogeneic spleen cells into LCMV persistently infected mice to generate cytotoxic T cells, while Cole (1978) and Doyle *et al.* (1978) used concanavalin A treatment of spleen cells harvested from mice persistently infected with LCMV to make LCMV virus-specific cytotoxic T cells. Dunlop and Blanden (1977) showed that cytotoxic T cells specific for LCMV were suppressed by a variety of approaches, all of which had in common the addition of either a high level of LCMV or LCMV-infected cells. Of interest was the correlation that the amount of virus present in mice persistently infected with LCMV was sufficient to inactivate cytotoxic T-cell activity. In related experiments using a different approach, Welsh and Oldstone (1977) implicated the generation of defective interferon virus (DIV) in the inhibition of cytotoxic T-cell-induced injury of cultured cells infected with LCMV. They noted that the expression of LCMV antigens on the surfaces of infected cells peaked 2–4 days after infection and precipitously declined thereafter with little or no viral antigen expressed on surfaces of persistently infected cells. The expression of viral antigens on the surfaces of infected cells was regulated by virus–cell interactions and closely associated with DIV interference. DI LCMV, *per se*, blocked the synthesis and cell-surface expression of LCMV antigens and abrogated the efficiency of cytotoxic

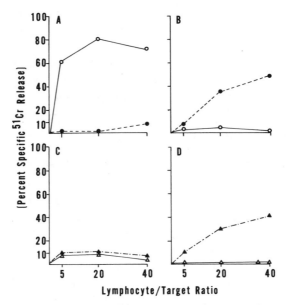

Fig. 4.   A,B: Specificity in the generation of cytotoxic T cells during arenavirus infections. Adult C3H/St mice (*H-2k*) given LCMV or Pichinde virus were sacrificed 7 days
later, and their spleen cells were harvested and tested against L929 (*H-2k*) target cells
infected with either LCMV (A) or Pichinde virus (B). Specific lysis quantitated by a
^{51}Cr release assay. O———O, Cytotoxic T cells generated during acute LCMV infection;
●----●, Cytotoxic T cells generated during acute Pichinde virus infection. C:
Demonstration of the difficulty in generating cytotoxic T cells to LCMV in adult
C3H/St mice persistently infected with LCMV and challenged with LCMV. D: In
contrast, cytotoxic T cells against Pichinde virus can be generated in adult C3H/St
mice persistently infected with LCMV after challenge with Pichinde virus. Targets are
L929 cells infected with LCMV (C) or Pichinde virus (D). △———△, Cytotoxic T cells
generated during acute LCMV infection; ▲·—·—·▲, cytotoxic T cells generated during
acute Pichinde virus infection. From M. Buchmeier, R. Ott, and M. Oldstone
(unpublished data).

T-cell killing (Table 3). Taken *in toto*, these reports suggest that
cytotoxic T cells are present in persistently infected mice and indicate
mechanisms whereby such cell-mediated immune responses can be
blocked.

5.4.   Retrovirus Models

The findings with experimental retrovirus infection parallel those
with LCMV infection in mice. The inability to detect antibodies free in
the circulations of animals persistently infected with retroviruses led to

the concept that immunological tolerance occurred (Gross, 1970; Volkert and Larsen, 1965). However, like LCMV, it was soon noted that antibody to Gross leukemia virus was in immune complexes that circulated in the blood and deposited in several tissues including glomeruli of the infected mice (Oldstone et al., 1972b). Several reports in the early 1970s showed that the immunoglobulin eluted and recovered from the infected animals' renal glomeruli contained specific antibodies to the cell-surface antigens of Gross leukemia virus and of the viral reverse transcriptase (Oldstone et al., 1972a; Hollis et al., 1974; Dore et al., 1970). Subsequent studies in which the eluted immunoglobulin recovered from immune complex deposits from infected animals' kidneys was incubated with radiolabeled polypeptides of retroviruses demonstrated the competency of B-cell responses to the major polypeptides of the retrovirus (Oldstone et al., 1976) (Fig. 5). Nowinski (1975) later confirmed these findings while investigating natural antibodies in leukemic mice. Other definitive studies showing anti-retrovirus antibody(ies) during natural infection have been reported by Ihle, Bolognesi, and their colleagues (Ihle et al., 1973; Ihle et al., 1976a,b). The generation of cytotoxic T cells has been reported during leukemia virus infection of mice (Wahren and Metcalf, 1970; Hirsh et al., 1975).

Although both B cells and T cells are responsive at times in mice

TABLE 3

Relationship between Defective Interfering Virus, Expression of Virus Antigens on the Cells' Surface, and Killing of Virus-Infected Cells by Immune-Specific Cytotoxic T Cells[a]

Treatment of cultured cells		Results of assay at 24 hr for		
First	Second	Infectivity ($\log_{10}$ PFU/ml)	% cells with surface LCMV	% ^{51}Cr released on addition of cytotoxic T cells
MEM	MEM	0	0	7 ± 0.2[b]
DI LCMV	MEM	0	0	7 ± 0.1
MEM	LCMV	7.5	33	66 ± 0.2
DI LCMV	LCMV	5.1	<1	10 ± 0.6

[a] DI LCMV (defective interfering LCMV) was obtained from supernatant fluids of BHK cells persistently infected with LCMV. Cultured L929 cells were incubated with $120\times$ concentrate DI LCMV (or MEM) for 1½ hr and then challenged with infectious LCMV, MOI 1 (or MEM), for 1½ hr. Methodology for determining surface viral antigens, infectious virus, DI LCM, and cytotoxic T-cell killing has been published (see Welsh and Oldstone, 1977, for experimental details).
[b] Mean of triplicate values $\pm$ 1 SD.

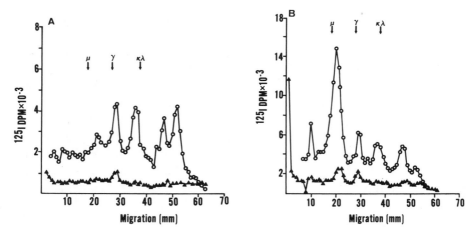

Fig. 5. A: SDS-polyacrylamide gel electrophoresis of MuLV (AKR) proteins that react with antibody from AKR kidney eluates. Radioiodinated MuLV (ARK) proteins were incubated with normal BALB/c serum or with normal BALB/c serum mixed with 0.75 μg of Ig isolated from renal glomeruli of AKR/J mice, and then goat antimurine Ig was added to precipitate all the murine Ig in the mixture. After washing, the immune precipitate was suspended in 8 M urea, 2% β-mercaptoethanol, and 1% SDS, heated, and then analyzed on 6% polyacrylamide gels. Specific precipitate: ^{125}I-labeled MuLV (AKR) proteins that reacted with antibodies from the AKR renal eluate (O). Trapping control precipitate: ^{125}I-labeled MuLV (AKR) proteins that were found in the normal murine Ig–goat anti-murine Ig precipitate (▲). Positions of μ, γ, and κλ marker proteins are indicated by arrows. B: SDS-polyacrylamide gel electrophoresis of MuLV (Scripps) proteins that react with antibody from AKR kidney eluates. Radioiodinated MuLV (Scripps) proteins were analyzed as described above. Specific precipitate: ^{125}I-labeled MuLV (Scripps) proteins that reacted with antibodies from the AKR eluate (O). Trapping control precipitate: ^{125}I-labeled MuLV (Scripps) proteins that were found in the normal mouse Ig–goat anti-mouse Ig precipitate (▲). See Oldstone et al. (1976) for experimental details.

naturally or experimentally infected with a variety of leukemic viruses, the overall picture is not complete. The recent findings of recombinant viruses (Kawashima et al., 1976; Hartley et al., 1977; Elder et al., 1977) and the increasing confusion over the cross-reactivity of specific antigenic determinants for these viruses leave some questions of B- and T-cell responses unresolved.

5.5. Unconventional Viruses

Over the last decade several viruses have been classified as unconventional because of the distinctive disease pattern they produce and their apparent failure to cause immune responses (Gajdusek and Gibbs, 1975). The disease these viruses produce include Jacob-Kreutzfeldt disease, kuru, scrapie, and mink encephalopathy. The tissue injury associated with infection by these viruses *in vivo* usually is not accompanied by inflammatory responses (Lampert *et al.*, 1972). At present there is insufficient information concerning the nature of these agents to distinguish whether B- and/or T-cell responses are operative. Conventional immunological assays have been unrewarding (Porter *et al.*, 1973). However, until the antigens are at hand and better detection methods are used, the question of immune unresponsiveness to the unconventional viruses remains an open issue.

6. CONCLUSION

Investigation of the events leading to the expression of immunity has led to an appreciation for the complexity of the immune system. Immune responsiveness is finely tuned by a network of factors that enhance or suppress its intensity. Hence both antibody formation and cell-mediated immune responses appear to be the end products of a collaboration among subsets of T cells, B cells, and macrophages under genetic control. There is increasing evidence that these cells of the immune system may be infected by viruses, which can persist in them during an animal's life. These immunologically competent cells and/or their products usually represent important factors in limiting the spread and thereby containing a virus infection. The inability of some infected hosts to rid themselves of virus or virus-infected cells has focused the attention of investigators on the possible unresponsiveness or tolerance of cells that normally generate immune responses. Sensitive assays indicate that an immune response frequently occurs but virus may still persist not because the immune system has failed but rather because of the location, density, or presentation of virus on the surfaces of infected target cells (Oldstone, 1977; Welsh and Oldstone, 1977). Table 4 lists several mechanisms whereby viruses can persist and escape the host's immune response.

Investigation of immunological competence during persistent LCMV infection in mice has indicated that the B cells are fully functional. Antibodies are made to all the known structural viral polypeptides. Of the T-cell subsets, cytotoxic lymphocytes specific for LCMV are found not at all or only with difficulty. Several studies suggest that stimulation by allogeneic spleen cells or with concanavalin A

TABLE 4

Mechanisms of Virus Persistence and Escape from Immune Surveillance

1. Viral properties favoring persistence
   a. Generation of defective interfering particles
   b. Generation of temperature-sensitive mutants
   c. Generation of other mutants
   d. Generation of recombinants
   e. Viral integration
   f. Nonimmunogenicity of virus
   g. Tropism for immune competent cells leading to the dysfunction or elimination of
       (1) Thymus-derived cytotoxic T lymphocytes
       (2) Thymus-derived helper lymphocytes
       (3) Bone-marrow-derived lymphocytes
       (4) Macrophages
2. Host or immune properties favoring persistence
   a. Antibody-induced modulation of viral antigens off surfaces of infected cells
   b. Antibody-induced immune selection
   c. Antibody-induced blocking factors
       (1) Non-complement-binding antibodies
       (2) Antigen–antibody complexes
   d. Defects in the complement system
   e. Generation of interferon
   f. Generation of suppressor cells
   g. Dysfunction of immunocompetent cells from a secondary source

results in generation of cytotoxic T cells. With retrovirus infections, B-cell and cytotoxic T-cell responses have been reported. Currently immune responses have not been detected during infections with the unconventional viruses. However, until specific antigens for Jacob-Kreutzfeldt disease or scrapie are described, the detection of such responses will remain an open issue.

ACKNOWLEDGMENTS

This is Publication No. 1625 from the Department of Immuno-pathology, Scripps Clinic and Research Foundation, La Jolla, California 92037.

This research was supported by U.S. Public Health Service Grants AI-07007, AI-09484, and NS-12428; National Foundation March of Dimes Grant No. 1-364; and Biomedical Research Support Program Grant No. 1 S07 RR-05514.

The author acknowledges the collaboration with colleagues at Scripps Clinic and Research Foundation, especially those in the Viral-Immunology Unit with whom it has been a continuing pleasure to work with over the years. Recognition is given to Drs. Michael Buchmeier, John Huddlestone, Michael Doyle, and Peter Lampert, who have contributed unpublished data to this chapter.

7. REFERENCES

Benacerraf, B., and McDevitt, H., 1972, Histocompatibility-linked immune response genes, *Science* **175**:273.

Bloom, B. R., and David, J. R., 1976, *In Vitro Methods in Cell-Mediated and Tumor Immunity*, Academic Press, New York.

Bloom, B., Senik, A., Stoner, G., Ju, G., Nowakowski, M., Kano, S., and Jimenez, L., 1977, Studies on the interactions between viruses and lymphocytes, *Cold Spring Harbor Symp. Quant. Biol.* **41**:128.

Brautigam, A. R., Olding, L. B., Dutko, F. J., and Oldstone, M. B. A., 1979, Pathogenesis of murine cytomegalovirus infection: The macrophage as a permissive cell for cytomegalovirus infection, replication and latency, *J. Gen. Virol.* (in press).

Brunner, T., Engers, H., and Cerottini, J. C., 1976, The ^{51}Cr release assay as used for the quantitative measurement of cell mediated cytolysis in vitro, in: *In Vitro Methods in Cell Mediated and Tumor Immunity* (B. R. Bloom and J. R. David, eds.), pp. 423–428, Academic Press, New York.

Buchmeier, M. J., and Oldstone, M. B. A., 1978, Virus induced immune complex disease: Identification of specific viral antigens and antibodies deposited in complexes during chronic lymphocytic choriomeningitis virus infection, *J. Immunol.* **120**:1297.

Buchmeier, M. J., Elder, J. H., and Oldstone, M. B. A., 1978, Protein structure of lymphocytic choriomeningitis virus: Identification of the virus structural and cell associated polypeptides, *Virology* **89**:133.

Burnett, F. M., 1959, *The Clonal Selection Theory of Acquired Immunity*, Vanderbilt University Press, Nashville, Tenn.

Burnett, F. M., and Fenner, F., 1949, *The Production of Antibodies*, Macmillan, New York.

Burns, W., Billups, L., and Notkins, A., 1975, Thymus dependence of viral antigens, *Nature (London)* **256**:654.

Chiller, J. M., and Weigle, W. O., 1972, Cellular basis of immunologic unresponsiveness, in: *Contemporary Topics in Immunobiology*, Vol. 1 (M. G. Hanna, Jr., ed.), pp. 119–142, Plenum Press, New York.

Chiller, J. M., and Weigle, W. O., 1973, Termination of tolerance to human gamma globulin in mice by antigen and bacterial lipopolysaccharide (endotoxin), *J. Exp. Med.* **137**:740.

Chiller, J. M., and Weigle, W. O., 1975, Biography of a tolerant state: Cellular parameters of the unresponsive state induced in adult mice to human gamma globulin. *J. Reticuloendo. Soc.* **17**:180.

Chiller, J. M., Habicht, G. S., and Weigle, W. O., 1970, Cellular sites of immunologic unresponsiveness, *Proc. Natl. Acad. Sci. USA* **65**:551.

Cihak, J., and Lehmann-Grube, F., 1978, Immunological tolerance to lymphocytic choriomeningitis virus in neonatally infected mice: Evidence supporting a clonal inactivation mechanism, *Immunology* **34**:265.

Cole, G. A., 1978, unpublished data.

Cole, G. A., Nathanson, N., and Prendergast, R. A., 1972, Requirement for θ-bearing cells in lymphocytic choriomeningitis virus-induced central nervous system disease, *Nature (London)* **238**:335.

Cole, G. A., Prendergast, R. A., and Henney, C. S., 1973, *In vitro* correlates of LCM virus-induced immune response, in: *Lymphocytic Choriomeningitis Virus and Other Arenaviruses* (F. Lehmann-Grube, ed.), pp. 61–71, Springer-Verlag, Berlin.

Coutinho, A., and Moller, G., 1975, Thymus-independent B-cell induction and paralysis, *Adv. Immunol.* **21**:113.

de Maeyer, E., de Maeyer-Guignard, J., and Vandeputte, M., 1975, Inhibition by interferon of delayed hypersensitivity in the mouse, *Proc. Natl. Acad. Sci. USA* **72**:1753.

de Maeyer-Guignard, J., Cachard, A., and de Maeyer, E., 1975, Delayed type hypersensitivity to sheep red blood cells: Inhibition of sensitization by interferon, *Science* **190**:574.

Dixon, F. J., Oldstone, M. B. A., and Tonietti, G., 1971, Pathogenesis of immune complex glomerulonephritis of New Zealand mice, *J. Exp. Med.* **134**:65s.

Doherty, P. C., and Zinkernagel, R. M., 1974, T-cell-mediated immunopathology in viral infections, *Transplant. Rev.* **19**:89.

Dore, J., Ajuria, E., and Mathe, G., 1970, Nonleukemic AKR mice are not tolerant to cells of leukemia induced by Gross virus, *Rev. Eur. Etud. Clin. Biol.* **XV**:81.

Doyle, M. V., and Oldstone, M. B. A., 1978, Interactions between viruses and lymphocytes. I. *In vivo* replication of lymphocytic choriomeningitis virus in mononuclear cells during both chronic and acute viral infections, *J. Immunol.* **121**:1262.

Doyle, M. V., Bloom, L., and Oldstone, M. B. A., 1978, unpublished data.

Dunlop, M., and Blanden, R., 1977, Mechanisms of suppression of cytotoxic T-cell responses in murine lymphocytic choriomeningitis virus infection, *J. Exp. Med.* **145**:1131.

Elder, J. H., Gautsch, J. W., Jensen, F. C., Lerner, R. A., Hartley, J. W., and Rowe, W. P., 1977, Biochemical evidence that MCF murine leukemia viruses are envelope (*env*) gene recombinants, *Proc. Natl. Acad. Sci. USA* **74**:4676.

Ferrarini, M., Moretta, L., Abrile, R., and Durante, M. L., 1975, Receptors for IgG molecules on human lymphocytes forming spontaneous rosettes with sheep red cells, *Eur. J. Immunol.* **5**:70.

Finkel, A., and Dent, P. B., 1973*a*, Abnormalities in lymphocyte proliferation in classical and atypical measles infection, *Cell. Immunol.* **6**:41.

Finkel, A., and Dent, P. B., 1973*b*, Virus-leukocyte interactions: Relationship to host resistance in virus infections in man, *Pathobiol. Annu.* **3**:47.

Fireman, P., Friday, G., and Kumate, J., 1969, Effect of measles vaccine on immunologic responsiveness, *Pediatrics* **43**:264.

Fujiwara, M., and Cinader, B., 1974, Cellular aspects of tolerance. V. The *in vivo* cooperative role of accessory and thymus derived cells in responsiveness and unresponsiveness of SJL mice, *Cell. Immunol.* **12**:194.

Gajdusek, D. C., and Gibbs, C. J., Jr., 1975, Slow virus infections of the nervous system and the laboratories of slow, latent and temperate virus infections, in: *The Nervous System*, Vol. 2 (D. B. Tower, ed.), pp. 113–135, Raven Press, New York.

Gershon, R. K., 1974, T cell control of antibody production, in: *Contemporary Topics in Immunobiology*, Vol. 3 (M. D. Cooper and N. L. Warners, eds.), pp. 1–40, Plenum Press, New York.

Gershon, R. K., Cohen, P., Hencin, R., and Liebhaber, S. A., 1972, Suppressor T cells, *J. Immunol.* **108**:586.

Gonatas, N. K., and Howard, J. C., 1974, Inhibition of experimental allergic encephalomyelitis in rats severely depleted of T cells, *Science* **186**:839.

Greaves, M. F., Owen, J. J. T., and Raff, M. C., 1974, *T and B Lymphocytes: Origins, Properties and Roles in Immune Responses*, Excerpta Medica, Amsterdam, American Elsevier, New York.

Gresser, I., and Chany, C., 1963, Isolation of measles virus from the washed leucocytic fraction of blood, *Proc. Soc. Exp. Biol. Med.* **113**:695.

Gross, L., 1970, *Oncogenic Viruses*, 2nd ed., Pergamon Press, New York.

Ha, T.-Y., Waksman, B. H., and Treffers, H. P., 1974, The thymic suppressor cell. I. Suppression of subpopulations with suppressor activity, *J. Exp. Med.* **139**:13.

Hartley, J. W., Wolford, N. K., Old, L. J., and Rowe, W. P., 1977, A new class of murine leukemia virus associated with development of spontaneous lymphomas, *Proc. Natl. Acad. Sci. USA* **74**:789.

Hirsh, M. E., Kelly, A. P., Proffitt, M. R., and Black, P. H., 1975, Cell-mediated immunity to antigens associated with endogenous murine C-type leukemia viruses, *Science* **187**:959.

Hollis, V. W., Aoki, T., Barrera, O., Oldstone, M. B. A., and Dixon, F. J., 1974, Detection of naturally occurring antibodies to RNA-dependent DNA polymerase of MuLV in kidney eluates of AKR mice, *J. Virol.* **13**:448.

Hotchin, J. E., and Cinits, M., 1958, Lymphocytic choriomeningitis infection of mice as a model for the study of latent virus infection, *Can. J. Microbiol.* **4**:149.

Huddlestone, J. R., Lampert, P. W., and Oldstone, M. B. A., 1979, manuscript in preparation.

Ihle, J. N., Yurconic, M., Jr., and Hanna, M. G., Jr., 1973, Autogenous immunity to endogenous RNA tumor virus, *J. Exp. Med.* **138**:194.

Ihle, J. N., Collins, J. J., Lee, J. C., Fischinger, P. J., Moennig, V., Schafer, W., Hanna, M. G., Jr., and Bolognesi, D. P., 1976a, Characterization of the immune response to the major glycoprotein (gp71) of Friend leukemia virus. I. Response in BALB/c mice, *Virology* **75**:74.

Ihle, J. N., Denny, T. P., and Bolognesi, D. P., 1976b, Purification and serological characterization of the major envelope glycoprotein from AKR murine leukemia virus and its reactivity with autogenous immune sera from mice, *J. Virol.* **17**:727.

Jerne, N. K., 1974, Towards a network theory of the immune system, *Ann. Immunol. Paris* **125C**:373.

Jerne, N. K., and Nordin, A. A., 1963, Plaque formation in agar by single antibody-producing cells, *Science* **140**:405.

Jondal, M., Klein, G., Oldstone, M. B. A., Bokisch, V., and Yefenof, E., 1976, Surface markers on human B and T lymphocytes. VIII. Association between complement and Epstein-Barr virus (EBV) receptors on human lymphoid cells, *Scand. J. Immunol.* **5**:401.

Joseph, B. S., Lampert, P. W., and Oldstone, M. B. A., 1975, Replication and persistence of measles virus in defined subpopulations of human leukocytes, *J. Virol.* **16**:1638.

Katz, D. H., 1977, *Lymphocyte Differentiation, Recognition, and Regulation*, Academic Press, New York.

Katz, D. H., and Benacerraf, B., eds., 1974, *Immunological Tolerance: Mechanisms and Therapeutic Applications*, Academic Press, New York.

Katz, D. H., Paul, W. E., Goidl, E. A., and Benacerraf, B., 1971, Carrier function in anti-hapten antibody responses. III. Stimulation of antibody synthesis and facilitation of hapten-specific secondary antibody responses by graft-versus-host reactions, *J. Exp. Med.* **133**:169.

Katz, S. L., and Enders, J. F., 1965, Measles virus, in: *Viral and Rickettsial Infections of Man* (F. L. Horsfall, Jr., and I. Tamm, eds.), pp. 784–801, Lippincott, Philadelphia.

Kawashima, K., Ikeda, H., Hartley, J. W., Stockert, E., Rowe, W. P., and Old, L. J., 1976, Changes in expression of murine leukemia virus antigens and production of xenotropic virus in the late preleukemic period in AKR mice, *Proc. Natl. Acad. Sci. USA* **73**:4680.

Lampert, P. W., Gajdusek, D. C., and Gibbs, C. J., 1972, Subacute spongiform virus encephalopathies: Scrapie, Kuru and Creutzfeldt Jakob disease, *Am. J. Pathol.* **68**:626.

Lennette, E. H., and Schmidt, N., 1979, *Diagnostic Procedures for Viral and Rickettsial Infections*, 5th ed., American Public Health Association, Washington, D.C., in press.

Lindahl, P., Leary, P., and Gresser, I., 1973, Enhancement by interferon of the expression of surface antigens on murine leukemia L1210 cells, *Proc. Natl. Acad. Sci. USA* **70**:2785.

Lindahl, P., Leary, P., and Gresser, I., 1974, Enhancement of the expression of histocompatibility antigens of mouse lymphoid cells by interferon in vitro, *Eur. J. Immunol.* **4**:779.

Lindahl, P., Gresser, I., Leary, P., and Tovey, M., 1976, Interferon treatment of mice: Enhanced expression of histocompatibility antigens on lymphoid cells, *Proc. Natl. Acad. Sci. USA* **73**:1284.

Lucas, C., Ubels-Postma, J., Rezee, A., and Galama, J., 1978, Activation of measles virus from silently infected human lymphocytes, *J. Exp. Med.* **48**:940.

Lukic, M. L., Cowing, C., and Leskowitz, S., 1975a, Strain differences in ease of tolerance induction bovine γ-globulin, *J. Immunol.* **114**:503.

Lukic, M. L., Wortis, H. H., and Leskowitz, S., 1975b, A gene locus affecting tolerance to BGG in mice, *Cell. Immunol.* **15**:457.

Lundstedt, C., 1969, Interaction between antigenically different cells: Virus induced cytotoxicity by immune lymphocytes in vitro, *Acta Pathol. Microbiol. Scand.* **75**:134.

Marchette, N., Halstead, S., and Chow, J., 1976, Replication of Dengue virus in cultures of peripheral blood leukocytes from Dengue-immune rhesus monkeys, *J. Infect. Dis.* **133**:274.

Marker, O., and Volkert, M., 1973, In vitro measurement of the time course of cellular immunity to LCM virus in mice, in: *Lymphocytic Choriomeningitis Virus and Other Arenaviruses* (F. Lehmann-Grube, ed.), pp. 207–216, Springer-Verlag, Berlin.

McDevitt, H., and Landy, M., eds., 1972, *Genetic Control of Immune Responsiveness*, Academic Press, New York.

Mims, C. A., and Subrahmanyan, T. P., 1966, Immunofluorescence study of the mechanism of resistance to superinfection in mice carrying lymphocytic choriomeningitis virus, *J. Pathol. Bacteriol.* **91**:403.

Mitchell, G. F., 1977, Observations and speculations of the influence of T cells in the cellular events of induction of antibody formation and tolerance *in vivo*, in: *The*

Lymphocyte: Structure and Function (J. J. Marchalonis, ed.), pp. 227–256, Dekker, New York.

Moretta, L., Webb, S. K., Grossi, C. E., Lydyard, P. M., and Cooper, M. D., 1977, Functional analysis of two human T-cell subpopulations: Help and suppression of B-cell responses by T cell bearing receptors for IgM or IgG, *J. Exp. Med.* **146**:184.

Nossal, G., and Ada, G., 1971, *Antigens, Lymphoid Cells, and the Immune Response*, Academic Press, New York.

Notkins, A., Mergenhagen, S., and Howard, R., 1970, Effect of virus infections on the function of the immune system, *Annu. Rev. Microbiol.* **24**:525.

Nowinski, R. C., 1975, Immune response to leukemia viruses in mice, in: *Viral Immunology and Immunopathology* (A. L. Notkins, ed.), pp. 237–260, Academic Press, New York.

Olding, L. B., Jensen, F. C., and Oldstone, M. B. A., 1975, Pathogenesis of cytomegalovirus infection. I. Activation of virus from bone marrow-derived lymphocytes by *in vitro* allogenic reaction, *J. Exp. Med.* **141**:561.

Olding, L. B., Kingsbury, D. T., and Oldstone, M. B. A., 1976, Pathogenesis of cytomegalovirus infection. Distribution of viral products, immune complexes and autoimmunity during latent murine infection, *J. Gen. Virol.* **33**:267.

Oldstone, M. B. A., 1973, Thymus dependent (T) cell competence in chronic LCM virus infection, in: *Lymphocytic Choriomeningitis Virus and Other Arenaviruses* (F. Lehmann-Grube, ed.), pp. 185–193, Springer-Verlag, Berlin.

Oldstone, M. B. A., 1975, Virus neutralization and virus-induced immune complex disease: Virus-antibody union resulting in immunoprotection or immunologic injury—Two different sides of the same coin, in: *Progress in Medical Virology*, Vol. 19 (J. L. Melnick, ed.), pp. 84–119, Karger, Basel.

Oldstone, M. B. A., 1977, Role of antibody in regulating virus persistence: Modulation of viral antigens expressed on the cell's plasma membrane and analyses of cell lysis, in: *Development of Host Defenses* (M. D. Cooper and D. H. Dayton, eds.), pp. 223–235, Raven Press, New York.

Oldstone, M. B. A., 1978, Virus–antiviral antibody immune complexes, p. 17, Abstracts of the Fourth European Immunology Meeting, Budapest, Hungary.

Oldstone, M. B. A., and Dixon, F. J., 1967, Lymphocytic choriomeningitis: Production of anti-LCM antibody by "tolerant" LCM-infected mice, *Science* **158**:1193.

Oldstone, M. B. A., and Dixon, F. J., 1969, Pathogenesis of chronic disease associated with persistent lymphocytic choriomeningitis viral infection. I. Relationship of antibody production to disease in neonatally infected mice, *J. Exp. Med.* **129**:483.

Oldstone, M. B. A., and Dixon, F. J., 1971, The immune response in lymphocytic choriomeningitis viral infection, in: *Sixth International Symposium of Immunopathology* (P. Miescher, ed.), pp. 391–398, Schwabe, Basel.

Oldstone, M. B. A., and Dixon, F. J., 1972, Disease accompanying in utero viral infection. The role of maternal antibody in tissue injury after transplacental infection with lymphocytic choriomeningitis virus, *J. Exp. Med.* **135**:827.

Oldstone, M. B. A., and Perrin, L. H., 1979, Assays of cell mediated immunity and immune complexes in virus infections, in: *Diagnostic Procedures for Viral and Rickettsial Infections*, 5th ed. (E. H. Lennette and N. Schmidt, eds.), American Public Health Association, Washington, D.C., in press.

Oldstone, M. B. A., Aoki, T., and Dixon, F. J., 1972a, The antibody response of mice to murine leukemia virus in spontaneous infection. Absence of classical immunologic tolerance, *Proc. Natl. Acad. Sci. USA* **69**:134.

Oldstone, M. B. A., Tishon, A., Tonietti, G., and Dixon, F. J., 1972b, Immune com-
    plex disease associated with spontaneous murine leukemia: Incidence and
    pathogenesis of glomerulonephritis, *Clin. Immunol. Immunopathol.* **1**:6.
Oldstone, M. B. A., Tishon, A., Chiller, J., Weigle, W., and Dixon, F. J., 1973, Effect
    of chronic viral infection on the immune system. I. Comparison of the immune
    responsiveness of mice chronically infected with LCM virus with that of
    noninfected mice, *J. Immunol.* **110**:1268.
Oldstone, M. B. A., Tison, A., and Chiller, J. M., 1974, Chronic virus infection and
    immune responsiveness, II. Lactic dehydrogenase virus infection and immune
    response to non-viral antigens, *J. Immunol.* **112**:370.
Oldstone, M. B. A., Welsh, R. M., and Joseph, B. S., 1975, Pathogenic mechanisms of
    tissue injury in persistent viral infections, *Ann. N.Y. Acad. Sci.* **256**:65.
Oldstone, M. B. A., Del Villano, B. C., and Dixon, F. J., 1976, Autologous immune
    responses to the major oncornavirus polypeptides in unmanipulated AKR/J mice,
    J. Virol. **18**:176.
Oldstone, M. B. A., Holmstoen, J., and Welsh, R. M. Jr., 1977a, Alterations of
    acetylcholine enzymes in neuroblastoma cells persistently infected with lympho-
    cytic choriomeningitis virus, *J. Cell. Physiol.* **91**:459.
Oldstone, M. B. A., Tishon, A., and Moretta, L., 1977b, Active thymus derived sup-
    pressor lymphocytes in human cord blood, *Nature (London)* **269**:333.
Owen, R. D., 1945, Immunogenetic consequences of vascular anastomoses between
    bovine twins, *Science* **102**:400.
Paterson, P. Y., 1977, Autoimmune neurological disease: Experimental animal systems
    and implications for multiple sclerosis, in: *Autoimmunity*, pp. 643–692, Academic
    Press, New York.
Pfizenmaier, K., Starzinski-Powitz, A., Rollinghoff, M., Dalke, D., and Wagner, H.,
    1977, T cell-mediated cytotoxicity against herpes simplex virus-infected target
    cells, *Nature (London)* **265**:630.
Popescu, M., 1978, Infectious lymphocytes in LCM virus carrier mice, Abstracts of the
    Fourth International Congress for Virology held at The Hague, The Netherlands,
    August 30–September 6.
Popescu, M., Lohler, J., and Lehmann-Grube, F., 1977, Infectious lymphocytes in mice
    persistently infected with lymphocytic choriomeningitis virus, *Z. Naturforsch.*
    32c:1026.
Porter, D. D., Porter, H. G., and Cox, N. A., 1973, Failure to demonstrate a humoral
    immune response to scrapie infection in mice, *J. Immunol.* **111**:1407.
Raff, M. C., 1977, Surface antigenic markers for distinguishing T and B lymphocytes
    in mice, *Transplant. Rev.* **6**:52.
Raff, M. C., Owen, J. J. T., Cooper, M. D., Lawton, A. R., Megson, M., and Gath-
    ings, W. E., 1975, Differences in susceptibility of mature and immature mouse B
    lymphocytes to anti-immunoglobulin-induced immunoglobulin separation *in vitro:*
    Possible implications for B-cell tolerance to self, *J. Exp. Med.* **142**:1052.
Rollinghoff, M., Starzinski-Powitz, A., Pfizenmaier, K., and Wagner, H., 1977,
    Cyclophosphamide-sensitive T lymphocytes suppress the *in vivo* generation of
    antigen-specific cytotoxic T lymphocytes, *J. Exp. Med.* **145**:455.
Rowe, W. P. 1954. Studies on pathogenesis and immunity in lymphocytic choriomenin-
    gitis infection of the mouse, *Res. Rep. Nav. Med. Res. Inst.* **12**:167.
Schreiner, G. F., and Unanue, E. R., 1976, Membrane and cytoplasmic changes in B
    lymphocytes induced by ligand-surface immunoglobulin interaction, *Adv.
    Immunol.* **24**:38.

Sidman, C. L., and Unanue, E. R., 1975, Receptor-mediated inactivation of early B lymphocytes, *Nature (London)* **257**:149.

Smithwick, E. M., and Berkovich, S., 1966, *In vitro* suppression of the lymphocyte response to tuberculin by live measles virus, *Proc. Soc. Exp. Biol. Med.* **123**:276.

Sullivan, J. L., Barry, D., Lucas, S. J., and Albrecht, P., 1975, Measles infection of human mononuclear cells. I. Acute infection of peripheral blood lymphocytes and monocytes, *J. Exp. Med.* **142**:773.

Taussig, M., Mozes, E., and Isac, R., 1974, Antigen-specific thymus cell factors in the genetic control of the immune response to poly-(tyrosyl, glutamyl)-poly-D;L-alanyl-poly-lysyl, *J. Exp. Med.* **140**:301.

Theofilopoulos, A. N., and Dixon, F. J., 1976, Immune complexes in human sera detected by the Raji cell radioimmune assay, in: *In Vitro Methods in Cell Mediated and Tumor Immunity* (B. R. Bloom and J. R. David, eds.), pp. 555–563, Academic Press, New York.

Traub, E., 1936a, Persistence of lymphocytic choriomeningitis virus in immune animals and its relation to immunity, *J. Exp. Med.* **63**:847.

Traub, E., 1936b, The epidemiology of lymphocytic choriomeningitis in white mice, *J. Exp. Med.* **64**:183.

Traub, E., 1960, Observations on immunological tolerance and immunity in mice infected congenitally with the virus of lymphocytic choriomeningitis, *Arch Gesamte Virusforsch.* **303**.

Virelizier, J., Virelizier, A., and Allison, A., 1976, The role of circulating interferon in the modifications of immune responsiveness by mouse hepatitis virus (MHV-3), *J. Immunol.* **17**:748.

Volkert, M., and Larsen, J. H., 1965, Immunological tolerance to viruses, *Prog. Med. Virol.* **7**:160.

von Pirquet, C., 1908, Das Verhalden der kutanen Tuberkulin-reakton wahrend der Masern, *Dtsch. Med. Wochenschr.* **34**:1247.

Wahren, B., and Metcalf, D., 1970, Cytotoxicity in vitro of pre leukemic lymphoid cells on syngeneic monolayers of embryo or thymus cells, *Clin. Exp. Immunol.* **7**:373.

Waldmann, T. A., Broder, S., Blaese, R. M., Durm, M., Blackman, M., and Strober, W., 1974, Role of suppressor T cell in pathogenesis of common variable hypo-gamma globulinemia, *Lancet* **2**:609.

Weigle, W. O., 1977, Cellular events in experimental autoimmune thyroiditis, allergic encephalomyelitis and tolerance to self, in: *Autoimmunity: Genetic, Immunologic, Virologic and Clinical Aspects* (N. Talal, ed.), pp. 141–170, Academic Press, New York.

Weiner, E., and Bandieri, A., 1974, The genetic control of immune response to different antigenic determinants within the synthetic polypeptide poly (His-Glu)-poly pro-poly lys, *Eur. J. Immunol.* **4**:463.

Welsh, R. M., and Oldstone, M. B. A., 1977, Inhibition of immunologic injury of cultured cells infected with lymphocytic choriomeningitis virus: Role of defective interfering virus in regulating viral antigenic expression, *J. Exp. Med.* **145**:1449.

Wheelock, F., and Toy, S. T., 1973, Participation of lymphocytes in viral infections, *Adv. Immunol.* **16**:123.

White, R. G., and Boyd, J. F., 1973, The effect of measles on the thymus and other lymphoid tissues, *Clin. Exp. Immunol.* **13**:343.

Williams, R., and Moore, M. J., 1973, Linkage of susceptibility to experimental allergic encephalomyelitis to the major histocompatibility locus in the rat, *J. Exp. Med.* **138**:775.

Wilson, A., Planterose, D., Nagington, J., Park, J., Barry, R., and Coombs, R. R. A., 1976, Influenza A antigens on human lymphocytes in vitro and probably in vivo, *Nature* (*London*) **259**:582.

Woodruff, J., and Woodruff, J., 1975, T lymphocyte interaction with viruses and virus infected tissues, *Prog. Med. Virol.* **19**:120.

Yefenof, E., Klein, G., Jondal, M., and Oldstone, M. B. A., 1976, Surface markers on human B- and T-lymphocytes. IX. Two-color immunofluorescence studies on the association between EBV receptors and complement receptors on the surface of lymphoid cell lines, *Int. J. Cancer* **17**:693.

Zinkernagel, R. M., and Doherty, P. C., 1973, Cytotoxic thymus-derived lymphocytes in cerebrospinal fluid of mice with lymphocytic choriomeningitis, *J. Exp. Med.* **138**:1266.

Zinkernagel, R. M., and Doherty, P. C., 1974, Indications of active suppression in mouse carriers of lymphocytic choriomeningitis virus, in: *Immunological Tolerance* (D. Katz and B. Benacerraf, eds.), pp. 403–411, Academic Press, New York.

Zinkernagel, R. M., and Welsh, R. M., 1976, *H-2* compatibility requirement for virus-specific T cell-mediated effector functions *in vivo*. I. Specificity of T cells conferring antiviral protection against lymphocytic choriomeningitis virus is associated with *H-2K* and *H-2D*, *J. Immunol.* **117**:1495.

Zinkernagel, R. M., Callahan, A., Althage, A., Cooper, S., Streilein, J. W., and Klein, J., 1978, The lymphoreticular system in triggering virus-plus-self-specific cytotoxic T cells: Evidence for T help, *J. Exp. Med.* **147**:897.

Zubler, H., and Lambert, P. H., 1976, The ^{125}I-C1q binding test for the detection of soluble immune complexes, in: *In Vitro Methods in Cell Mediated and Tumor Immunity* (B. R. Bloom and J. R. David, eds.), pp. 565–572, Academic Press, New York.

Zweiman, B., Pappagianis, D., Maibach, H., and Hildreth, E. H., 1971, Effect of measles immunization on tuberculin hypersensitivity and *in vitro* lymphocyte reactivity, *Int. Arch. Allergy Appl. Immunol.* **40**:834.

CHAPTER 2

Interaction of Viruses with Neutralizing Antibodies

Benjamin Mandel

Department of Virology
The Public Health Research Institute of the City of New York, Inc.
New York, New York 10016

1. INTRODUCTION

Possibly the earliest published expectation and demonstration of the neutralizing capacity of humoral antibody is contained in the report of Sternberg (1892). He suspected that the blood of an individual recently recovered from a viral infection contained an "antitoxine" that could nullify the infectious capability of the causative agent. He then demonstrated that the serum of a calf recently vaccinated with cowpox (?) virus neutralized the infectivity of this virus when the two were mixed prior to inoculation. The validity of this result was corroborated, and extended, by Béclère *et al.* (1898) in their studies involving a different host, man, and a different virus, variola. Worthy of note is the empirical aspect of these speculations and experimentations since the nature of antibody as well as virus was at that time unknown.

Studies of this phenomenon were pursued in the early 1900s with animal viruses, e.g., vaccinia and herpes cultivated in rabbit testicular

The following abbreviations will be used to designate specific viruses (V): EAV, equine abortion; FLV, Friend leukemia; IBV, infectious bronchitis; JEV, Japanese encephalitis; LDV, lactic dehydrogenase; NDV, Newcastle disease; RSV, respiratory syncitial; TMV, tobacco mosaic; VEV, Venezuelan encephalitis; VSV, vesicular stomatitis; WEV, Western encephalitis; WNV, West Nile.

tissue or in the chorioallantoic membrane of chicken embryo, and bacterial viruses specific for strains of *Escherichia* or *Staphylococcus*. Of
particular relevance are the studies of Andrewes and Burnet and their
colleagues. Many of their observations have provided parameters and
interpretations that are still valid, and, of the many questions they had
posed, some have since been answered and others are still relevant and
still elusive.

Early in the studies of viral neutralization the question of
mechanism of action was investigated. In several instances the
interpretation favored the direct interaction of virus and antibody (e.g.,
Smith, 1930), whereas other interpretations favored the concept that
antibody reacted with the target cell, rendering it resistant (e.g., Long
and Olitzky, 1930; Sabin, 1935*a,b*). However, subsequent studies
established beyond doubt that virus and homologous antibody interact
to form a complex that can vary with respect to the quantity of each
reactant according to their respective valences, and according to their
relative concentrations in the reaction mixture.

The gross nature of antibody was shown to be protein of the γ-
globulin class (Tiselius and Kabat, 1939). Subsequent intensive studies
on the nature of antibody have resulted in classifications of antibody
according to physicochemical characteristics (e.g., molecular size, sedimentation constant), according to antigenicity (e.g., iso-, allo-,
idiotype), and according to biological function (e.g., neutralizing, complement fixing, sensitizing). These studies have revealed the broadly
heterogeneous nature of this group of substances and have resulted in
subclassifications based on subtle distinctions (see the review of
Spielberg, 1974). In like manner, studies on the physicochemical and
antigenic characteristics of viruses have revealed a wide diversity of
complexity. Some contain a single surface antigenic determinant, some
contain more than one, some contain multiple determinants including
surface as well as internal. Viruses characterized by lipoprotein
envelopes contain, in addition to virus-specific determinants, host-
specific determinants as constituents of the envelope. Since not all
antigens are essential for infectivity, the interaction of antibody with a
viral antigen does not inevitably result in neutralization. Hence, with
respect to neutralization, antigenic sites can be distinguished as critical
or noncritical. Although perhaps not directly relevant to the essence of
this chapter, it is worth noting that with some double-stranded viruses,
antibodies in immunized rabbits are specific for the double-stranded
viral genome (e.g., see Ikegami and Francki, 1973).

A common denominator in all studies on neutralization is the use
of serum (i.e., antibody). As indicated above, antibody is a generic

representation of a group of diverse molecules. Diversification is related to many variable factors: animal species, characteristics of the immunogen, conditions of immunological stimulation such as dose, regimen, and use of adjuvants, and elapsed time after stimulation (e.g., see Nicklin and Stephan, 1973; Petty and Steward, 1977). Also, results can vary according to conditions of handling of serum since it has been shown that some antibodies function in conjunction with accessory serum factors that may be thermolabile. In many studies on viral neutralization the characteristics of antisera in use were simply described as, e.g., "hyperimmune rabbit antiserum." Since the immune response is time dependent with respect to both class and binding affinity of antibody, a definitive interpretation of results would require identification of the antibody under investigation.

The quantitative analyses of bacteriophage neutralization by Kalmanson et al. (1942) and Delbrück (1945) and of animal virus neutralization by Dulbecco et al. (1956) initiated a renewed interest in virus–antibody interaction. The studies of Dulbecco et al. not only defined various parameters of the system but also delineated several basic problems. A further impetus to studies of viral neutralization was the incisive critique and reinterpretation by Fazekas de St. Groth and Reid (1958) of the data of Dulbecco et al. (1956).

The studies of Eisen and Karush (1949), Epstein et al. (1956), and Karush (1956) laid the conceptual and methodological groundwork for defining antibody–hapten interactions in thermodynamic and kinetic terms. By substituting equilibrium filtration for equilibrium dialysis, Fazekas de St. Groth and Webster succeeded in deriving thermodynamic and kinetic parameters for the interaction of influenza virus and antibody (Fazekas de St. Groth, 1961; Fazekas de St. Groth and Webster 1961, 1963a,b).

A survey of recent literature pertaining to viral neutralization reveals that several problems essential to a complete understanding of this phenomenon have yet to be answered (e.g., see Dudley et al., 1970; Burns and Allison, 1975; Daniels, 1975; Della-Porta and Westaway, 1978; Yoshino and Isono, 1978; Mandel, 1976, 1978).

2. METHODS

Details for conducting neutralization experiments vary widely and will not be reviewed. However, the methods will be distinguished according to the underlying principle and the parameter to be evaluated.

2.1. Static (End-Point) Methods

In static (end-point) methods the concentration of serum/antibody capable of neutralizing a specified fraction of a given input of virus under a given set of conditions is determined.

2.1.1. Quantal Method

When whole animals, or occasionally cell cultures, serve as host, the quantal method is used. This is based on the qualitative response of replicate test subjects. The concentration of antiserum required to reduce the infectivity of a given dose of virus to 50% of the test subjects is calculated by a statistical method (e.g., Kärber, 1931; Reed and Muench, 1938) from data obtained by the use of a wide range of antiserum concentrations.

2.1.2. Enumerative Method

Where viral infectivity can be assayed by quantitation of plaques, pocks, foci, or leaf lesions, antibody can be assayed in terms of 50% (or other percentage) reduction in count.

2.2. Kinetic Method

The rate of the reaction between virus and antibody is both time and concentration dependent. Consequently, by adjusting the concentrations of virus and antibody appropriately, the rate of the reaction can be measured as a function of time. It has been seen generally that a constant fraction of virus is neutralized per unit of time, conforming to the equation for a first-order reaction (Kalmanson *et al.*, 1942) and therefore can be expressed mathematically:

$$V_t/V_0 = e^{-kt/D} \tag{1}$$

where V_t and V_0 are the concentrations of infectious virus at times t and 0, respectively, D is the dilution factor of serum, and k is the reaction rate constant. The value of k is an empirical measure of the neutralizing potency of the serum and has the dimensions of $\min^{-1}$ usually, or if the molar concentration of antibody is known and substituted for $1/D$, k has the dimensions of $\mathrm{mol}^{-1}\ \min^{-1}$.

The implications of the various methods should be noted. In a quantal assay with an intact animal as the test host four competing dynamic systems will be generated: (1) The interaction between virus and antibody, initiated *in vitro*, may continue after inoculation but probably at a reduced rate. (2) Susceptible cells will compete with antibody for virus not yet neutralized. (3) Infected cells will eventually release progeny virions which will react with antibody that may still be present. (4) If the animal is immunocompetent, viral antibody will be synthesized. Under such conditions a quantitative expression of antibody-neutralizing activity represents the net result of the above competing and overlapping interactions. A further complication arises if replicate assays are conducted in various hosts, or by different routes of inoculation, as exemplified in Fig. 1. Simplification of the assay system, e.g., use of cell cultures instead of whole animals, reduces the number of imponderables and permits a more accurate determination of the state of a reaction at a given time, or under a given set of conditions. It is of course obvious that extrapolation of results under a simplified situation to the real situation may be fraught with a new set of imponderables.

3. ANTIBODY

Studies of the nature, origin, and function of antibody have evolved as one of the major intellectual achievements of modern biological science. No attempt will be made to review the vast literature

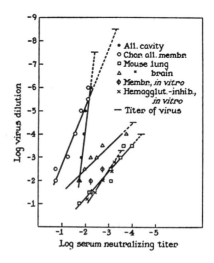

Fig. 1.   Results of neutralization experiments with NWS (single pool of infected allantoic fluid) and one immune serum in five host-cell systems. Log virus dilution used is given on the vertical axis. The titer of the virus found in each host-cell system is represented by the horizontal line at the top of each curve. The slopes for the various host-cell systems are chorioallantoic membrane 2.6, allantoic cavity 4.7, mouse brain 1.0, mouse lung 1.2, and hemagglutination-inhibition *in vitro* 1.3. From Tyrrell and Horsfall (1953), with permission of the publisher.

describing these achievements. Rather, those salient aspects that are relevant to viral neutralization will be indicated.

3.1. Physicochemical Characteristics

Five major classes of antibody have been identified, IgG, IgM, IgA, IgD, and IgE. These immunoglobulins (Ig) are distinguishable by the antigenic characteristics of their heavy polypeptide chains as well as by their physicochemical characteristics. The IgD and IgE classes have not yet been implicated in neutralization of viruses and will not be discussed.

3.1.1. IgG (7 S, 150,000 Daltons)

IgG, formerly designated γG, is the most abundant humoral antibody. As represented in Fig. 2, it consists of four polypeptide chains, two identical heavy (H) and two identical light (L) chains joined by disulfide linkages. In addition to the interpeptide disulfide linkages, there are intrapeptide disulfide linkages which contribute to the tertiary structure. All chains have the same orientation with respect to terminus. The binding sites are represented by the two H-L chain pairs at the *N*-terminus. (It has been found that almost all terminal amino groups are blocked by pyrrolidone carboxylic acid.) The primary structure of the *N*-terminal regions is variable and endows the molecule with specificity (i.e., affinity for the antigenic determinant responsible for its induction). The molecule is composed of three functional domains, two Fab domains, which contain the antigen-combining sites, and one Fc domain. The Fc region has little or no direct role in neutralization but has effector functions such as complement fixation and recognition of cell-surface receptors.

As suggested by the schematic representation (Fig. 2) the molecule has a Y-shaped configuration. The hinge region just above the junction of the arms of the "Y" imparts flexibility, a characteristic that has considerable significance for neutralization when multimeric antigens are involved. Electron microscopic studies have indicated variability in the normal angle of the arms, as well as the angle when antibody is complexed with antigen. In some cases the angle may be as great as 180° (Crothers and Metzger, 1972). Studies on rabbit IgG in solution (Werner *et al.*, 1972) have indicated that the minimum angle between the two arms is 80–90°, and the binding sites are located at or very near the tips. Therefore, at the minimum angle, the binding sites are about 9 nm apart. Yguerabide *et al.* (1970) have shown that the Fab portions of the molecule can rotate over an angle of 33° within nanosecond periods. Other studies (e.g., Feinstein and Rowe, 1965; Valentine and Green, 1967) have suggested that when bound to antigen the angular dimension may differ from that of the free molecule. These studies suggest that within the limitations imposed by its geometry and mobility an IgG molecule may possibly adjust its binding sites to accommodate simultaneously two determinants that are within 9–20 nm apart. That this flexibility is not characteristic of all IgG molecules has been indicated by Crothers and Metzger (1972) and by Green (1969).

The anatomy of the molecule was discerned through controlled enzymatic digestion (Porter, 1959; Nisonoff *et al.*, 1960; Putnam *et al.*, 1962). Under reducing conditions, papain cleaves the molecule above the hinge region, liberating three fragments: two Fab and one Fc. The two monovalent Fab fragments retain their antigen-binding capacity.

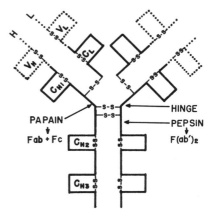

Fig. 2. Schematic representation of a molecule of IgG antibody. The molecue is symmetrical about the vertical axis. The two heavy (H) chains are joined by inter-peptide disulfide linkages. The light (L) chains are joined to the H-H chains by interpeptide disulfide bonds. Each chain consists of distinct homology domains delimited by intrapeptide disulfide bonds. The amino-terminal domains (·····) consist of variable amino acid sequences (V_H and V_L) which represent the specific antigen recognition and binding sites. The carboxyl-terminal domains (——) consist of constant amino acid sequences ($C_{H1,2,3}$ and C_L). Short sequences at the juncture of the H chains impart flexibility to the "arms" of the molecule. Enzymatic cleavage results in specific fragments. Pepsin severs the molecule below the inter-H disulfide bonds, yielding a fragment $(Fab')_2$ that is bivalent and functional. Reduction of $(Fab')_2$ releases two monovalent functional fragments, Fab'. Treatment of the intact molecule with papain cleaves the H chains above the juncture and releases three fragments: two Fab and one Fc. The Fab fragments are monovalent and functional. The Fc fragment is not involved in antigen recognition or binding. The distinction between Fab and Fab' is the increased length of H chain of the latter. Occasionally the H chains of these fragments are referred to as Fd and Fd' , respectively. Fab fragments fall into two classes designated Fab I and Fab II. These are derived from different IgG molecules: Fab I from early antibody, probably γ_1-globulin, and Fab II from late antibody, probably γ_2-globulin. From Palmer *et al.* (1962).

Pepsin cleaves the molecule below the hinge region, yielding one F(ab')$_2$ fragment and oligopeptides. In contrast to the Fab fragment, the F(ab')$_2$ is divalent and is dissociable by reducing agents into two mono-valent Fab' fragments. Under carefully controlled reducing conditions, the interpeptide disulfide bonds of the intact molecule can be disrupted, yielding the four constituent polypeptides. The careful dismemberment of the molecule has proved to be exceedingly informative for elucidating certain aspects of antigen–antibody interactions.

3.1.2.   IgM (19 S, 900,000 Daltons)

IgM is a covalently linked pentamer of IgG. The five monomers are joined by —S—S— linkages between the hinge region and the C-terminus. A third distinct polypeptide, J, has been identified. Although there are theoretically ten binding sites, the molecule binds five ligands. Possibly the binding at one site of a monomer sterically precludes binding at the second site. Exposure to reducing conditions releases the monomers, but they are no longer capable of binding. Studies by electron microscopy have indicated that the molecules may acquire configurations described as "flat," "staple," "loop," "spider," "angular" structures (e.g., see Feinstein and Munn, 1966; Almeida et al., 1967; Chesebro et al., 1968; Svehag et al., 1968) depending on whether they are free or bound to flat or curved structures. The implication of these observations is that IgM possesses flexibility, although in some studies it has been considered that the degree is less than that of IgG.

3.1.3.   IgA [(7 S)$_n$, (150,000)$_n$ Daltons]

IgA may occur as a monomer, dimer, or trimer of a 7 S monomer. As IgM, the monomers are polymerized by —S—S— linkages since it has been shown that mild reducing conditions will dissociate the multi-meric forms. Of pertinent interest is the observation that some forms of the IgA antibody may be found in secretions of exocrine glands. In contrast to humoral IgA, the antibody found in secretions has an additional glycoprotein moiety (secretory protein). Brandtzaeg (1978) has shown, for example, that the secretory component is present on the surface of epithelial cells of the gut. Polymeric IgA, formed by plasma cells vicinal to the glandular epithelial cells, binds through its J polypeptide to the secretory component and acquires the property necessary for its concentration in glandular secretions. In like manner

IgA antibody is concentrated in secretions such as saliva, milk, tears, and mucus. Localization of neutralizing antibody in such regional fluids very likely serves a defense purpose. Karl and Thormar (1971) have reported that immunization of rabbits (not a natural host) with visna virus resulted in the appearance of antibodies detectable by passive hemagglutination, complement fixation, and immunofluorescence. However, neutralizing antibody was not detectable. In contrast, sheep (a natural host) produced neutralizing antibody. These investigators suggested that the neutralizing antibody was of the IgA class which rabbits are incapable of synthesizing.

3.2. Heterogeneity

It has become increasingly evident that antibodies are an exceedingly and subtly diverse group of molecules. Since it is considered that each specifically distinct molecule represents a clonally derived family of antibody-producing cells, the attendant question of origin—germ line vs. somatic mutation—is of current interest (Cohn, 1971; Haurowitz, 1973; Wigzell, 1973; Cunningham, 1974; Cunningham and Pilarski, 1974; Copra and Kehoe, 1974; Seidman *et al.*, 1978) but outside the scope of this chapter.

3.2.1. Binding Affinity

From the functional standpoint, heterogeneity is a reflection of variable binding strength. As described in Svehag's discussion (1966), diversity can be approximately assessed by examining various aspects of virus–antibody interaction with loss, or recovery, of infectivity as indicator. Such studies elicit overall (i.e., avidity) rather than definable parameters. In order to evaluate specific parameters such as affinity and heterogeneity, various characteristics of the system must be known precisely. An example of the hazards of attempting to measure fundamental parameters is illustrated in studies of tobacco mosaic virus (TMV) (Mamet-Bratley, 1966). TMV was selected because of its relative simplicity and because of its known structure—namely, a capsid composed of 2130 equivalently situated helically arranged structural units. Each unit was assumed to represent one effective antigenic site. Fab fragments, prepared from purified rabbit anti-TMV antibody, were interacted with TMV at low antibody multiplicity. Calculations of free and bound antibody, and the assumed total valence of TMV, were analyzed by the method of Scatchard (1949) (see Section 4.1.1). Extrapolation of the plot of r/c as a function of r (r is moles of viral subunits per mole Fab; c is moles of viral subunits not covered) indicated a valence for Fab of approximately 0.8. Discrepancy with the theoretical valence of 1.0 was attributed to the presence of nonfunctional Fab. Further analysis of the data by the method of Karush (1962) yielded heterogeneity indices varying from 0.95 to 0.99 for antibody from four different sera and from one pool of several sera. The almost perfect index of homogeneity, as well as the linearity of the Scatchard plot, was presented as evidence of a homogeneous antibody population.

This conclusion was challenged by Hardie and van Regenmortel (1975) on the grounds of an erroneous value (2130) for antigen valence. They determined a valence of 800, consistent with previously reported values of 650–950 (Rappaport, 1965; van Regenmortel, 1966). Scatchard plots employing 800 as total effective antigen valence indicated a deviation from linearity and therefore evidence for heterogeneity.

The determination of several parameters of the interaction of influenza virus with antibody has been reported (Fazekas de St. Groth, 1961; Fazekas de St. Groth and Webster, 1963a,b). Subsequent analysis of their data by Day (1972) has indicated other possible interpretations with respect to number of antigenic sites, maximum number of molecules that can bind to one virion, degree of homogeneity of the antibody population in a given serum, and the ambiguity of the valence of antibody.

3.2.2. Chronology of Synthesis and Persistence of Different Classes of Antibody

The distribution in serum of antibodies of various classes at a given time in the immune response is variable. Studies with animal and bacterial viruses as immunogens in nonsusceptible animals have shown that the class of antibody, as well as the rate of synthesis is dependent on dose of immunogen (Uhr *et al.*, 1962; Uhr and Finkelstein, 1963; Uhr, 1964; Svehag and Mandel, 1962, 1964a,b; Svehag, 1966). Based on neutralizing activity it was seen that, with low doses, immunogens induced the production of IgM antibody only and that the duration of synthesis was short-lived. With high doses, IgM and IgG antibodies were produced, the IgM antibody preceding the IgG. Whereas IgM synthesis soon terminated, IgG persisted for a long time. It has been suggested (Hornick and Karush, 1972; Cowan, 1973; Osler, 1976) that IgG antibody may be synthesized concurrently with or preceding IgM. Because of the greater avidity of IgM, methods other than neutralization would be required for the detection of IgG antibody in the presence of IgM in very early sera. It would appear, therefore, that the very early IgG is of such low affinity as to be irrelevant for neutralization. However, with respect to the kinetics of antibody synthesis and antibody maturation, the presence of such antibody is indeed of pertinent interest. The above results, obtained under the "artificial" conditions of the laboratory, were found to have their counterpart in the field among previously infected or immunized persons (Ogra *et al.*, 1968, 1975; McKercher and Giordano, 1967, Graves *et al.*, 1964; Brown *et al.*, 1964).

3.2.3. Activity

On the basis of their biological effects, antibodies have been categorized as neutralizing, complement fixing, precipitating, agglutinating, etc. In recent studies on virus–antibody interaction, it has been observed that virus–antibody complexes may occur that retain infectivity. However, on addition of a third component, e.g., complement, infectivity is neutralized. Under such circumstances antibody has been designated as sensitizing, complement requiring, etc. (see reviews by Notkins, 1971; Majer, 1972). The original observation of this phenomenon (Mandel, 1958) in a cell culture system was seen to have its parallel in animal (Notkins *et al.*, 1966) as well as bacterial systems (Stemke and Lennox, 1967). The pathological sequelae of such circulating virus–antibody complexes have been recognized and are of sufficient importance to have earned the name of "immune complex diseases," to which a branch of immunopathology is devoted (see Oldstone, 1975).

Extensive studies by Yoshino and his colleagues have shown that sensitizing antibodies to herpesvirus appear early and they may be either of the IgM or the IgG class. With time they are superseded by IgG antibodies that neutralize independently (Yoshino and Taniguchi, 1964, 1965a; Shinkai and Yoshino, 1975a,b). Basically similar results were described by Hampar *et al.* (1968) and Stevens *et al.* (1968) for herpesvirus and by Hajek (1966, 1968, 1969) and Hajek and Mandel (1966) for antibacteriophage T2 antibodies.

3.2.4. Summary

Immunogenic stimulation induces the synthesis of several classes of antibodies. The rate of production and the duration of both production and antibody survival (i.e., half-life) are unique for each class. Within each class there is a distribution of antibodies capable of neutralizing, of antibodies capable of reacting but requiring assistance for neutralization, and possibly of antibodies capable of reacting but unreceptive to assistance. Of most relevance perhaps is the variation in binding affinity. Studies (Eisen and Siskind, 1964) have shown that for a given dose of antigen the average affinity (association constant) increased between 100- and 250-fold from the second to the eighth week after stimulation. It would be of interest to determine if the transition from complement requirement for neutralization to independence paralleled the transition from a lower to a higher level of binding affinity. Finally, the functional activity of antibody induced in a given animal will vary according to such conditions as the dosage and physical state of the immunogen, frequency of stimulation, route of inoculation, use of adjuvants of varying composition, and elapsed time after immunogenic stimulation. This topic has been reviewed analytically by Macario and Conway de Macario (1975).

4.   ANTIGEN–ANTIBODY INTERACTION

The union of antigen and antibody is mediated by noncovalent interactions. Probably, the initial affinity is generated by coulombic attractions supplemented by additional short-range forces (apolar, H-bond, van der Waals) as the distance between the reactants decreases. The inhibitory and dissociative effects of high ionic concentrations and of pH extremes attest to the nature of the antigen–antibody interaction. Although an increase in temperature favors the reaction with respect to reaction rate ($Q_{10} \cong 1.5$), a decrease in temperature favors the formation of the complex because of an accompanying decrease in enthalpy. Also, an increase in entropy (i.e., release of bound water) favors the forward reaction. Szweczuk and Mukkur (1977) have suggested that the relative contributions of the changes in enthalpy and entropy to the forward reaction vary with temperature. At low temperature the enthalpy change is the principal driving force whereas at high temperature (37°C) the change in entropy is more significant.

4.1.   Hapten–Antibody Interaction

The interaction of antibody and a complex protein antigen initially involves the specific antibody-combining site and the specific determinant group of the antigen. Subsequent interactions may occur between the nonspecific domains of each reactant. In order to measure the interaction parameters related only to site-specific binding, studies were carried out with haptens reacting with antibody that was induced by homologously haptenated proteins.

4.2. Studies

4.2.1. Kinetic Aspects

The reversible reaction between a monovalent hapten and a free antibody binding site results in a hapten–antibody complex:

$$[H] + [A] \underset{k_2}{\overset{k_1}{\rightleftharpoons}} [HA] \tag{2}$$

At equilibrium the intrinsic association constant is represented by

$$K_a = \frac{k_1}{k_2} = \frac{[HA]}{[H] + [A]} \text{ liter mol}^{-1} \tag{3}$$

where K_a is the intrinsic association constant, [H], [A], [HA], are, respectively, the concentrations of hapten, antibody, and the complex, and k_1, k_2 are, respectively, the forward and reverse reaction rate constants. For some purposes it has been found more useful to determine the average (or standard) intrinsic association constant, K_0:

$$K_0 = \frac{1}{c} \text{ liter mol}^{-1} \tag{4}$$

where c is the concentration of free hapten when 50% of the effective antibody sites are occupied, determined at 25°C. Based on the analysis described by Scatchard (1949), equation (3) can be restated as

$$\frac{r}{c} = nK_a - rK_a \tag{5}$$

where r is the number of bound hapten molecules per antibody molecule, n is the maximum effective valence of antibody, and c is the concentration of free hapten. It can be seen that equation (5) is equivalent to equation (4) when r is equal to $n/2$. The twofold usefulness of equation (5) is apparent when r/c is plotted as a function of r. First, the value of n (antibody valence) is indicated when the value of r/c approaches zero (i.e., $nK_a = rK_a$) and $n = r$. Second, since the plot depends on the activity (K_a) of antibody determined at various concentrations, deviation from linearity is indicative of the heterogeneity of antibody. A quantitative evaluation of degree of heterogeneity is obtained from the equation (Sips distribution function)

$$\log \frac{r}{n - r} = a \log K_a + a \log c \qquad (6)$$

The slope of the curve (i.e., a) when $\log [r/(n - r)]$ is plotted as a function of $\log c$ is a measure of heterogeneity. A value of 1.0 indicates a nonheterogeneous (within a Gaussian distribution) dispersion. However, the validity of conclusions based on such an analysis is limited by the reliability of each parameter of the system. As indicated in Section 3.2.1, the use of two different values for the maximum valence of TMV led to divergent conclusions pertaining to the homogeneity of antiviral antibody.

The studies of Day et al. (1962, 1963) revealed that the reaction of hapten and antibody was extremely rapid, necessitating measurements of the order of milliseconds. To reduce the rate to a more conventional level would have required too extreme a reduction in the concentrations of the reactants. With the methods devised by Day et al., reactions of antibody with the hapten DNP (dinitrophenyl) were characterized and showed a forward rate of 8×10^7 mol^{-1} sec^{-1}, a dissociation rate of 1.4 sec^{-1}, and an equilibrium constant of 5.7×10^7 mol^{-1}. Consistent with these data are the results (Froese, 1968; Froese and Sehon, 1965; Froese et al., 1962) of other studies of hapten–antibody reactions showing 1.8×10^8 mol^{-1} sec^{-1}, 760 sec^{-1}, and 2.4×10^5 mol^{-1} for the forward and reverse reaction rates and the equilibrium constant, respectively. The above as well as other studies have shown that the forward reaction rates for various hapten–antibody reactions are quite similar, although the equilibrium constants vary. Hence the equilibrium constant (i.e., the affinity constant) reflects primarily the tendency for the complex to undergo dissociation.

4.2.2. Effect of Antibody Valence on Binding Affinity

Because of the multivalency of antibody (i.e., IgG $= 2$, IgM $= 10$, IgA ≥ 2) and the multivalency of viruses, the effect of multivalent binding is of particular relevance to neutralization. The quantitative aspect was illustrated in studies by Hornick and Karush (1969, 1972) and Gopalakrishnan and Karush (1974a,b) and reviewed recently by Karush (1976). Earlier studies (Klinman et al., 1967) indicated that bivalent antibody was more effective in neutralizing bacteriophage than the cleaved monovalent antibody fragment. More definitive studies were made possible by the discovery (Haimovich and Sela, 1966; Mäkelä, 1966) that bacteriophages can be coupled to haptens and that such bacteriophages can be neutralized by antibody that is specific for the hapten. Hornick and Karush (1969) studied the effect of multivalent binding on the neutralization of bacteriophage ϕX174 labeled with DNP. An attractive feature of this system was the ability to measure the rate of dissociation as well as association. The measured equilibrium constant of 3.5×10^{11} mol^{-1} was in good agreement with the calculated value of 1.1×10^{11} mol^{-1} derived from values of 3.7×10^7 mol^{-1} sec^{-1} and 3.4×10^{-4} sec^{-1} for the forward and reverse rates, respectively. Since the intrinsic association constant (the monovalent reaction) was 6×10^6 mol^{-1}, the functional association constant (the multivalent reaction) showed an enhancement of $> 10^4$. The validity of these results was substantiated in later studies (Hornick and Karush, 1972) when the neutralizing activities of bivalent 7 S, bivalent 5 S, monovalent 3.5 S, and monovalent hybrid 7 S antibodies were compared. An enhancement factor of the order of 10^3 was seen. In still another study on the neutralization of ϕX174 coupled to a lactoside hapten, Gopalakrishnan and Karush (1974b) observed a 10^4 enhancement due to multivalent binding.

Similar studies on the effect of multivalency on the neutralizing activity of IgM antibody (Hornick and Karush, 1972) disclosed that the intrinsic affinity was lower than that of IgG. However, since the functional affinities of the two classes of antibody were similar, the enhancement factor was of the order of 10^6. In the view of the authors it is likely that at least three antigenic sites per virion were bound by one molecule of IgM antibody. Representative kinetic and thermodynamic data are shown in Tables 1 and 2.

The significance of multivalent binding was stressed by Crothers and Metzger (1972). They pointed out that the net affinity is the summation of (1) the intrinsic association constant, (2) the number of determinants per antigen, (3) the relative geometries of the interacting sites, and (4) the degree of flexibility or mobility of the interacting structures. With respect to the last consideration, these authors, as well as Green (1969), have indicated that the degree of flexibility of antibody may vary for the same class of antibody (e.g., IgG) when derived from

TABLE 1
Kinetic Data for Several Hapten–Antibody and Virus–Antibody Reactions

| Hapten or virus | Rabbit antibody[a] | | Rate constants for | | Association constants for | | References[b] |
	Type	Molarity	Association $(mol^{-1} sec^{-1})$	Dissociation (sec^{-1})	Neutralization (mol^{-1})	Ligand binding (mol^{-1})	
DNP	7 S	4.7×10^{-7}	8.3×10^7	1.1	—	7.6×10^6	1
$\phi\text{-AsO}_3\text{H}^{-}$ [c]	—	—	2×10^7	50	—	4×10^5	2
$\phi\text{-NO}_2$ [d]	7 S	—	1.8×10^8	7.6×10^2	—	2.4×10^5	3
DNP	2 wk	—	—	—	—	$0.32 \times 10^6\text{–}1.6 \times 10^6$	4
	5 wk	—	—	—	—	$1.5 \times 10^6\text{–}3.2 \times 10^7$	
	8 wk	—	—	—	—	$2 \times 10^7\text{–}2.5 \times 10^8$	
DNP	7 S	1×10^{-6}	—	—	—	6×10^6	5
DNP-ϕX174 [e]		1.5×10^{-11}	3.7×10^7	4.3×10^{-4}	1.1×10^{11}	—	
DNP	7 S	4.5×10^{-7}				1.8×10^7	6
DNP-ϕX174		1.4×10^{-10}	6×10^6	3.3×10^{-4}	2×10^{10}	—	
DNP-ϕX174	5 S	1.2×10^{-10}	9.6×10^6	2.9×10^{-4}	3.3×10^{10}	—	
DNP	3.5 S					1.0×10^7	
DNP-ϕX174		9.5×10^{-9}	—	—	4.7×10^8	—	

DNP	19 S	—	—	—	—	<10⁶	—
DNP-φX174		5 × 10⁻¹²	—	—	2.4 × 10¹¹	—	
DNP	19 Sᵃ	—	—	—	—	2 × 10²	
DNP-φX174	7 S	1 × 10⁻⁷	—	—	1 × 10⁷	—	
Lactᶠ		—	—	—	—	2.4 × 10⁵	7
Lact-φX174ᶠ		4 × 10⁻¹⁰	7 × 10⁵	8 × 10⁻⁴	8.7 × 10⁹	—	
Influenza							
Mel		—	—	—	9.2 × 10¹⁰	—	8
Lee		—	—	—	5.3 × 10¹¹	—	
SW		—	—	—	1.4 × 10¹¹	—	
Phage f2	7 S	2.12 × 10⁷	—	—	—	—	9
	5 S	0.44 × 10⁷	—	—	—	—	
	3.5 S	0.16 × 10⁷	—	—	—	—	
Phage f2	7 S	2.01 × 10⁷	—	—	—	—	10
	5 S	0.95 × 10⁷	—	—	—	—	
	3.5 S	0.15 × 10⁷	—	—	—	—	

ᵃ In all instances antibody was obtained from immunized rabbits except in these two experiments in which human serum was the source.

ᵇ References: 1, Day et al. (1963); 2, Froese et al. (1962); 3, Froese and Sehon (1965); 4, Eisen and Siskind (1964); 5, Hornick and Karush (1969); 6, Hornick and Karush (1972); 7, Gopalakrishnan and Karush (1974b); 8, Fazekas de St. Groth and Webster (1963b); 9, Rowlands (1967); 10, Dudley et al. (1970).

ᶜ p-Azophenylarsonic acid.

ᵈ 4,5-Dihydroxy-3-(p-nitrophenylazo)-2,7-naphthalene disulfonic acid.

ᵉ DNP coupled to bacteriophage φX174.

ᶠ Lactoside coupled to bacteriophage φX174 or lactoside used as hapten.

TABLE 2

Thermodynamic Data for Several Hapten–Antibody and Virus–Antibody Reactions

Hapten or virus	Antibody Source[a]	Antibody Class	E_a (kcal/mol)	$-\Delta H$ (kcal/mol)	$-\Delta F$ (kcal/mol)	ΔS (eu/mol)	Reference[b]
DNP	Rb	IgG[c]	4	9.5	7.7	—	1
DNP	Rb	—	—	19.6	10.9	30.4	2
ϕ-AsO$_3$H^{-d}	Rb	IgG[c]	—	—	7.7	—	3
Arsanilic acid	Rb	IgG	—	0.8	7.4–8.3	22 ($\pm$9)	4
D-Ip[e]	Rb	IgG[c]	—	—	6.7–7.8	0	5
WEV	Rb	IgG[c]	6	—	—	—	6
Poliovirus	Hu	IgG	8.5	—	—	—	7
VEV	Mk	—	9	—	—	—	8
ϕX174	Rb	IgG[c]	9.6	—	—	—	9
f2	Rb	IgG	7.3	6.7	7.8	−4	10
		(Fab')$_2$	8.6	8.0	8.3	−0.9	
		Fab'	13.9	13.3	9.4	12	

[a] Source of antibody: Rb, rabbit; Hu, human; Mk, monkey.
[b] References: 1, Day *et al.* (1963); 2, Eisen and Siskind (1964); 3, Eisen and Karush (1949); 4, Epstein *et al.* (1956); 5, Karush (1956); 6, Dulbecco *et al.* (1956); 7, Philipson (1966); 8, Hahon (1969); 9, Bowman and Patnode (1964); 10, Dudley *et al.* (1970).
[c] The class of antibody was not actually established. However, based on the described immunization procedure, it is considered very likely that the class is as indicated.
[d] *p*-Azophenylarsonic acid.
[e] Azohapten phenyl-[*p*-(*p*-dimethylaminobenzeneazo)-benzoylamino]acetate.

different species of animals. Also, they indicated that the degree of flexibility of IgG is greater than that of IgM. However, it should be borne in mind that the fivefold higher valence of the IgM molecule may more than compensate for its lesser flexibility.

5. NEUTRALIZATION

Neutralization refers to the phenomenological consequence of the interaction of virus and neutralizing antibody without any implication of mechanism. Analyses of various situations have shown that the loss of infective capability may be the result of several distinguishable phenomena (e.g., see Svehag, 1968; Daniels, 1975; Burns and Allison, 1975). With respect to the underlying mechanism, neutralization may be classified as either an intrinsic, an extrinsic, or a pseudo-phenomenon.

5.1. Intrinsic Neutralization

5.1.1. Primary

The binding of the minimum number of molecules of antibody to a critical site of a single virion results in the nullification of infectivity. The initial event, i.e., the formation of the complex, may not be the event *per se* that causes neutralization but rather the initiating reaction of a multiphasic phenomenon.

5.1.2. Mediated

In spite of the initial interaction with antibody, a virion may retain its infective capability. Addition of a third specific component, e.g., complement, consummates the neutralization reaction. Infectious virus–antibody complexes have been referred to as sensitized virus.

5.1.3. Multiphasic

Structurally differentiated viruses, e.g., adenovirus, may have two or more antigenic sites involved in neutralization. Interaction of a quasicritical site with antibody is prerequisite for the activation of a critical site, possibly through a conformational rearrangement of the capsomeric subunits (e.g., see Kjellén and Pereira, 1968).

5.2. Extrinsic Neutralization

The binding of antibody to noncritical sites may, under certain conditions, result in neutralization.

5.2.1. Steric Hindrance

The topological disposition of critical and noncritical sites may allow for steric interference of critical-site function when antibody at high multiplicity binds to noncritical sites. Unlike intrinsically neutralized virus, extrinsically neutralized virus has not undergone the critical neutralization reaction. At low antibody multiplicity, binding of

antibody to noncritical sites may result in sensitization and susceptibility to mediated neutralization due to steric effects.

5.2.2. Virolysis

Enveloped viruses may contain antigenic determinants characteristic of the host cell. Interaction of these noncritical antigens with
antibody in the presence of complement results in discrete lytic lesions
in the envelope (Berry and Almeida, 1968; Almeida and Waterson,
1969; Radwan *et al.*, 1973). Such lesions may (Oroszlan and Gilden,
1970; Oldstone, 1975) or may not (Schluederberg *et al.*, 1976) result in
the spontaneous egress of the viral genome.

5.3. Pseudoneutralization

Under conditions of equivalent concentrations, the binding of antibody to noncritical sites may lead to secondary interactions such as
aggregation. Although the individual virions are not *per se* neutralized,
each multimeric aggregate registers as one infectious unit.

6. VIRAL NEUTRALIZATION

By virtue of their data, their critical interpretations, and their dis-
cernment of various problems, Andrewes and Elford (1933*a,b*) and
Burnet *et al.* (1937) laid the groundwork for future studies of viral neutralization. The underlying assumption on which these studies were
based was that direct combination of virus and antibody was the initial
and necessary event for neutralization. Several prior investigations were
in conflict with this assumption, which, however, was subsequently
firmly validated.

The "percentage law," first described by Andrewes and Elford
(1933*a*) in their studies on bacteriophage neutralization, was shown by
Burnet *et al.* to apply to animal viruses as well. The "law," as described
by Andrewes and Elford, specifies that "over a very wide range a given
dilution of serum neutralized in a given time an approximately constant percentage of phage, *however much phage was present*. This
phenomenon we refer to for convenience as the 'percentage law.'" In
addition to this result, kinetic studies disclosed that the reaction was
time dependent, that the reaction proceeded immediately, that the

initial relatively rapid rate was succeeded by a steadily diminishing rate, and that the rate of the reaction was proportional to the concentration of serum (i.e., antibody). In some instances it was shown by Burnet *et al.* that at very low concentrations of serum a short lag preceded the course of inactivation.

The tendency for the reaction to terminate prior to complete neutralization was a puzzling feature which was investigated without success. Although several hypotheses were found untenable, both groups considered a reasonable explanation for survival to be related to viral heterogeneity.

Neutralization is essentially a chemical reaction subject to the laws of mass action. Early studies on the reversibility of the reaction resulted in diverse conclusions ranging from freely reversible to irreversible. Examination of this problem by Andrewes and Elford led them to conclude that once the bacteriophage–antibody complex had formed, it was not spontaneously dissociable even when highly diluted. Similar studies led Burnet *et al.* to conclude that whereas the bacteriophage–antibody complex was irreversible, the complex involving animal viruses was readily reversible by dilution of the reaction mixture. However, Burnet *et al.* obtained evidence that suggested a very slow transition to an irreversible state. It is of interest that although the reaction of bacteriophage and antibody was viewed as being irreversible, Burnet *et al.* envisioned the possibility that the reaction reached an equilibrium state, which, however, was not experimentally demonstrable.

That the neutralization phenomenon was not simply an all-or-none effect was recognized when "intermediate" events were observed. Studies on bacteriophage revealed that survivors in virus–antiserum mixtures formed abnormally small plaques. This was considered to reflect infectious virus–antibody complexes that required additional time to initiate infection. It was found that virus–antibody complexes retained the capacity to adsorb to cells, although some of the complexes could not initiate infection. The infective status of virus–antibody complexes varied according to the host as well as the route of inoculation. Studies on the activity of various antisera led Burnet *et al.* to suspect that antibody synthesized early in the immune response was of "low grade," a suspicion that was substantiated 20 years later (Jerne and Avegno, 1956).

As to the mechanism of viral neutralization, Burnet *et al.* speculated that several distinct phenomena might be represented: (1) Virus may be prevented from attaching to a cell. (2) Virus may attach but is prevented from "entering" the cell. (3) Several particles may aggregate, thereby reducing the number of infectious units from several to one. Because of the resistance of infectious virus–antibody complexes to inactivation by PIA (phage-inactivating agent, an extract of susceptible bacteria, probably containing receptor substance), Burnet *et al.* postulated that neutralization required the binding of more than one molecule of antibody per virion. Andrewes and Elford suggested that neutralization entailed two stages, a rapid first stage followed by a second stage. The first stage represented a weakly bound complex that could be reversed by dilution. With some antisera, antibody was of a quality that allowed the first stage to be completed very rapidly.

It is also of relevance that several early investigations implicated the participation of a third factor in viral neutralization. The studies of Mueller (1931), which corroborated several previous observations, led him to propose that the third factor was alexin (i.e., complement) and that it acted in conjunction with certain classes of antibody. Subsequent studies confirmed the validity of this proposal.

In 1956 Dulbecco *et al.* reported the results of extensive studies of the neutralization of two animal viruses. These studies confirmed and amplified some of the earlier studies as well as defined additional parameters and problems. Technological developments in virology, e.g., plaque assay, purification methods, and radioisotopic labeling, and in immunology, e.g., isolation and purification of antibody, fractionation to obtain monovalent fragments, and methods for determining thermodynamic and kinetic parameters, stimulated a renewed interest in the neutralization reaction.

6.1. Kinetics of the Neutralization Reaction

The rate at which viral infectivity diminishes is usually measured as a function of time, as illustrated, for example, in Fig. 3. the procedure entails the use of appropriate concentrations of virus and antibody (as whole serum or purified antibody) so that the reaction is readily measured as a function of time, e.g., minutes. It has been indicated that the reaction of antibody and hapten is so rapid that measurements require millisecond intervals (Day *et al.*, 1962, 1963). However, the reaction with virus, utilizing infectivity as the measurable parameter, is extremely sensitive. Hence concentrations of virus on the order of 10^{-15} to 10^{-17} M are ordinarily used with sufficiently diluted antibody (e.g., 10^{-8} to 10^{-9} M) to allow for reactions with a half-life between 1 and 10 min. The extreme sensitivity of this system was emphasized by Sarvas and Mäkelä (1970). They showed that with 10^{-17}

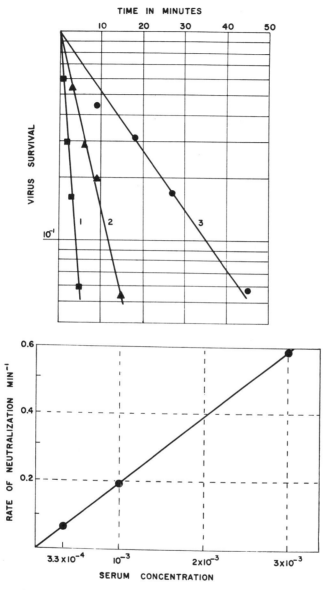

Fig. 3. Dependence of the slope of the kinetic curve on the concentration of the anti-serum. The kinetic curves were determined by using P1 virus (Brunhilde wild type) at the concentration of 3.6×10^5 PFU/ml. The general procedure was as follows: virus and serum were prewarmed, mixed at $t = 0$, and incubated at 37°C. At various sub-sequent times a sample of 0.1 ml was blown into cold PBS to ensure correct timing and then assayed for active virus. The concentration of the antiserum (rabbit) was 3×10^{-3} for curve 1, 10^{-3} for curve 2, and 3.33×10^{-4} for curve 3. From Dulbecco *et al.* (1956), with permission of the publisher.

M haptenated bacteriophage about 10^{-13} M antibody could be detected. Reaction rate constants can therefore be accurately determined in units of seconds or minutes.

When plotted on semilogarithmic coordinates, the decrease in infectious virus follows a linear course for a certain time, then the rate decreases slowly or abruptly. The extent of the linear portion varies with the state of maturity of the antibody. Ozaki (1968) compared the neutralizing activity of several antisera derived from the same rabbit at various times after immunogenic stimulation. Each serum was diluted to contain equal activity units (based on a 50% static end-pont assay). It can be seen in Fig. 4 that the early linear course was similar for all reactions to about 10% survival but thereafter they diverged markedly. The divergence is indicative of antibody heterogeneity with respect to binding affinity; the earlier the serum, the greater the extent of heterogeneity. Jerne and Avegno (1956) demonstrated the transition from weakly binding to firmly binding antibody at increasing times

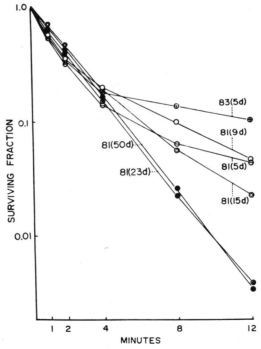

Fig. 4. Comparison between dose–response curves of different sera. Five-tenths milliliter of each diluted serum was mixed with an equal volume of Mahoney strain and incubated at 37°C for 3 hr. The surviving virus was titrated. The virus concentration was $10^{7.6}$ PFU/ml. From Ozaki (1968), with permission of the publisher.

after immunization of horses with bacteriophage T4. Following this demonstration, an extensive literature has accrued on the subject of antibody diversity and antibody maturation with respect to viral neutralization (see Svehag, 1965a,b, 1966, 1968).

Close examination of the kinetics of neutralization in general has revealed that the early course of the reaction may actually be very slightly curvilinear. The reaction rate may decelerate continuously, eventually approaching a zero level in spite of the presence of excess antibody and infectious virus. One possible explanation for this result is the presence of antibodies of varying affinities, those with lower affinity forming complexes that may dissociate during the assay procedure. In order to circumvent this event, Jerne and Avegno (1956) devised the "decision" assay method. In essence, complexes that fail to dissociate within a set period of time after dilution are prevented from doing so by a second addition of antiserum in high concentration. A comparison of the kinetics of neutralization of bacteriophage T4 by an early antiserum by the direct plating method and by the "decision" plating method showed a considerably higher rate and tendency to a more linear course by the latter method by a late antiserum (Jerne and Avegno, 1956). A similar analysis of the neutralization of bacteriophage $Q\beta$ (Hale et al., (1969) showed somewhat different results. When assayed by two different "decision" methods, the rates of neutralization were higher than in the direct assay. However, the nonlinear character of the curves remained. Since independent evidence for dissociation could not be obtained, and there was no evidence for viral heterogeneity, the authors proposed that a finite probability existed that the interaction of bacteriophage and antibody may result in a complex that retains infectivity and also resists neutralization.

Krummel and Uhr (1969) have also reported deviation from linearity in the course of neutralization of ϕX174 bacteriophage by guinea pig antiserum. A higher rate and a tendency toward a more linear course of neutralization were seen by the "decision" method compared to the direct method. Since they found that the slight extent of dissociation that occurred could not account for the difference, they postulated that the formation of infectious virus–antibody complexes was the critical factor for the deviation. To test this proposal they developed a "complex inactivation" method which included a "decision" stage followed by inactivation of infectious complexes through the use of antibody directed against the antiviral antibody. Under these conditions the course of inactivation remained linear for more than 99% loss of infectivity. Another cause for deviation from linearity was described by Bowman and Patnode (1964). Whereas highly purified bacteriophage ϕX174 showed an extensively linear course, less purified viral preparations showed a distinctly curvilinear course.

The studies of Hale *et al.* (1969) and Krummel and Uhr (1969) on bacteriophage neutralization, and the studies of Dulbecco *et al.* (1956) on animal virus neutralization, as well as the results described by Andrews and Elford (1933*a*) and Burnet *et al.* (1937), typify the kinetic aspects of viral neutralization: namely, a rapid linear course that eventually diminishes in rate because of the formation of stable, neutralization resistant virus–antibody complexes. It is of interest that tobacco mosaic virus shows the same general features of neutralization (Rappaport, 1957, 1965). The difficulties encountered in plant virus studies requiring infectivity as the assay system have been stressed by Rappaport.

6.2. Kinetics of Reactivation

It has been shown for several animal, bacterial, and plant viruses that the neutralizing effect of antibody can be reversed. Procedures that have been employed for reactivation have been previously described (Mandel, 1971*a*). Analyses of the kinetics of neutralization and reactivation of hapten-coupled ϕX174 bacteriophage have been reported (Hornick and Karush, 1972; Gopalakrishnan and Karush, 1974*b*). As seen in Figs. 5 and 6, the forward and reverse reactions were both kinetically characteristic of a single-event phenomenon. A similar result was seen in the reactivation of neutralized poliovirus (Mandel, 1961) by a different procedure (Fig. 7). Although it seemed possible that two critical sites might be involved, more than two appeared to be extremely unlikely (Gopalakrishnan and Karush, 1974*b*). These investigators have interpreted the data for the forward as well as the reverse reaction as evidence that one or possibly two, but not more than two, antigenic sites were critical for infectivity. Interaction of this site(s) with antibody resulted in neutralization.

6.3. Single-Hit and Multihit Reactions

The stoichiometric aspect of viral neutralization has received considerable attention, as will be discussed later (see Section 10.4.3). The problem revolves around the interpretation of kinetic data. A plot of the course of inactivation on semilogarithmic coordinates as a function of time may show an immediate decline in survivors, or a decline

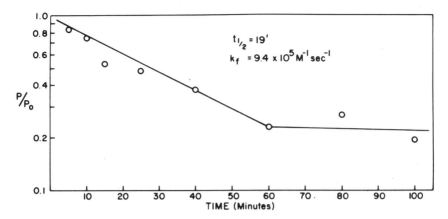

Fig. 5.   Neutralization of PAPL-ϕX174 by anti-PAPL antibody (fraction I of rabbit 1491 antibody) at 25°C. Concentration of antibody was 5×10^{-10} M. Note: PAPL is *p*-aminophenyl-β-lactoside. From Gopalakrishnan and Karush (1974*b*), with permission of the publisher.

only after a finite time has elapsed. The immediate decline has been taken as evidence for the inactivation of one virion by one molecule of antibody. The occurrence of a lag period has been taken as evidence that inactivation of one virion requires the participation of more than one molecule, the number being proportional to the extent of the lag period.

Burnet *et al.* (1937) observed that when a given antibacteriophage serum was used at low concentration the reaction was multihit in contrast to single-hit when used at a threefold higher concentration. Because of a short lag, Kalmanson *et al.* (1942) estimated that neu-

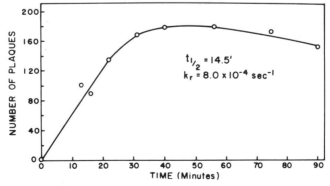

Fig. 6.   Kinetics of reactivation of neutralized PAPL-ϕX174 at 25°C in presence of 0.02 M lactose. Note: PAPL is *p*-aminophenyl-β-lactoside. From Gopalakrishnan and Karush (1974*b*), with permission of the publisher.

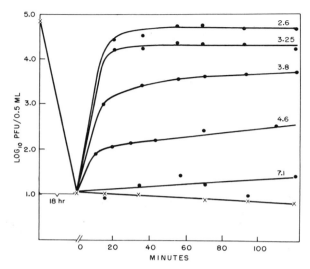

Fig. 7.   Variation in the kinetics of the dissociation reaction as a function of pH. Virus and antiserum were allowed to react at pH 7 for 18 hr; then aliquots were diluted in buffers of the pH's shown on each curve. An aliquot of the original virus–antiserum mixture was held without dilution. The increase in titer of infectious virus at the various pH's (●) and the titer of the undiluted original mixture (×) are shown as a function of time. From Mandel (1961), with permission of the publisher.

tralization of bacteriophage required two or three molecules of anti-body. Lafferty (1963a) observed single-hit or multihit kinetics when influenza virus was neutralized by serum at twenty- or fortyfold dilu-tion, respectively. An estimation by extrapolation indicates that perhaps three to five molecules of antibody may be required. A multihit reaction was also seen with rabbit pox virus (Lafferty, 1963a). Philipson (1966) reported that the interaction of poliovirus with IgM antibody showed a lag. However, in these studies neutralization was not the parameter for the reaction but rather the change in the distribution properties of the virus in an aqueous polymer system consisting of poly-ethylene glycol and sodium dextran sulfate.

     Although one interpretation for a time lag is the requirement for multiple interactions, it may be worthwhile to keep in mind other possi-bilities. For example, it was shown (Sagik, 1954) that bacteriophage T2 showed a brief rise in titer on reacting with T2 antiserum preceding the linear decline. Sagik showed that an inhibitor was present that could mask viral infectivity and was removed by the antiserum. Mixing virus and serum initiated two concurrent opposing reactions, one resulting in an increase in infectivity, the other in a decrease. Similarly, but perhaps for a different reason, certain viruses (e.g., rabbit pox, Murray Valley encephalitis) showed an increase preceding a decrease in infectivity on reacting with antibody (Hawkes, 1964; Hawkes and Lafferty, 1967). If the two opposing reactions proceeded initially at similar rates, the kinetic curve could simulate in appearance a truly multihit curve. In studies on the neutralization of bacteriophage ϕX174, Bowman and Patnode (1964) demonstrated that deviation from truly exponential inactivation was related to the presence of contaminants.

6.4. Reversibility of the Virus–Antibody Reaction

The question of the reversibility of the reaction of virus with neutralizing antibody has been debated almost from the time of the first demonstration of neutralization. Reversibility in the present context refers to an equilibrium state between reactants and reaction product. Demonstration of such an equilibrium is usually based on dilution of the reaction mixture, which should reequilibrate according to the equilibrium constant for the system. One result of reequilibration is the appearance of reactivated virus. Early studies with animal and bacterial viruses resulted in opposing conclusions for different viruses, or when the same viruses were compared by different investigators. Andrewes and Elford (1933a) proposed that the neutralization of bacteriophages was essentially irreversible. Burnet et al. (1937) concurred in this conclusion, and in addition proposed that, unlike bacteriophages, animal viruses formed readily reversible complexes. Kalmanson et al. (1942) speculated that, with regard to reversibility, there should be no distinction between bacterial and animal viruses. More detailed studies led to the realization that the neutralization reaction may be more complicated than the simple immediate binding of antibody to virion. It was seen (Andrewes and Elford, 1933a; Burnet et al., 1937) that the degree of reversibility diminished the longer the reaction was allowed to proceed. Gard (1955, 1957) presented data in support of this phenomenon that he designated "immunoinactivation." Lafferty (1963a) showed that for a brief time (about 20 min at 0°C) the complex of influenza virus and specific antibody was completely reversible by dilution. There then followed a period of time during which the fraction of reversibly neutralized virus diminished to about 0.1% at 150 min. The transition to irreversibility was a consequence of the formation of a second monogamous bond as shown by electron microscopy (Lafferty and Oertelis, 1963).

In their studies of the neutralization of poliovirus and WEV,

Dulbecco *et al.* (1956) concluded that the reaction was irreversible. Similar conclusions were drawn for NDV (Rubin, 1957; Rubin and Franklin, 1957; Granoff, 1965), poliovirus (Mandel, 1961; Ketler *et al.*, 1961; Keller, 1965; Wallis *et al.*, 1973), adenovirus (Kjellén, 1957, 1962), visna virus (Thormar, 1963), herpesvirus (Yoshino and Taniguchi, 1965*b*; Ashe and Notkins, 1967), and VEV (Hahon, 1969). It was reported that, to a small degree, reversibility occurred with JEV (Hashimoto and Prince, 1963; Iwasaki and Ogura, 1968*b*), herpesvirus (Ide and Yoshino, 1974), and WNV (Westaway, 1965*a*). Fazekas de St. Groth and Reid (1958) and Fazekas de St. Groth and Webster (1963*a*) viewed the reaction of viruses with antibody as an example of a mass action equilibrium system that therefore should proceed in either direction in accordance with the affinity constant for a specific system.

A more intimate understanding of viruses, antibodies, and the nature of their interaction indicates that there is no fundamental difference among the various interpretations. It has been shown for several animal, bacterial, and plant viruses (see Mandel, 1971*a*, for a general discussion) that neutralized virus can be reactivated as a result of either dissociation of the complex or degradation of the antibody. Hence the potential for dissociation exists. The role of two parameters in viral neutralization has been shown to be of exceeding importance to the problem of reversibility: (1) Inasmuch as antibody and virus can bind via multivalent linkages the binding energy can be of a very high order of magnitude (see Section 4.1.2). Association constants of the order of 10^{11} mol^{-1} indicate that the forward reaction is extremely favored. Although, literally, the reaction is reversible (by dilution), practically, the rate of dissociation can be neglected (Krummel and Uhr, 1969). (2) Antibodies may vary considerably in their binding affinity. It has been shown that maturation of antibody is time dependent. Early synthesized antibodies have a low binding affinity, in contrast to those appearing later. Eisen and Siskind (1964) showed, for example, that antibody to 2,4-DNP collected on the fifth week after immunization had a sixfold higher association constant than antibody collected on the second week. On the eighth week there was another fortyfold increase compared with the fifth week. Of interest also are their data showing the high degree of variability in antibody quality derived from several rabbits subjected to the same program of immunogenic stimulation. Variation in the affinity of antibody to poliovirus was described by Svehag (1965*b*) based on the dissociation of the virus–antibody complex at various H$^+$ concentrations. Distinct classes of antibody of increasing affinity were detected before 3 days, between 3 and 5 days, and between 5 and 14 days, and a final class 14 days after stimulation of rabbits. A similar conclusion emerged from the studies of the effect of salt concentration on the stability of the poliovirus–antibody complex (Svehag, 1965a). Antibody induced in guinea pigs to bacteriophage ϕX174 showed time-dependent maturation toward high affinity when examined by the "decision tube" method of neutralization (Finkelstein and Uhr, 1966).

On the basis of available data, it would appear reasonable to consider the reaction formally reversible in the light of quantitative data. From the practical point of view when high-affinity (late, 7 S) antibody reacts under conditions that favor multimonogamous binding to virus, the bond strength is of an order of magnitude that renders the complex not demonstrably reversible.

7. THE NONNEUTRALIZED FRACTION (NNF)

Several early reports (e.g., Andrewes and Elford, 1933a; Burnet et al., 1937) had shown that usually a small fraction of a viral population escaped neutralization in spite of the presence of excess antibody. However, it was the later studies of Dulbecco et al. (1956), and the dissenting interpretation of their data by Fazekas de St. Groth and Reid (1958), that focused attention on this problem. At about this time it was shown that the fraction of virus that remained infectious in the presence of excess antibody could be neutralized by the secondary addition of antibody specific for the antiviral antibody (i.e., antiglobulin) (Mandel, 1958). This result implied that the surviving virus had reacted with antibody and that the reaction had imparted to the virion a state of refractoriness. Subsequent investigations disclosed that this was a common phenomenon among a wide array of viruses (Wallis and Melnick, 1967; see Majer, 1972, for a review).

The biological implications of this phenomenon were emphasized when it was shown that infectious virus coexisted with neutralizing antibody in the blood of visna-virus-infected sheep (Gudnadóttir and Pálsson, 1965) and in H1-virus-infected hamsters (Toolan, 1965). Direct evidence was presented for the occurrence of infectious virus–antibody complexes in lactic-dehydrogenase-virus-infected mice (Notkins et al., 1966) and in Aleutian-disease-virus-infected mink (Porter and Larsen, 1967). Subsequent recognition of the wide variety of virus–host systems showing this phenomenon has elevated it to the status of an area of major medical concern (Oldstone, 1975).

7.1. Explanatory Hypotheses

Several hypotheses have been proposed to explain the nonneutralized state. These fall into two basically different concepts. One concept rejects the actual existence of infectious virus–antibody complexes.
It has been proposed that because of the reversible nature of the
virus–antibody complex, and because of the inescapable dilution
inherent in the assay procedure, the reactivation of originally neutralized virus simulates the existence of a nonneutralized fraction
(Fazekas de St. Groth *et al.*, 1958; Fazekas de St. Groth and Reid,
1958).

All other hypotheses consider antibody to be a contributing factor.
It has been shown that when virus particles exist as aggregates—due to
cross-linking by antibody or by other factors—such aggregates cannot
be completely neutralized. Presumably the sheltering effect of particles
at the periphery precludes the neutralization of every particle (Wallis
and Melnick, 1967, 1970). A variation of this idea was proposed by
Rappaport (1970). He observed that the small RNA phage MS2, with
presumably 180 antigenic sites, could bind only about 80 molecules of
antibody. Because of the presence of free sites, the complex was still
infectious, with, however, a greatly diminished probability for a produc-
tive infection.

Lafferty (1963*a,b*) has proposed two different antibody-dependent
nonneutralized states. One is induced by antibody of low avidity and is
readily undone by dilution of the virus–antibody complex. This is the
"reversibly protected" state. The other is induced by avid antibody,
producing an "irreversibly protected" state. In the latter case protection is not absolute since the amount of protected virus varies according
to the host cells composing the assay system. Hence the latter has been
designated the "cell-dependent protected fraction." Some differences
were observed between rabbit pox and influenza viruses in respect to the
different protected states (Lafferty, 1963*a,b*).

Other studies implicate antibody heterogeneity. McNeill (1968)
has considered the existence of an "interfering" antibody capable of
inducing the nonneutralized state in vaccinia virus. No suggestions
about the nature of such antibody were presented. Studies with
poliovirus have implicated the degree of maturation of antibody. When
antisera were collected at various times after immunization of rabbits,
the nonneutralized level was lower with sera that were collected later, as
seen in Fig. 8 (Ozaki, 1968; Lewenton-Kriss and Mandel, 1972).
Attempts to isolate a class of antibody uniquely involved in inducing
the nonneutralized state were unsuccessful (Lewenton-Kriss and

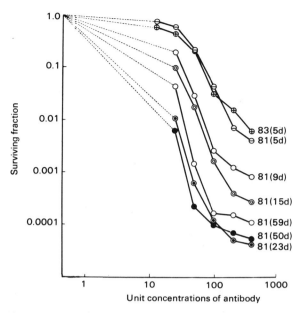

Fig. 8. Neutralization kinetic curves of Mahoney strain in sera obtained at different times during the course of immunization. Five-tenths milliliter of each diluted antiserum was mixed with an equal volume of Mahoney strain containing $10^{7.6}$ PFU/ml and incubated at 37°C. At various intervals, 0.1 ml was diluted in 9.9 ml of chilled phosphate-buffered saline. The surviving virus was titrated. Antibody concentrations: 81(5d), 81(9d), 81(15d), 81(23d), and 81(50d), 200 units; 83(5d), 400 units. From Ozaki (1968), with permission of the publisher.

Mandel, 1972). Several fractionation procedures—rate zonal sedimentation in sucrose density gradients, molecular sieving in Sephadex gels, and isoelectric focusing electrophoresis—were employed. In no instance were antibodies isolated that could only induce the nonneutralized state or only neutralize.

A role for the host cell was indicated in early studies and reemphasized by the striking difference in the levels of nonneutralized VSV depending on whether avian or mammalian cells were used (Kjellén and Schlesinger, 1959). Quantitatively less impressive results of this effect were shown in studies of rabbitpox (Lafferty, 1963a,b). Bradish et al. (1962) also described a host-dependent variation in studies on neutralization of FMD virus. A different role of the host cell was shown with poliovirus that was derived from either HeLa cells or monkey kidney cells. The nonneutralized virus level with HeLa-grown virus was about a hundredfold higher than with kidney-cell-grown virus when the assays were done in HeLa cells (Lewenton-Kriss and Mandel, 1972).

The above résumé shows that each component of the system—

virus, antibody, cell—participates actively, and possibly variably, in the ultimate result of virus–antibody interaction.

7.2. Mediated Neutralization

The enhancement of the degree of neutralization of animal viruses by an extraneous factor was suspected as early as 1925 (Gordon, 1925) and somewhat later by Douglas and Smith (1930) and Mueller (1931). In these studies (as well as later studies not cited here) it was observed that a thermolabile serum factor increased the extent of neutralization. Mueller suspected that complement was the participating factor, a suspicion that was subsequently documented. The enhancing effect of complement was also shown to apply to bacterial viruses (Barlow et al., 1958; Cowan, 1962; Toussaint and Muschel, 1962; Pernis et al., 1963; Adler et al., 1971).

Mediation of the neutralization reaction can also be implemented by antibody directed against the antiviral antibody in the case of animal viruses (Mandel, 1958; Notkins et al., 1966; Ashe and Notkins, 1967; Kjellén and Pereira, 1968; Keller and Dwyer, 1968; Majer and Link, 1970, 1971; Hahon, 1970; Radwan and Burger, 1973a,b) and bacterial viruses (Goodman and Donch, 1965; Krummel and Uhr, 1969; Dudley et al., 1970; Adler et al., 1971).

Still other serum components have been implicated as mediators of neutralization. Rheumatoid factor, an IgM molecule that appears in the circulatory system as a consequence of certain pathological conditions, has been shown to be active as a mediator (Ashe et al., 1971; Gipson et al., 1974; Markenson et al., 1975). Its mode of action is, however, somewhat cryptic since it, per se, does not mediate the reaction but is a link between the infectious virus–antibody complex and either complement or antiantibody.

Styk et al. (1958) described the mediating effect of a serum factor in the neutralization of influenza virus. As a result of extensive studies by this group (Styk, 1965; Styk and Hana, 1965a,b) it was concluded that this substance, probably a lipoprotein, was not part of the complement system. It was reported that nonimmune serum from various species of animal was effective in mediating the neutralization of Semliki Forest virus by antiserum from guinea pig (Way and Garwes, 1970). Neither its nature nor its mode of action was described.

Protein A, derived from staphylococci, was reported to be effective in mediating neutralization of herpesvirus and vaccinia virus (Austin and Daniels, 1974). It functions either directly or as an intermediary component.

Kulberg and Pervikov (1976) reported the occurrence in unimmunized animals of a factor that mediates the neutralization of infectious complexes of poliovirus and Fab' fragments. Interestingly, this report indicates that the factor is inactive against complexes of poliovirus and intact IgG.

Örvell and Norrby (1977) have shown that, *in vitro*, antibody that is specific for the VP2 protein (i.e., the hemagglutinin–neuraminidase spike structure) of Sendai virus neutralizes infectivity. In contrast, antibody that is specific for the VP4 protein (i.e., the fusion spike structure) does not neutralize. However, *in vivo*, passively administered anti-VP4 antiserum has a protective effect. A possible explanation for this result, in the opinion of the authors, is the presence in serum of a factor that can mediate neutralization of the virus–anti-VP4 complex.

7.2.1. Mediation by Antiglobulin Antibody

Notkins *et al.* (1966) demonstrated the existence of infectious virus–antibody complexes. Infectious virus was obtained from the blood of mice chronically infected with LDV in spite of the fact the blood of these mice contained antibody. Exposure of the virus to antiserum that was induced in goats with mouse γ-globulin resulted in neutralization. Subsequently, it was shown by Notkins and his colleagues that herpesvirus, too, can exist as an infectious virus–antibody complex that is sensitive to an antiserum directed against the viral γ-globulin. Notkins and his colleagues investigated this phenomenon (Notkins *et al.*, 1966, 1968, 1971; Ashe and Notkins, 1966, 1967; Ashe *et al.*, 1968, 1969; Hampar *et al.*, 1968).

The literature frequently contains the expression "antiantibody" for antiserum prepared in one species of animal employing γ-globulin of another species of animal or in the same species of animal but of different allotype. Such sera will hereafter be designated as antiglobulin with the understanding that the serological reaction involves the two antibodies—namely, the antiviral antibody and the antibody induced by the intact or fractionated globulin fraction of the same species as the antiviral antibody. Notkins *et al.* adopted the term "sensitization" for the process of formation of infectious virus–antibody complexes that can be neutralized secondarily by such reagents as complement and antiglobulin (see Section 7.2). Until a better-defined understanding of this phenomenon evolves, the same connotation is being assigned to such expressions as "sensitized virus," "persistent fraction," "nonneutralizable fraction," "nonneutralized fraction," and "protected fraction."

A study by Notkins and his colleagues showed that when LDV was sensitized by mouse antibody, virus could be neutralized by antisera induced in rabbits with either mouse whole γ-globulin, mouse IgG, or mouse IgA but not with antiserum to mouse IgM. A further study was made of the activity of papain digested fragments of goat antiglobulin. Compared with the undigested antibody, the Fab fragment was active, but to a lesser degree, while the Fc fragment was inactive. Of interest is their observation that interaction with the Fab fragment in some instances occurred without causing neutralization. This was discerned by the increased resistance to neutralization by intact bivalent antibody.

Shifting to herpesvirus, Notkins and colleagues examined direct neutralization, sensitization, and mediated neutralization, with the results shown in Table 3. The neutralization of virus that was sensitized by bi- or monovalent antibody was readily mediated by bivalent antiglobulin. Virus that was sensitized by monovalent antibodies was less efficiently neutralized by antimonovalent globulin, particularly Fab II. When virus was sensitized with early antibodies of the 19 S or 7 S class, only the latter were neutralized by antiglobulin. In contrast, with late antibodies, both classes produced antiglobulin-sensitive complexes.

An examination of the allotypic specificity of mediated neutralization was carried out with rabbit sera. For example, antiviral serum was induced in rabbits of *a3b4* allotype and γ-globulin from these rabbits was used to induce antibody in rabbits of *a1b5a2b5* allotype. These sera were effective in sensitizing and mediating neutralization, respectively. As reviewed by Kindt (1975), the *a* and *b* allotype markers reside respectively in the variable region of the heavy chains, and in the light (κ) chain.

Several other studies have involved togaviruses. These are enveloped virions with surface glycoproteins, one of which has hemagglutinating capacity. These viruses, formerly known as arboviruses, are subdivided into alphavirus and flavivirus subgroups.

Ozaki and colleagues (Ozaki and Tabeyi, 1967; Ozaki and Kumagai, 1969; Ozaki *et al.*, 1974) studied mediated neutralization of JEV, a flavivirus. Exposure to early serum (i.e., IgM antibody) resulted in neutralization to a survival of about 3%. Treatment with anti-IgM globulin reduced the level to about 0.01%, whereas anti-IgG globulin was without effect. When virus was exposed to late (i.e., IgG) antibody,

TABLE 3

Virus Sensitization as Measured by Papain-Derived Fragments of Sheep Anti-Rabbit γ-Globulin[a]

Rabbit anti-HSV	Sensitization as measured by sheep anti-rabbit γ-globulin (virus survival, $\log_{10}$)		
	Undigested	Fab I	Fab II
γ-Globulin (undigested)	−2.1	−0.8	−1.3
Fab I	−1.9	−0.9	−0.6
Fab II	−0.9	−0.4	−0.5

[a] Approximately 10^6 PFU/ml of HSV was sensitized with 0.14 mg/ml of undigested or papain-derived fragments of rabbit anti-HSV γ-globulin for 2 hr at 37°C. Each reaction mixture then was diluted 1:10 or 1:100 and incubated with undigested sheep anti-rabbit γ-globulin (0.42 mg/ml) or its papain-derived fragments (Fab I, 0.75 mg/ml; Fab II, 0.58 mg/ml). From Ashe *et al.* (1968).

the surviving level was about 0.03% and was reduced slightly (0.01%) by anti-IgG but not at all by anti-IgM globulin. It was also reported that sensitization by IgM rendered virus resistant to late anti-viral IgG antibody. Also of interest is their observation that when sensitized virus was adsorbed to cells it could still be neutralized by the appropriate antiglobulin. The quantitative data of these studies indicated that the proportion of virus that became sensitized rather than neutralized was considerably greater with early IgM than with late IgG antibody.

Iwasaki and Ogura (1968*b*) also explored antiglobulin-mediated neutralization of JEV. Kinetic analysis of the neutralization by antiviral mouse serum showed single-hit exponential inactivation to about 1% survival, with no further decline. Mediated neutralization of the NNF was examined kinetically with either heterologous antiglobulin or allotypic antiglobulin prepared, respectively, with γ-globulin from mice of (BALB/c) strain in rabbits or in mice of (A/JAX) strain. As in direct neutralization, mediated neutralization with both antiglobulins showed single-hit exponential inactivation (Fig. 9). The allotypic determinants involved in these studies reside in the Fc domain of the antibody molecule.

Studies on the neutralization of VEV, a flavivirus, were described by Hahon (1970). Although prior filtration reduced the level of the NNF, use of antiglobulin was effective in mediating still further neutralization. Hence aggregation was considered to be a contributing, but not the principal, cause for the occurrence of the NNF. No differences

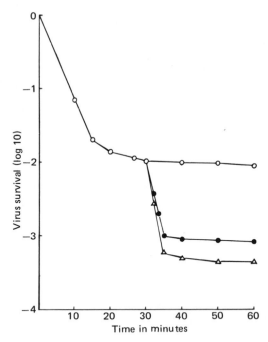

Fig. 9. Kinetics of neutralization of the resistant virus fraction by heterotype or allotype antibody. Equal volumes of virus (5 × 10⁶ PFU/ml) and anti-JEV antibody (1:10) were mixed. The mixtures were incubated at 37°C. After 30 min incubation, heterotype antibody (1:10) or allotype antibody (1:10) was added to each mixture. After various intervals samples were removed and assayed. O, Titer of the mixture consisting of JEV and anti-JEV antibody; ●, titer of the mixture consisting of the resistant virus fraction and heterotype antibody; △, titer of the mixture consisting of the resistant virus fraction and allotype antibody. From Iwasaki and Ogura (1968b), with permission of the publisher.

were observed in the level of the NNF when five different host cells were used for assay. In mediating neutralization, anti-IgG was more effective than anti-IgA. Anti-IgG, anti-Fab, and anti-Fc were effective in decreasing order. Anti-IgM had no effect. It should be mentioned that in these studies the assay for viral activity was based on enumeration of cells showing immunofluorescence.

Still another togavirus, EAV, possibly an alphavirus, was studied by Radwan and colleagues (Radwan and Burger, 1973a,b; Radwan et al., 1973). As in other studies, evidence for dilution–dissociation was not demonstrable, nor did the complex undergo reactivation when subjected to ultrasonic vibration. The interesting observation was reported that whereas complement or antiglobulin could mediate neutralization of the NNF, treatment of the NNF with trypsin rendered the complex insensitive to complement but not to antiglobulin. This result distinguished the targets for mediated neutralization as the Fc region for complement, and the Fab region for antiglobulin. Mediation by antiglobulin was considered to be the result of a nontraumatic change in the virus–antibody complex. However, a more complex situation pertained to the effect of complement. At low temperature the effect was nontraumatic, but at 37°C the physical integrity of the virion was impaired as a result of the lytic effect on the viral envelope (i.e., virolysis).

Infectious virus–antibody complexes of Sindbis virus, an alphatogavirus, resulted from interaction of each of the two surface glycoproteins with homotypic antibody (Symington et al., 1977). In each case, neutralization was mediated by antiglobulin. It is of interest that antibody induced by the intact virion was more effective than antibody induced by each of the isolated glycoproteins, when these were used individually or in combination.

Studies on mediated neutralization of vaccinia and influenza viruses were described by Majer and Link (1970, 1971, 1972). The NNF of vaccinia virus resulting from interaction with human antiserum was effectively neutralized by sheep anti-human globulin. In studies on influenza virus, advantage was taken of the availability of specific antisera for each of the two surface glycoproteins—the hemagglutinin and the neuraminidase. Antiserum to the hemagglutinin had a neutralizing effect and could not be extended by use of antiglobulin. The reverse was seen with the neuraminidase antiserum, namely, no direct neutralization but effective mediated neutralization. Hence the hemagglutinin was considered critical and the neuraminidase noncritical. Binding of the antiglobulin to the complex of virus with the neuraminidase antibody resulted in steric interference with hemagglutinin function, in the opinion of these investigators.

Adenoviruses are structurally complex, containing three antigenically distinct units—the hexon, penton, and fiber. Hexons vary according to their location, which affects their assembly with neighboring hexons, e.g., on the face, or edge, or vertex of the icosahedral capsid. It has been suggested by Shortridge and Biddle (1970) and Shortridge (1972) that the serological specificity of the antigenic units in the capsid may not be identical with that of the isolated units. Hence the conformation of the assembled capsid substructures represents the native specificity.

Wadell (1972) compared the serological reactions of several adenovirus groups. Homotypic antihexon antisera efficiently neutralized groups I and II, but group III was neutralized poorly. Efficiency was evaluated as the ratio of neutralizing to complement-fixing activity. Neutralization of group III was mediated by antiglobulin. Wadell considered the possibility that with this group the hexon critical antigen may be less accessible than in the case of groups I and II. A similar interpretation was proposed by Kjellén and Pereira (1968) as a result of studies on type 5 adenovirus. Subsequent to interaction with homotypic antiserum, neutralization could be enhanced by any of several heterotypic antisera (e.g., types 1,2,12). They have suggested that the homotypic reaction promotes a conformational change in the structure that makes accessible antigenic determinants common to the other serotypes.

Studies on the NNF of poliovirus showed that sensitized infectious virus could be neutralized by antiglobulin (Mandel, 1958). In these experiments, mediated neutralization was achieved after sensitized virus had adsorbed to host cells. Further studies with poliovirus (Lewenton-Kriss and Mandel, 1972) showed that when virus propagated in HeLa cells or monkey kidney cells the level of the NNF was 2 logs lower with the latter virus. When HeLa or monkey kidney cells were used as the assay system, the results of direct neutralization were the same, also observed by Dulbecco *et al.* (1956). However, mediated neutralization was demonstrable only with HeLa cells. These results indicate a host influence on mediated neutralization with respect to the virus *per se* and the assay system. Studies on the mechanism of mediation revealed that the antiglobulin combined with the virus–antibody complex rather than caused its dissociation. The latter possibility was considered since such an event would expose the virus to possible direct neutralization. Dissociation of a complex of bacteriophage ϕX174 with early IgM by antiglobulin was mentioned by Krummel and Uhr (1969). Attempts to isolate a uniquely sensitizing antibody from early and late sera by several fractionation procedures were unsuccessful. The 19 S and 7 S antibodies in the antiglobulin sera were separated, and each was found to be active in mediating neutralization (Lewenton-Kriss and Mandel, 1972).

The participation of antibody fragments in sensitization of poliovirus was investigated by Keller (1968) and Keller and Dwyer (1968). Virus was neutralized by IgG and then reactivated by pepsin digestion followed by sulfhydryl reduction. The resulting infectious virus was shown to be complexed to the Fab' fragment by virtue of its neutralization by antiglobulin. In a second interesting (because of its relevance to a natural *in vivo* situation) report, Keller and Dwyer examined the state of poliovirus and antibodies in the stools of children and adults following known, or presumed, exposure to vaccine strains of poliovirus. The predominant class of antibody found was IgA. Although the presence of neutralized virus in the stools was demonstrated, it was seen that a considerable amount of sensitized virus also was present as revealed by mediation with anti-IgA globulin. More detailed analysis indicated the likelihood that the sensitization involved the light chain of the antibody molecule.

Sensitization of reovirus by rabbit antibody and mediated neutralization by antiglobulin were described by Huggett *et al.* (1972). In these studies aggregation was found not to be a contributing factor either prior to or subsequent to treatment with antiviral antibody.

A number of studies on the neutralization of bacteriophages involved antiglobulin-mediated neutralization. These studies focused more on the mechanism of the neutralization reaction than on the nature of sensitization. Goodman and Donch (1965) demonstrated that the L chain polypeptide of rabbit anti-T1 antibody reacted with T1 bacteriophage without causing neutralization. The complex was sensitive to neutralization by goat anti-L-chain antibody. In a somewhat similar study, Stemke and Lennox (1967) observed that direct neutralization of bacteriophages T2 and T5 could be achieved by whole antibody, less effectively by Fab II, and least effectively by Fab I. Mediation by the corresponding antiglobulins showed enhanced neutralization in reverse order; Fab I was enhanced most, then Fab II, and IgG least. The interesting speculation was raised that possibly mediable neutralization represents antibody bound to a site different from the site that leads to direct neutralization.

Krummel and Uhr (1969) resorted to mediated neutralization in order to evaluate the true reactivity of antisera, "true" being a measure of all interactions—neutralization as well as sensitization. In these studies it was shown that the mediated reaction revealed more virus–antibody complexes than were detected by both direct and decision tube methods. The latter recognizes dissociable complexes. The deviation from first-order kinetics seen in direct neutralization was essentially eliminated in the mediated reaction.

The need for a highly sensitive neutralization test impelled Adler *et al.* (1971) to consider mediated neutralization. Since their studies dealt with "early" antibody, they used rat anti-rabbit IgM for the mediated neutralization assay. Extension of end-point titers was on the order of a thousandfold. In addition, they demonstrated the specificity of the mediated reaction through the use of allotype sera. In these tests titers were extended as much as a hundredfold. The authors were impressed by the positive results in view of the fact that the allotypic determinants are located in those regions of the antibody molecule concerned in binding antigen. Effective mediated neutralization was achieved involving allotype markers 1,3,4,5.

In studies on the neutralization of the small icosahedral RNA bacteriophage f2, Dudley *et al.* (1970) observed a threefold enhancement in rate constant in the mediated reaction. The same result was obtained when virus reacted with intact IgG, or F(ab')$_2$, or Fab', and mediated neutralization was by either anti-IgG or anti-5 S fragment. Dudley *et al.* observed that addition of the mediating antibody completely obliterated activity of the uncombined antiviral antibody. It is reasonable, therefore, to infer that antiglobulin functions by interacting with the infectious virus–antibody complex, rather than "exposing" the virion to extraneous neutralizing antibody.

7.2.2. Mediation by Complement

Mueller (1931) suspected the involvement of complement in the neutralization of animal viruses based on his own studies, as well as previously reported work of other investigators. Substantiation was provided by the results of Leymaster and Ward (1949), who used chick embryos as host for assaying NDV neutralization. The unique feature of these experiments was the use of a complement-free host, in contrast to previous studies. Extension of this role for complement to bacterial viruses was shown in several reports (Van Vunakis *et al.*, 1956; Barlow *et al.*, 1958; Cowan, 1962; Harris *et al.*, 1962; Toussaint and Muschel, 1962; Pernis *et al.*, 1963; Adler *et al.*, 1971).

Detailed analyses of this phenomenon have revealed that it varies according to the characteristics of the virus in question, the class of antibody, the development stage within a given class of antibody, the temperature of the reaction, and the components of the complement system responsible for the result. A detailed review of the various reports dealing with the above aspects will not be undertaken.

7.2.2a. Dependence on Type of Antibody

Bacteriophage T2 antibody in normal human serum, or in rabbit sera shortly after immunization, required complement for neutralization. However, sera from the same rabbits after intensive immunization neutralized and could not be further mediated by complement

(Toussaint and Muschel, 1962; Muschel and Toussaint, 1962). Similarly, Hajek and Mandel (Hajek, 1966, 1968, 1969; Hajek and Mandel, 1966) observed a pronounced mediating effect of complement with early T2 rabbit antibodies of 19 S and 7 S classes. The effect was reduced with late antibody and entirely absent after secondary stimulation for both 19 S and 7 S antibodies. Other studies involving bacteriophage T2 (Pernis *et al.*, 1963; Adler *et al.*, 1971) were in agreement: early rabbit antibody of the 19S class was partially or entirely complement dependent.

Studies involving animal viruses have resulted in a less consistent concept. The transition from early complement-dependent to late complement-independent neutralizing antibody has been reported for herpesvirus (Yoshino and Taniguchi, 1964; Heineman, 1967; Hampar *et al.*, 1968; Stevens *et al.*, 1968), for NDV (Linscott and Levinson, 1969), and for EAV (Radwan and Burger, 1973a; Hyllseth and Pettersson, 1970; Maess, 1971). Several investigations on cytomegalovirus have yielded discordant results (Ablashi *et al.*, 1969; Martos *et al.* 1970; Graham *et al.*, 1971; Minamishima *et al.*, 1971; Andersen, 1971, 1972). In some instances results varied when several strains were compared, or when sera from different species of animal were used. In one study, for example, two strains showed the usual result—namely, transition to independence—while two other strains remained dependent. Reasonable clues to account for the different results were not evident. Rawls *et al.* (1967) reported that antibodies to rubella virus were complement dependent in individuals newly infected as well as in individuals long (5 years) after infection. These sera were obtained from human subjects. Other reports also dealt with some of the ramifications in complement-mediated neutralization of rubella virus (Neva and Weller, 1964; Parkman *et al.*, 1964; Leerhøy, 1968).

Shinkai and Yoshino (1975a) compared herpesvirus antibodies from immunized rabbits and guinea pigs. Early rabbit antibodies (i.e., IgM, IgG1, IgG2) as well as early guinea pig antibodies effectively sensitized and were mediated by complement. The transition to complement-independence occurred sooner in the rabbits than the guinea pigs. A possible explanation may be related to their observation that the half-life of IgM was longer in the guinea pig than in the rabbit.

An interesting observation was described by Iwasaki and Ogura (1968a) in studies of JEV. Two specifically distinguishable antibodies, each complement dependent, were present in sera of immunized rabbits. One was specific for a viral antigen, the other for a host antigen that is a component of the lipoprotein viral envelope. In contrast to these results, Hashimoto and Prince (1963) had reported that antibody to

JEV was unequivocally completely independent. Still a third investigation employing the same virus, JEV (Ozaki and Tabeyi, 1967), described mediation by complement. Details of these several studies indicate the strong likelihood that differences in viral strains and, probably more relevant, differences in the culture histories contributed to the contradictions, which may not be real. Examination of the susceptibility of two other togaviruses, West Nile and Murray Valley encephalitis, to complement-mediated neutralization revealed that neutralization was slightly enhanced (Westaway, 1965a).

Other viruses for which complement-mediated neutralization has been reported are RSV (Baughman et al., 1968) and FLV (Bendinelli et al., 1974). In the case of Friend leukemia virus, the authors expressed some uncertainty about this interpretation inasmuch as they used sera from several species of unimmunized animals and they had no independent evidence for the participation of antibody. Oldstone (1975) has referred to preliminary evidence for a neutralizing effect of complement (C1 component) in the absence of antibody.

7.2.2b. Involvement of Components of the Complement System

Dozois et al. (1949) removed by chemical fractionation the constituents of the complement system from serum of rabbits immunized with WEV. Complement-mediating activity was restored by addition of components C2, C3, and C4. There was some uncertainty whether C1 was entirely nonessential or was required in trace concentrations. Based on current understanding of the complement system, it is very likely that C1 was involved since all subsequent stages in the complement cascade are initiated by the activation of the C1 component. Almost the same conclusion was reported by Taniguchi and Yoshino (1965). They selectively removed each of the first four components of complement from guinea pig serum. Removal of any one eradicated mediating activity. Hence they concluded that all four were essential. Daniels et al. (1970) considered these results unreliable for technical reasons. Based on their results, Daniels et al. concluded that neutralization by dependent IgM antibody could be mediated by components C1 and C4 acting jointly. However, they also observed that if the concentration of C4 was low, addition of C2 and C3 accelerated the reaction. The possible participation of the later components, C5–C9, was investigated by Linscott and Levinson (1969) with NDV. A serum from a C6-deficient rabbit was fully active in mediating neutralization. Hence there was no requirement for any components after

C5. Loss of mediating ability resulted from treatment with cobra venom, indicating a dependence on C3. Addition of individual components to decomplemented serum revealed the requirement for each of the first four components.

It should be noted that all animal viruses thus far studied for complement-mediated neutralization were enveloped viruses. Oldstone *et al.* (1972, 1974) have explored this phenomenon with polyoma virus, a nonenveloped virus. This work along with other related considerations has recently been reviewed by Oldstone (1975). When polyoma virus had reacted with an average of two molecules of antibody per virion, the complex was infectious and neutralization was mediated by (1) the complete complement system, (2) a C6-deficient system, (3) the C1q component, and (4) the combination of C1, C2, C3, and C4. Therefore, the first four components were essential, implicating a crucial role for C3 since the order of addition is C1, C4, C2, C3. The positive result with C1q was attributable to its ability to cross-link the complexes as revealed by sedimentation analysis.

Two studies have attempted to relate laboratory findings to an *in vivo* role for complement-mediated neutralization. Strunk *et al.* (1977) infected C4-deficient and normal guinea pigs with HSV. Assessment of the levels of C1 and C3 to C9 showed no differences when the two groups were compared or when pre and post levels in sera were compared. Moreover, no discernible clinical differences were evident. Since the classic pathway apparently was not involved, the possibility was considered that the alternative pathway (i.e., the properdin system) may have been activated.

Leddy *et al.* (1977) examined the mediating activity of human sera when used in conjunction with antiviral human or guinea pig serum vs. VSV or vaccinia virus. Their results were consistent with previously described *in vitro* results: namely, components C5–C9 did not participate, whereas the first four components were required. These studies were based on the effect of the complement components on the rate of *in vitro* neutralization. Concerning the *in vivo* significance, Leddy *et al.* considered that for most viruses complement participation may play a helpful but not a major defense role. With more "occult" viruses that have been implicated in persisting chronic infections, Leddy *et al.* envisioned a possibly more significant disease-abating role for complement.

Unlike the general results described in studies with animal viruses, Schrader and Muschel (1975) have concluded that whereas mediation of neutralization by early rabbit IgM required C1 and C4, IgG required only C1. Moreover, they observed a higher efficiency of C1 compared with whole guinea pig complement. Perhaps the report of Miller (1977) is of interest in this context: addition of complement to antigen (bovine serum albumin) complexed to mouse IgG promoted the dissociation of antibody.

7.2.3. Mediation by Other Substances

Several reports have described the mediating activity of rheumatoid factor on the neutralization of herpesvirus (Ashe *et al.*, 1971), vaccinia virus (Gipson *et al.*, 1974), and hepatitis B virus (Markenson *et al.*, 1975). However, unlike antiglobulin or complement, rheumatoid factor does not consummate the neutralization reaction. Addition of complement or antirheumatoid factor antibody is needed. In a slightly different manner, protein A of staphylococci can by itself, or with the aid of protein A antibody, mediates the neutralization of sensitized herpes and vaccinia viruses (Austin and Daniels, 1974).

A rather unusual instance of mediated neutralization was described by Kulberg and Pervikov (1976). Normal rabbit sera contain a substance, designated "homoreactant," that mediates the neutralization of infectious complexes of poliovirus and antibody. "Homoreactant" was considered to be an antiglobulin substance and, oddly, did not mediate the neutralization of poliovirus complexed with whole IgG but only with Fab'.

A quite extensive investigation has been described by Styk and colleagues on a serum component, designated "cofactor," which mediates the neutralization of sensitized influenza virus (for the more recent aspects of these studies, see Styk, 1965; Styk and Hana, 1965*a,b*). "Cofactor" was considered to be a β-globulin unrelated to any component of the complement system. Since it did not interact with virus, the presumption was that it reacted with the antibody of the sensitized virus. A similar finding was described by Smorodintsev and Yabrov (1963).

8. NEUTRALIZATION BY ANTIBODY FRAGMENTS

Enzymatic dissection of antibody has enabled an assessment of the functional role in neutralization of the various domains of the antibody molecule (see Section 3.1.1). The ability to alter the size of the molecule without changing the valence (i.e., 7 S → 5 S), or size and valence (5 S → 3.5 S), or valence and not size (hybrid 7 S), or to compare early and late fragments (Fab I and Fab II), or the constituent chains (H and L), has made possible an experimental approach to evaluating the above parameters (i.e., size and valence) in respect to neutralization.

Kjellén's (1964) attempts to neutralize adenovirus with fragments Fab I and Fab II were unsuccessful. However, he observed that Fab II did combine with virus since neutralization by intact antibody was blocked. In a second study (Kjellén, 1965a) it was seen that the bivalent fragment F(ab')₂ was relatively ineffective in neutralizing adenovirus. These data indicated to Kjellén the possibility of a role in neutralization for the Fc structure, perhaps its absence resulted in a fragment that "lacked the quality . . . of transforming infective virus–antibody complexes into a non-infective state."

Cremer et al. (1964, 1975), Vogt et al. (1964), Keller (1966, 1968), and Philipson and Bennich (1966) used poliovirus in studies with antibody fragments. In each study, neutralization with monovalent Fab I and II fragments was reported, although at various levels of efficiency. One cause for reduced efficiency was considered to be low binding affinity and therefore increased tendency for dissociation. Vogt failed to detect dissociation by dilution. Keller, on the other hand, observed a tendency for Fab', and to a lesser extent F(ab')₂, to undergo dissociation. This tendency was inversely related to the length of time that virus and fragment had interacted. Keller considered the possibility of a stabilizing effect of Fc on the virus–antibody complex. Cremer et al. (1964) observed neutralization of poliovirus and WEV by Fab' in cell cultures. However, when mouse protection was examined with WEV, Fab' failed to neutralize. Dissociation seemed an unlikely reason since neither dilution nor sonication appeared capable of dissociating the complex. The possibility was suggested that in the case of WEV a cell-mediated mechanism is required for neutralization and for this event the Fc moiety would be necessary.

Keller (1968) examined the interaction of poliovirus and Fab' in a "reverse" manner. Following neutralization of virus with intact antibody, he used pepsin to convert antibody to the bivalent 5 S state. The virus remained neutralized. The 5 S fragment was then reduced to the monovalent 3.5 S (Fab') state, resulting in restoration of infectivity. That restoration was not due to dissociation was shown by subsequent mediated neutralization with antiglobulin. Similarly, reactivation of adenovirus did not require dissociation of the complex (Kjellén, 1965b).

By means of a phase distribution procedure, Philipson and Bennich (1966) observed that whereas intact antibody affected the distribution characteristics of poliovirus, neither Fab I nor Fab II had this effect, although these fragments neutralized. Further studies showed that the separated light and heavy chains had no effect either by distribution or by infectivity assays.

Similar studies on the role of size and valence were conducted with bacteriophage model systems. Goodman and Donch (1964, 1965) concluded that molecular size was a determinant in neutralization efficiency. Efficiency was proportional to size, namely, 7 S, 5 S, 3.5 S, in neutralizing bacteriophages T1 and T6. A comparison of Fab I and Fab II indicated the latter to be somewhat more effective. The neutralizing capacity of separated chains was examined. Some activity, in decreasing order, was seen with H, L, and Fd chains. However, additional neutralization by each was mediated by anti-fragment III, anti-fragment I, and anti-fragment I, respectively. Goodman and Donch considered these results consistent with their view of the role of molecular size in neutralization. It should be borne in mind that failure to neutralize was not due to failure to bind. It has been seen in several studies that relatively poor neutralization is accompanied by a relatively high level of mediated neutralization.

The role of binding affinity was evaluated in other studies. Rowlands (1967) measured neutralization rates of bacteriophage f2 using IgG, F(ab')$_2$, and Fab'. Since the rates were 2.12, 0.44, and 0.16 $\times$ 10^{-12} molecule^{-1} ml min^{-1} for each, the discrepancy between rate and size compelled Rowlands to conclude that steric (i.e., size) effects were not the sole factor in determining neutralization efficiency. Klinman *et al.* (1967) similarly relegated size to a secondary role. Rates of neutralization of bacteriophage R17 by 7 S and 5 S bivalent antibodies, and by monovalent 7 S, 5 S, and 3.5 S antibodies, were found to be thirtyfold higher for the bivalent antibodies. A similar conclusion evolved from the studies of Stemke and Lennox (1967) and Stemke (1969) when they observed equal competence to neutralize bacteriophages T2 and T5 by Fab' and F(ab'$_1$, ab'$_2$). In these studies it was also seen that Fab II neutralized more efficiently than Fab I. However, by antiglobulin-mediated neutralization, Fab I showed a twofold higher degree of enhancement than Fab II. This result indicates that although binding is an essential prerequisite for neutralization, neutralization is not an inevitable result. More likely, the binding energy is of crucial significance.

Rosenstein *et al.* (1971) briefly reviewed the literature on this subject. Some of the divergent results, in their opnion, represented the effect of reagents of different activities, specifically the degree of maturity of antibody. To demonstrate the significance of antibody maturation, they obtained antibodies to ϕX174 bacteriophage early and late in immunogenesis. With late antibody, monovalent 3.5 S and bivalent 7 S neutralized equally well. With early antibody, 3.5 S showed little capability to neutralize, unlike 7 S antibody. Dissociation appeared not to be a factor since all four categories of antibody formed firm complexes with virus. Therefore, it was considered that neither molecular size nor the presence of Fc was important. On the other hand, binding affinity was the major consideration. With early antibody, bivalence compensates for low affinty.

Generally similar results were described by Shinkai and Yoshino (1975b) for herpesvirus. Antisera were obtained at early, intermediate, and late times after immunization. Neutralization and binding without neutralization (i.e., sensitization) were determined. Early F(ab')$_2$ neutralized poorly, but survivors were sensitive to antiglobulin mediation. Although intermediate F(ab')$_2$ neutralized well, the Fab' fragment neither neutralized nor sensitized. Late Fab' neutralized moderately well, and when subjected to antiglobulin mediation the extent of neutralization was comparable to that of intact antibody. Consistent with these results was Shinkai and Yoshino's observation that late Fab II was more effective than late Fab I.

A divergent situation was described by Lafferty (1963a). Monovalent antibody was prepared from serum of rabbits hyperimmunized to influenza virus. Although the fragment was able to neutralize, it bound to virus via a readily reversible bond. Moreover, after prolonged incubation the complex was still fully dissociated by dilution

9. VIROLYSIS

In 1968 Berry and Almeida described an effect on a virus that is the counterpart of immune hemolysis. Exposure of avian infectious bronchitis virus to unheated immune serum from fowl (homotypic) or rabbit (heterotypic) resulted in neutralization. If the sera were heated there was a considerable reduction in neutralization. Activity was restored by addition of the unheated respective sera. Examination of these events in the electron microscope revealed that with unheated homotypic serum antibody had reacted with the surface projections. With the unheated heterotypic serum, antibody was seen attached to the projections and also to the viral envelope. In addition, discrete regions of lysis of the envelope were visible. A similar result was described with a mouse leukemia virus (Oroszlan and Gilden, 1970), EAV (Radwan et al., 1973), Moloney leukemia virus (Oldstone, 1975), rubella virus (Schluederberg et al., 1976), and myxovirus (Haukenes, 1977). Under the same conditions that resulted in virolysis of the above enveloped viruses, no evidence for a lytic effect was seen with polyoma, a nonenveloped virus, (Oldstone *et al.*, 1974). This phenomenon has been discussed at length by Almeida and Waterson (1969).

Some consequences of the virolytic effect have been described. Release of genomic RNA was reported by Oroszlan and Gilden as well as by Oldstone. However, Oroszlan and Gilden suspected the presence of contaminating ribonuclease since the RNA was in the form of oligonucleotides, while in Oldstone's experiments the liberated RNA was still digestible by RNase. Radwan *et al.* reported that a considerable amount of virion RNA was released, and treatment with RNase resulted in further release. Schluederberg *et al.* found that only after treatment with RNase was there release of RNA.

The morphological appearance of rubella virus subjected to the virolytic effect of antibody plus complement differed from that of avian infectious bronchitis and influenza viruses. Whereas the latter two viruses displayed well-defined membrane craters or holes, rubella virus appeared to have shed its outer envelope (Almeida and Laurence, 1969).

Of relevant interest is the observation that in every instance where examined, virolysis was not a necessary or sole mechanism for neutralization.

10. MECHANISMS

It would be a source of gratification if at this point it were possible to coordinate all relevant studies and extract therefrom a unified concept of viral neutralization. Regrettably, it is not yet possible. One difficulty arises from the negativity of the phenomenon, since neutralization is manifested by a loss of function. Without direct examination of the nonfunctional virion, the nature of the effect of antibody can only be surmised. As indicated previously (Section 5) several distinctly different pathways may lead to the same end result. Recognition of this plurality has led to discussions of "mechanisms" of neutralization (Burnet *et al.*, 1937; Svehag, 1968; Daniels, 1975; Burns and Allison, 1975). A critical examination of the various fundamental mechanisms reduces the number of putative processes to two: (1) Neutralization is solely a steric phenomenon. The presence of antibody on the surface of a virion physically obstructs viral function. (2) Neutralization is an active process. The interaction of two proteins—viral capsid and antibody—induces chemical modifications in each. The modification in the viral capsid represents the neutralization process. Since it depends in part on the host, neutralization can be envisioned as a conditional process; i.e., a virus–antibody complex may be recognized by one cell as being unchanged but by another cell as being neutralized. Recent studies on antigen–antibody interaction as an active process have yielded data that lend support to this hypothesis. Most of these studies have involved antigens other than viruses. In some cases, evidence for a conformational change was sought in the antibody, while in other studies the antigen was probed.

10.1. Conformational Change in Antibody Induced by Antigen

It had been observed long ago that antibodies can react with complement only after they have combined with antigen. This phenomenon has prompted inquiries into the nature of the change induced in the antibody molecule. It has also been known that interaction with complement is via the Fc region whereas interaction with antigen is via the Fab regions. Hence the speculation arose that interaction with antigen could induce a change in the remote Fc region through cooperative transitional effects. However, other speculative models have been considered. In his review of this topic, Metzger (1974) has proposed three models for consideration: (1) The allosteric model involves overall conformational alterations of the antibody molecule that result from interaction with antigen. (2) The distortive model involves geometric changes when antibody reacts with a multivalent antigen. These changes may either expose or cover reactive sites. (3) The associative model represents the formation of a multivalent substrate from a univalent structure simply due to aggregation. Consideration of available knowledge has led Metzger to tentative preference for the associative model.

Somewhat similarly, Hoffman (1976a,b,c) has considered possible model systems with the judgment that, as yet, no final decision can reasonably be made. Allosteric and aggregative influences were proposed as viable alternatives. However, some recent studies have emphasized the conformation hypothesis. Jaton *et al.* (1975) reported conformational changes in antibody on interaction with homologous antigen. Comparison of the differences in the degree of change in circular polarization of luminescence induced in IgG, F(ab')$_2$ and Fab on binding antigen has indicated that the Fc portion contributes to the change. The contribution by the Fc region was attributed to the result of a conformation change in the antibody molecule initiated at the Fab site and transmitted to the Fc region.

Brown and Koshland (1975) have also presented data in support of a conformational change following interaction with antigen. In order to segregate the respective contributions of aggregation and conformational change to activation of Fc functions, studies involved the interaction of IgM antibody with antigen. Although hapten did not activate Fc, monovalent antigen effectively induced Fc activity. It has been known that activation of the Fc region of IgG antibody requires aggregation. Brown and Koshland have therefore suggested that aggregation is necessary for "effective signal transmission." Since the IgM molecule is normally an aggregate (a covalently linked pentameric form of IgG), the interaction with the antigen initiates the "transmissible signal."

A somewhat more complex situation was described by Drake and Mardiney (1975) concerning the effect of complement. Antibodies to the surface antigens of a mouse lymphoma (EL4) interact specifically with the homologous antigens and possibly, if at all, cross-react with normal tissue antigens. When, however, complement is present the heterologous reaction is quite pronounced. Their interpretation of this result is that "functional complement results in a change in antibody and/or antigen conformation allowing for a firmer union."

10.2. Conformational Change in Antigen Induced by Antibody

Numerous examples of conformational changes in antigens (many are enzymes) resulting from reaction with antibody have been reported. A few will be reviewed to illustrate the kinds of observations that have been strongly suggestive of such antibody-induced effects (for additional examples, see Cinader, 1966).

Rotman and Celada (1968) reported that antiserum to β-D-galactosidase markedly enhanced enzyme activity of a defective enzyme extracted from *Escherichia coli* mutants. Stabilization against thermal inactivation as the basis for activation was considered less likely than a conformational change induced by the bound antibody.

Enzyme activity of L-amino acid oxidase can be nullified by heating or freezing (Zimmerman *et al.*, 1971). Concomitantly, the electrophoretic behavior is altered. Treatment of inactive enzyme with antibody specific for native enzyme restored enzyme activity as well as the characteristic electrophoretic behavior. Since antibody did not inhibit activity of native enzyme, the antibody binding site must have been distinct from the enzyme active site.

The effect of antibody on defective catalase from mutant mice was studied by Feinstein *et al.* (1971). The defect in the catalase molecule is at or near the catalytic site but removed from the antigenic site. When the defective enzyme reacted with antibody specific for the native enzyme, full activity was observed. In contrast, with homologous antibody the enzyme remained inactive. The authors postulated that (1) the mutant enzyme actually was functional but, because of a structural change, had become inordinately thermolabile, (2) "restoration" of activity was in fact "restoration" of thermostability, and (3) the heterologous antibody (i.e., for native enzyme) induced a conformational change in the mutant enzyme consistant with the structure of native enzyme. The homologous antibody (i.e., for mutant) did not induce such a change.

Stabilization against thermal inactivation was described by Foti *et al.* (1975) for an acid phosphatase enzyme when complexed with specific antibody. It was considered either that antibody was bound to a site that directly protected the enzyme site or that antibody "maintains a more optimal tertiary structure."

Erickson (1974) postulated that inhibition of trypsin activity by antibody was related to antibody binding affinity. Studies with antibody obtained under different immunization protocols supported his expectation; there was a positive correlation between binding affinity and trypsin-inhibiting activity. Studies on the thermal stabilization of human hexosaminidase by antibody resulted in the interpretation that antibody does not stabilize the catalytic site directly but rather stabilizes "an overall conformation" (Ben-Yoseph *et al.*, 1975).

In a review of the various mechanisms that underlie inhibition of enzyme function, Arnon (1971) proposed that the inhibitor (antibody, for our purpose) could act in three ways: (1) By binding at, or close to, the active site of the enzyme, it could sterically obstruct access of substrate or egress of product. (2) It could polymerize several molecules of enzyme, thereby making active sites inaccessible. (3) By binding at a locus other than the active site, a conformational change could be engendered that would inactivate a functional enzyme or, conversely, activate one that is nonfunctional. Closely analogous to the above mechanisms are the modes of neutralization of viral infectivity previously outlined (Section 5). There can be little doubt that antibody can deprive virus of its ability to function as a result of obstruction or reduce the potential activity of virus as a result of aggregation. On the other hand, there are at present also a few instances where conformational influences have been shown, or have been suspected, to be the underlying decisive factor in neutralization.

Andrewes and Elford (1933*b*) proposed that virus could be "altered," and Burnet *et al.* (1937) referred to virus under certain conditions as "partly neutralized." More directly, Bowman and Patnode (1963) reported that specific antibody rendered bacteriophage ϕX174 incapable of infecting *E. coli*. However, protoplasts of *E. coli* could be infected. They also showed that a lupus erythematosus serum (i.e., anti-DNA) could prevent infection of the protoplasts. These results indicated that antiviral antibody, in the course of neutralizing ϕX174, has inflicted a change in the capsid which made it permeable—namely, for allowing passage of the viral DNA into protoplasts or for passage of anti-DNA antibody into the virion.

Carthew (1976) examined the accessibility of the viral polypeptides of a bovine enterovirus to external labeling with ^{125}I. VP1 was labeled heavily, VP2 and VP3 were labeled very lightly, and VP4 was labeled not at all. However, after neutralization, VP4 was labeled readily. This result represents a reorganization of the capsid polypeptide arrangement instigated by antibody. The isoelectric points of the three poliovirus serotypes were shown to be markedly altered after interacting with antibody (Mandel, 1971*b*, 1976). In other studies with poliovirus it was reported that the affinity of neutralized poliovirus for HeLa cell receptor was enhanced as shown by an increased capacity to adsorb and a decreased tendency to elute (Mandel, 1967*a,b*). In related studies (Mandel, unpublished) a marked increase was seen in adsorption affinity for solid and semisolid substrates such as polyacetate, agar, and starch. A change in the interaction with affinity gels as a result of neutralization was described by Thomssen (1963).

Kjellén and Pereira (1968) proposed that interaction of adenovirus hexon antigen with type-specific antibody induced "conformational changes" which exposed critical sites common to group members. Hawkes and Lafferty (1967) described the enhancement of infectivity by homologous antiserum. They attributed this result to an alteration in the capsid by antibody so that the virion in effect had a "new protein coat." The conditional effect of antibody on FMD virus, depending on the cell system, prompted Bradish *et al.* (1962) to refer to virus–antibody complexes as having "amphoteric" properties.

Although supporting data were not presented, Dudley *et al.* (1970) deemed worthy of consideration the possibility that an overall conformational change was the consequence of the interaction with antibody. On the other hand, Hornick and Karush (1969) and Gopalakrishnan and Karush (1974*b*) considered such a change to be unlikely but not to be ignored.

10.3. Mechanisms Pertaining to the Nonneutralized Fraction

Some investigators have alluded to a distinction between sensitized infectious virus–antibody complexes and nonneutralizable infectious virus–antibody complexes. The basis for this was solely operational. The fraction of a NNF that is subject to mediated neutralization was considered sensitized, while the remaining fraction that survived was considered nonneutralizable. Since there is general agreement that virus surviving exposure to excess antibody is in the form of infectious virus–antibody complexes, and since little is known about the molecular aspects or the diversity of these complexes, it is preferable at present to equate the two designations.

Two general mechanisms have been proposed to explain the formation of the NNF: (1) Aggregation of viral particles either prior to or as a result of exposure to antibody allows for the occurrence of functional critical sites under a protected status. Such critical sites, although not accessible to intact or fragmented antibody, are supposedly sufficiently exposed to interact with viral receptors on the cellular surface. (2) The interaction of monodispersed virus with intact or fragmented antibody results in monodispersed infectious virus–antibody complexes. The refractory state has been attributed either to a solely physical mechanism, namely steric hindrance of critical sites by juxtaposed antibody, or to an active subversion of viral function. Subversion may be the result either of the failure of a multistage reaction to attain completion or of a reaction proceeding via an aberrant pathway. The subversive mechanisms induce a state of resistance to further antibody interaction but not negation of infectivity. With respect to the aggregation mechanism, it has been reported that prior filtration yielded monodispersed virions that showed no NNF (Wallis and Melnick, 1967, 1970; Wallis, 1971), or a reduced NNF (Hahon, 1970), or the same NNF but enhanced kinetics of neutralization (Baughman et al., 1968; Lewenton-Kriss and Mandel, 1972), or little or no difference (Ashe et al., 1969; Hyllseth and Pettersson, 1970; Majer and Link, 1971, Huggett et al., 1972).

Each component of the system has been implicated in the formation or expression of the nonneutralized state. The same virus when replicated in different hosts has shown different propensities for sensitization (Ozaki and Kumagai, 1969; Lewenton-Kriss and Mandel, 1972). When assayed in different hosts, the same virus–antiserum mixture may show markedly different levels of the NNF (Kjellén and Schlesinger,

1959). Antibodies derived from a single animal, but varying with respect to maturation (i.e., affinity) or to molecular class, reacting with aliquots of a single virus preparation will result in different surviving levels in the presence of excess antibody (Ozaki, 1968). It has, for example, been reported that immature antibody can sensitize virus but, because of the low avidity of such antibody, desensitization is readily accomplished by simple dilution-sponsored dissociation (Lafferty, 1963a).

Recognition of sensitized virus has been achieved through the procedure of mediated neutralization—prinicipally by the complement system or by the use of antibody specific for the sensitizing immune globulin. Various studies have been reported concerning the mechanism of complement mediation. In one respect, there is considerable agreement. Of the total components of complement, C5–C9 are not involved. Of the first four components, reports have indicated, for example, that all four (Linscott and Levinson, 1969; Oldstone, 1975), or C1 alone (Schrader and Muschel, 1975), or C1 and C4 (but C2 and C3 can substitute for C4, Daniels et al., 1970), or C1q alone (Oldstone, 1975) can mediate neutralization of sensitized virus. This effect is achieved either through the amassing of protein molecules on the virus–antibody complex or by the formation of lattice structures by cross-linking.

Some interesting experiments have been described pertaining to mediated neutralization by antiglobulin. Kinetic studies of neutralization followed by antiglobulin-mediated neutralization have shown that both processes show single-hit, first-order kinetics (Iwasaki and Ogura, 1968b) (see Fig. 9), suggesting that either there is only one site responsible for sensitization or, if there are more than one, interaction of antiglobulin with any one is sufficient. It has also been shown that virus can be sensitized with monovalent fragments, and such sensitized virus can be secondarily neutralized by intact or monovalent antiglobulin (Table 3). These results establish the competence of monvalent antibodies for both sensitization and mediated neutralization, and therefore establish these phenomena as being independent of aggregation. It has also been shown in several studies that adsorbed sensitized virus is susceptible to mediated neutralization. In one study (Radwan and Burger, 1973b) it was shown that neutralization of sensitized virus was achieved with either complement or antiglobulin. However, following pepsin digestion of the bound sensitizing antibody, complement was no longer effective. Hence the essentiality of Fc for complement mediation and of Fab for antiglobulin mediation was demonstrated.

10.4. Mechanisms Pertaining to Intrinsic Neutralization

Under conditions of extremely low concentration, virus particles encountering neutralizing antibody are apt to be neutralized. It is reasonable to exclude secondary effects such as aggregation as the cause of reduction in titer. Neutralization is therefore the direct consequence of the union of a virion with one or more molecules of antibody. It is this intrinsic loss of infectivity, rather than the loss due to secondary phenomena (see Section 5), that is of greatest interest. Two problems pertaining to intrinsic neutralization have received investigative attention but without as yet general concurrence as to interpretation of data. (1) Studies of the neutralization of bacterial and animal viruses by kinetic analysis have led to the conclusion that neutralization is a single-hit phenomenon. In one study with a plant virus, a similar interpretation was offered (Rappaport, 1957). However, there has been opposition to this interpretation on the grounds that (a) some examples have been presented where kinetic analysis indicates a multihit phenomenon, (b) even when a single-hit curve is seen it has been proposed that the complexity of the neutralization phenomenon does not warrant so naive an interpretation, and (c) a few studies on the stoichiometric aspects of the reaction have shown that several molecules of antibody are bound to one virion at the moment it has been neutralized. (2) The other problem concerns the molecular basis for the loss of infectious capability.

Recently, several concepts have been offered in an effort to integrate the various scattered data into a unified theory that could explain the essential nature of viral neutralization (Mandel, 1976; Della-Porta and Westaway, 1978; Yoshino and Isono, 1978). Basically the hypotheses fall into two major categories: (1) Viral function is negated when antibodies in sufficient numbers bind to strategic sites on the viral surface. If a virus is multifunctional (e.g. hemagglutinin, enzyme activity), each function is dealt with individually. (2) The interaction with antibody leads to noncovalent physicochemical alterations in the viral capsid that modify the characteristics of normal virus–cell interaction. Consequently, an essential stage in the viral replication cycle is inhibited or subverted.

10.4.1. The Antibody-Sensitive Stage

A number of investigations have focused on the replication stage that is affected by virus. Direct irreversible denaturation of viruses by antibody is a rare event since it has been shown that neutralized virus can be restored to an infectious condition by a variety of procedures (Mandel, 1971a). It is also clear that antibody is without influence once virus has penetrated and uncoated. Hence the target stage must be one or more of the early phases of virus cell interaction—adsorption, penetration, uncoating.

The effect of antibody on viral adsorption to host cells has been described. Smith *et al.* (1961) and Morgan *et al.* (1968) have noted that the adsorptive capacity of vaccinia virus and herpesviruses is considerably curtailed when they are combined with antibody. Rubin and Franklin (1957) reported that the capacity of NDV to adsorb is a function of antibody multiplicity. When few molecules are bound to a viral particle, adsorption is not impaired. At higher multiplicities, adsorption diminishes.

Adsorption of virus–antibody complexes to cells has been described for bacterial viruses (Lanni and Lanni, 1953; Nagano *et al.*, 1952; Nagano and Mutai, 1954; Tolmach, 1956) and for animal viruses (Hultin and McKee, 1952; Rubin and Franklin, 1957; Mandel, 1958; Mannweiler, 1963; Dales and Kajioka, 1964; Joklik, 1964; Granoff, 1965; Stinski and Cunningham, 1970; Radwan and Burger, 1973a; Ozaki *et al.*, 1974). In studies of the adsorption of neutralized poliovirus to HeLa cells (Mandel, 1967a), it was seen that "lightly" neutralized particles showed an enhanced capacity to adsorb. Moreover, the enhancement increased with time when neutralized virus was held at 5°C. In various studies evidence for adsorbed neutralized virus has been based on direct examination by microscopy, by use of radioisotopically labeled virus, by use of ferritin-coupled viral antibody, and by reactivation of viral infectivity by exposure of the virus–cell–antibody complex to mild acid treatment. The inability of virus to initiate replication in spite of having adsorbed to a cell has also been shown by a modified procedure. When native virus adsorbs at low temperature, penetration and uncoating do not ensue. Virus can then be neutralized in this externally adsorbed state. This phenomenon has been observed with many different viruses. The above results thus far indicate that neither irreversible denaturation nor failure to adsorb represents the sole mechanism for neutralization.

Several studies have inquired into the fate of adsorbed neutralized virus. Three possibilities were considered, and were observed with different systems: (1) Antibody promotes elution of virus. (2) Antibody enhances binding to the cell membrane, and, as a result, virus neither elutes nor penetrates. (3) Virus penetrates and either does not uncoat or uncoats aberrantly. The tendency for adsorbed neutralized virus to elute was seen with rabbit pox virus (Joklik, 1964), NDV (Silverstein and Marcus, 1964), and influenza virus (Dourmashkin and Tyrrell, 1974). The reactions with influenza virus were studied in some detail. When antibody specific for the hemagglutinin was used, virus was found at a distance from the cell to which it had been attached. In contrast, when neuraminidase-specific antibody was used, adsorbed virus appeared, by electron microscopy, to be more firmly adherent than unneutralized virus (Dourmashkin and Tyrrell, 1974). Enhanced binding was also observed with poliovirus. The tendency for native poliovirus to elute has been described by Joklik and Darnell (1961) and by Fenwick and Cooper (1962). When virus was neutralized, the percentage of virus that eluted was markedly reduced (Mandel, 1967b). This effect is consistent with the previously described observation that the poliovirus–antibody complex shows a greater affinity for host cells than does native virus (Mandel, 1967a). Stinski and Cunningham (1970) noted that there was no difference between neutralized and unneutralized IBV with respect to elution.

The effect of antibody on the penetration of adsorbed virus has been investigated. The influenza–antineuraminidase antibody complex failed to undergo penetration (Dourmashkin and Tyrrell, 1974). Morgan and Rose (1968) similarly observed this effect, noting that it required "very few molecules necessary to prevent penetration" of influenza virus. In this study a rather intriguing observation (or interpretation?) was described. When a virion has begun to penetrate, antibody failed to react, suggesting that "during entry the antibody-combining sites at the surface of the virus distal to the cell become altered." Evidence for penetration of poliovirus–antibody complexes was described (Mandel, 1967b) based on the time-dependent decrease in ability to reactivate virus by acid treatment. Electron microscopic studies have shown penetration of some virus–antibody complexes of vaccinia virus (Dales and Kajioka, 1964), rabbit pox virus (Joklik, 1964), and NDV (Silverstein and Marcus, 1964).

Several studies have described the intracellular fate of neutralized virus. Based on EM analysis Joklik (1964) stated that rabbit pox virus underwent incomplete uncoating, while Dales and Kajioka (1964) observed degradation of vaccinia virus within phagocytic vesicles as opposed to the release of intact cores from vesicles seen with native virus. Silverstein and Marcus (1964) were impressed by the close proximity of intracellular neutralized NDV to cytoplasmic organelles that may have a "lytic function." Biochemical studies were described for poliovirus (Mandel, 1967*b*) and for IBV (Stinski and Cunningham, 1970) with essentially similar results. With both native and neutralized virus, a certain fraction of intracellular viral nucleic acid was degraded (i.e., acid soluble). With native virus a fraction (about 10–15%) of the viral RNA was conserved (i.e., acid insoluble) but little or no conserved RNA was present with neutralized poliovirus or IBV.

A summation of the preceding observations indicates that any of the early events may be interfered with by antibody. There is an implication that the fewer the number of bound molecules of antibody, the farther the virion can proceed in the replication cycle before neutralization manifests itself. Under these conditions, uncoating becomes the sensitive state. With some systems there appears to be aberrant uncoating, and in other cases uncoating is incomplete or absent. Studies with poliovirus focused on the effect of antibody on uncoating, utilizing an *in vitro* system capable of initiating the uncoating process (De Sena and Mandel, 1976). It was found that neutralized poliovirus was not sensitive to the system (Mandel, 1976). This result is consistent with the previous observation that intact viral RNA was not detectable in cells exposed to neutralized virus albeit virus had adsorbed and penetrated (Mandel, 1967*b*).

10.4.2. Theories of Neutralization

Recently several reports have appeared that have attempted to integrate available information of neutralization into a unified hypothesis. The basic postulates fall into either of two categories: (1) antibody obstructs viral functions because of its physical presence at crucial sites on the surface of the virion, or (2) the interaction between virus and antibody results in a molecular perturbation of the capsid structure, rendering the virion noninfectious (Mandel, 1976; Della-Porta and Westaway, 1978; Yoshino and Isono, 1978). It has also been indicated by Trautman (1976) and Trautman and Harris (1977) that an explanation of the neutralization phenomenon requires a knowledge of the various complexes, both infectious and noninfectious, that are generated during virus–antibody interaction. Also, they state that it is essential to determine the number of critical sites that must remain free for a virus–antibody complex to remain infectious for a specific host, involving a given class of antibody. A computer-assisted mathematical analysis for obtaining such information has been described (Trautman, 1976).

Inextricably bound to an explanation of neutralization is an explanation of the role of antibody multiplicity, namely, single-hit vs multihit. The single-hit concept can be further distinguished as to whether a virion possesses only one critical antigenic site or several, any one of which can lead to neutralization.

10.4.3. Single-Hit vs. Multihit Mechanism

The proposal that neutralization of a virion can be the result of binding one molecule of antibody has been based on kinetic analyses. Mathematically, the number of target sites that must be hit for inactivation of the virion is expressed by

$$\frac{V_t}{V_0} = 1-(1-e^{-kt/D})^n \qquad (7)$$

where V_t and V_0 are the concentrations of virus at times t and 0, k is the reaction rate constant, t is time, D is the dilution factor of the serum, and n is the number of critical targets. When $n = 1$, equation (7) reduced to

$$\frac{V_t}{V_0} = e^{-kt/D} \qquad (8)$$

which, graphically, is represented by (1) an exponential decline in viral infectivity as a function of time and (2) an immediate decline in surviving virus. When $n > 1$ there is an exponential decline but only after a delay which is proportional to the value of n. Based on the absence of a lag period in the survival curve when $\ln V_t/V_0$ is plotted as a function of t, it has been considered that one molecule of antibody can inactivate one viral particle. This interpretation has been applied to bacterial viruses (Cann and Clark, 1954; Stemke and Lennox, 1967; Stemke, 1969; Hornick and Karush, 1969, 1972; Dudley et al., 1970; Rohrmann and Krueger, 1970; Gopalakrishnan and Karush, 1974b), to animal viruses (Dulbecco et al., 1956; Rubin and Franklin, 1957; Mandel, 1960; Thormar, 1963; Granoff, 1965; Philipson, 1966), and to a plant virus (Rappaport, 1957). Based on the occurrence of a lag period preceding inactivation, a multihit mechanism was proposed (Kalmanson et al., 1942; Lafferty, 1963a; Philipson, 1966; Burnet et al., 1937). In some instances the demonstration of the multihit mechanism necessitated special conditions, e.g., use of a low concentration of antibody or a reaction temperature of about 5°C, or the use of IgM as opposed to

IgG antibody. Further support for the single-hit mechanism has been the common experience that the reaction rate constant is directly proportional to antibody concentration (e.g., see Fig. 3). On the other hand, it has been argued that antigen–antibody reactions are extremely rapid processes and the methods used for rate measurements of neutralization do not indicate true rates. However, as was discussed previously (see Section 6.1), reference to the great rapidity of antigen–antibody reactions has been directed at analyses of hapten–antibody interactions which involved concentrations of reactants one or more orders of magnitude greater than ordinarily used in neutralization studies. For example, Day *et al.* (1963) determined the rate of interaction of DNP lysine with rabbit antibody using approximately $2-5 \times 10^{-7}$ M concentrations of each. Forward reaction rates of the order of 8×10^{7} mol^{-1} sec^{-1} were calculated, necessitating sample determinations over millisecond intervals. Hornick and Karush (1969) reported a rate constant of about 4×10^{7} mol^{-1} sec^{-1} for the neutralization of DNP haptenated bacteriophage ϕX174 by rabbit antibody. At a concentration of 3×10^{-11} M of antibody 10 min was required for the neutralization of 50% of the initial viral concentration of about 2500 PFU/ml ($\simeq 10^{-16}$ M). The extremely lower concentrations of reactants normally used in neutralization studies would be expected to be reflected by correspondingly slower reaction rates.

10.4.4. Mechanism of Neutralization

A hypothesis was proposed that attempted to coordinate several aspects of the neutralization of poliovirus into a unified concept (Mandel, 1976). More recently two other reports have appeared that attempted to generalize the neutralization phenomenon (Della-Porta and Westaway, 1978; Yoshino and Isono, 1978). Two fundamentally different concepts are envisioned: (1) The effect of antibody on virus is to induce alterations in the structure of the capsid that render the virion "unrecognizable" at least to some host cells, if not all (Mandel, 1976; Yoshino and Isono, 1978). (2) The specific sites at which antibodies bind to the viral surface are crucial because of obstructive effects (Della-Porta and Westaway, 1978). A consequence of the different putative mechanisms is the compatibility of a single-hit mechanism in the first instance, whereas in the second instance a multihit mechanism alone can account for the effect of antibody.

Studies on the electrophoretic characteristics of poliovirus revealed that the capsid was capable of existing in either of two conformational states. These states were interconvertible and at neutral pH were in a state of equilibrium (Mandel, 1971*b*). When homologous antibody reacted with virus, the capsid was stabilized in one of the conformational states. Further studies (Mandel, 1976) on the quantitative relationship between conformational stabilization and neutralization yielded two results deemed significant: (1) Irrespective of the multiplicity of antibody per virion, only two populations of particles with respect to isoelectric point were seen. One represented unneutralized virus, the other neutralized virus. (2) The correlation between stabilization and neutralization was good. These results (Fig. 10) imply that stabilization in the noninfectious conformation is an all-or-none phenomenon. The minimum amount of antibody capable of neutralizing one particle is also capable of inducing the full transformation of the capsid from the infectious (i.e., isoelectric point of about 7) to the noninfectious conformation (i.e., isoelectric point of about 5). Accepting the single-hit hypothesis, it would appear that one molecule of antibody has the capability of modifying the overall characteristics of the capsid. In support of this interpretation, it was proposed (Mandel, 1971*b*, 1976) that the metastability of the viral capsid reflects the capability of the structural subunits to undergo allosteric transitions consistent with the model of Monod *et al.* (1965). Therefore, the hypothesis has been proposed that the effective binding of one molecule to an antigenic site can stabilize the structural subunit in which that site resides. Since the icosahedral architecture requires noncovalent bonding between adjacent substructures, these substructures are sensitive to mutual molecular constraints. Hence stabilization of one substructural unit can, through cooperative conformational transitions, stabilize adjacent units. The net result will be stabilization of all units. Electrophoretically this was manifested with poliovirus by the maximum change in isoelectric point, and biologically by the loss of infectivity. Both effects are the result of an effective interaction of one virion with one molecule of antibody.

As a result of their extensive studies on the neutralization of herpesvirus, Yoshino and colleagues have proposed a hypothesis that encompasses the nature of neutralization, sensitization, and complement-mediated neutralization (Yoshino and Isono, 1978). The foundation of this hypothesis is that neutralization is the end result of a series of physicochemical modifications in the virion inducible by one molecule of antibody. As represented in Fig. 11, the class and quality of antibody determine whether the reaction will proceed to the final stage, i.e., neutralization, or terminate prematurely, i.e., sensitization. In the latter case completion can be mediated by complement. This hypothesis

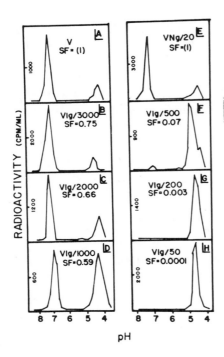

Fig. 10. Isoelectric focusing of virus and virus–antibody mixtures. γ-Globulin was precipitated from a normal (Ng) and from an immunized (Ig) rabbit by one-third saturation with ammonium sulfate. Virus was mixed with Ig at various dilutions and supplemented with Ng so that all mixtures contained 0.05% total protein. One preparation, in addition, contained no Ig, and one preparation contained no globulin. After 2 hr at 25°C and several days at 5°C, each mixture was assayed for infectivity, which is expressed as surviving fraction (SF) relative to the viral controls. Each mixture was characterized electrophoretically by isoelectric focusing. After collection, each fraction was assayed for pH and for radioactivity. Virus titer, as cpm/ml, is plotted as a function of pH. The results for the two virus controls are contained in panels A and E. The results obtained with increasing concentrations of Ig are contained in panels B, C, D, F, G, H. From Mandel (1976), with permission of the publisher.

(Yoshino and Isono, 1978) attempts to coordinate various observations within the provisions of their hypothesis: (1) the differential capability of different classes of antibody, and antibodies of different affinity, to initiate the minimal alteration in the virion necessary for neutralization; (2) the dependence on time and temperature for completion of the sequential changes; and (3) the role and quantitative requirements for mediation by complement. Since their basic concept envisions a mechanism akin to that described for poliovirus, they have raised the question of the manner whereby conformational changes can be transmitted in a virus such as herpes which has a lipoprotein envelope. They have considered as possibility that either within the envelope or adherent to the inner surface of the envelope there is a highly ordered array of protein subunits from which the surface antigenic proteins emanate. Such a contiguous arrangement, they speculate, could allow for extensive cooperative conformational transitions resulting from the initiation by one molecule of antibody binding to one surface antigen.

The hypothesis proposed by Della-Porta and Westaway (1978) is the outcome of studies by Westaway (1965a,b 1968) and colleagues on the neutralization of togaviruses involving comparisons of homologous and heterologous systems. The effect of antibody on both infectivity

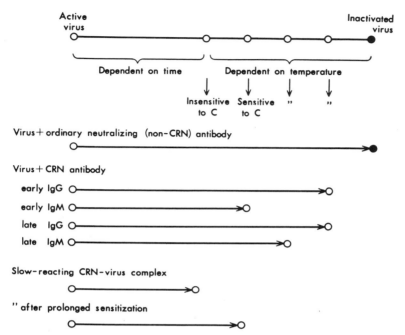

Fig. 11. Scheme to explain the mechanisms of neutralization and sensitization of herpes simplex virus. From Yoshino and Isono (1978), with permission of the publisher.

and hemagglutination enters into the proposed model. Essentially, inhibition of viral functions depends on the specific sites occupied by bound antibodies. Moreover, the hypothesis accounts for the variable effects of antibody when different host cells are used and also provides for a mechanism for mediated neutralization. This hypothesis is represented in Figs. 12 and 13. The crux of this proposed mechanism is that the disposition of antibody must conform to a definite pattern in order to inhibit function. Inhibition of each function (e.g., infectivity, hemagglutination) when examined with reference to a given cell may require a unique pattern. With respect to infection, this hypothesis stipulates that involvement of a critical area results in "the prevention of infection without any implication of damage to the virus particle." According to Della-Porta and Westaway (1978) the following phenomena are incompatible with a single-hit mechanism but can be explained satisfactorily on the basis of their multihit hypothesis: (1) In some cases multihit kinetics have been described. (2) Reaction rate constants that have been reported are not reliable because of the extremely rapid reaction rates reported for haptens with antibodies. (3) NNF and neutralization by mediators such as complement and anti-

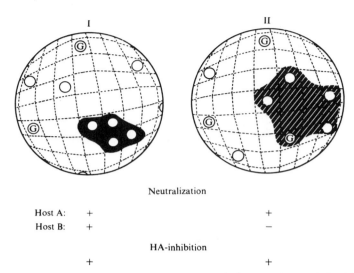

Neutralization

Host A: +   +
Host B: +   −

HA-inhibition
              +   +

Fig. 12.   Model for multihit mechanism for neutralization of virus infectivity by antibody. Homologous antibody system: O, antibody molecule attached to a type-specific
determinant; Ⓖ , antibody attached to a group-specific determinant. The shaded area
represents a critical area of attached antibody, sufficient to produce neutralization
(Westaway, 1965b). The requirements for neutralization are more stringent for cells of
host B. Although in case II the virus–antibody complex is still infectious for host B, it is
sensitized and could be neutralized by addition of anti-γ-globulin. From Della-Porta
and Westaway (1978), with permission of the publisher.

globulin occur. (4) The outcome of virus–antibody interaction is cell
dependent. (5) Synergistic effects resulting from antibodies bound to
different sites are in some instances necessary.

In the various studies on neutralization, it has been inferred that
the binding of antibody to virus is *per se* not a sufficient event for loss
of infectivity. In one domain, the host cell may have the power of decision. In another domain, the effect(s) on the viral capsid may be the
deciding parameter. The suggestion that neutralization may be the
culumination of sequential changes in the virus–antibody complex has
been made by Andrewes and Elford (1933a,b), Burnet *et al.* (1937),
Gard (1957), Lafferty, (1963a,b), Svehag (1963), Philipson (1966),
Dudley *et al.* (1970), Lewenton-Kriss and Mandel (1972), Mandel
(1976), and Yoshino and Isono (1978). Recent studies on mediated neutralization may be relevant. Kinetic analyses by direct and antiglobulin-
mediated neutralization have shown that infectious virus–antibody complexes are detectable shortly prior to neutralization and throughout the
course of the reaction. The observation has led to the inference that

sensitization precedes neutralization (Dudley *et al.*, 1970; Hahon, 1970; Krummel and Uhr, 1969; Lewenton-Kriss and Mandel, 1972; Philipson, 1966; Radwan and Burger, 1973*b*; Yoshino and Isono, 1978). Dudley *et al.*, for example, reported that the rate of neutralization of bacteriophage f2 by mediated neutralization was threefold higher than by direct neutralization with 7 S, 5 S, and 3.5 S antibodies. A similar result was shown by Krummel and Uhr (1969) for the neutralization of bacteriophage ϕX174 by 7 S antibody. Since sensitization appears also to be a single-hit phenomenon, and since it precedes neutralization, the possibility is suggested that sensitization is an essential forerunner stage in the neutralization reaction. The mediated reaction may therefore represent either (1) an acceleration of a reaction which is already in progress (Yoshino and Isono, 1978) or (2) the activation of a reaction

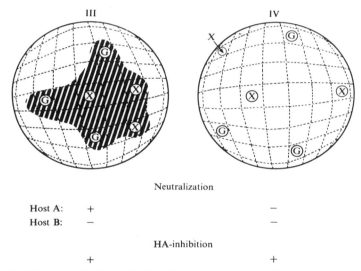

Neutralization

Host A:	+	−
Host B:	−	−

HA-inhibition

+   +

Fig. 13.   Model for multihit mechanism for neutralization of virus infectivity by antibody. Heterologous antibody system: Ⓖ, antibody molecule attached to a group-specific determinant; Ⓧ, (cross-reacting) antibody to a subgroup determinant, which functions as a type-specific determinant in homologous reactions. The shaded area represents a "critical area" of attached antibody which in case III produces neutralization in host A but is inadequate to produce neutralization in host B. The probability of attachment of cross-reacting antibody to subgroup determinants is lower than in the homologous reaction, and hence critical areas are formed less readily. For example, in case IV the attached antibody molecules are too dispersed on the surface of the virion to complete a "critical area" for either host but sufficient to (sterically) inhibit hemagglutination (HA). From Della-Porta and Westaway (1978), with permission of the publisher.

which was not destined to go to completion. In the latter case, the implication is that on the average several molecules of antibody combine with one particle but only one will be independently effective. However, one or more of the others may be activated by a mediator. The studies of Dudley *et al.* (1970) on the neutralization of bacteriophage f2 may be relevant. Among the various thermodynamic parameters for the neutralization of f2 by rabbit antibody, they reported energy of activation values of 7.3, 8.6, and 13.9 kcal/mol for 7 S, 5 S, and 3.5 S antibodies. These values were considered to be in excess of a process which is simply diffusion controlled, i.e., 4–5 kcal/mol. These and other thermodynamic data for this system (see Table II) indicated to Dudley *et al.* that they are "exactly opposite to what would have been anticipated were neutralization to depend on simple steric factors."

11. GENERAL CONCLUDING COMMENTS

The two main purposes of this chapter have been to collate salient information about the neutralization phenomenon and to delineate some of the unanswered problems. It becomes increasingly evident as one reads general discussions from past years (Schultz, 1928; Burnet *et al.*, 1937; Fazekas de St. Groth, 1962; Svehag, 1968; Daniels, 1975; Burns and Allison, 1975; Della-Porta and Westaway, 1978; Mandel, 1978) that the interaction of virus and antibody is a complex phenomenon. Complexity derives from the fact that virus and antibody each represent families of related but broadly variable constituents. The resulting variable interactions are further compounded by the variable responses of different cells to a given virus–antibody complex. Still another dimension of complexity has been added with the discovery that other components, e.g., complement and the product(s) of autoimmune responses, can participate in the neutralization reaction.

The interaction *in vivo* of a presumably "simple" virus such as a picornavirus with antibody of high affinity represents one end of the complexity spectrum. The interaction of an enveloped virus having critical and noncritical antigens with the respective antibodies of low affinity and requiring mediation by complement represents the opposite end of the complexity spectrum of neutralization. One can envision still another complication (outside the scope of this chapter) with the participation of killer T cells.

Whether a single particle of every known virus, reacting with the minimum number of molecules of neutralizing antibody, is neutralized by the same basic mechanism cannot as yet be answered. Whether the various forms of antibody, and accessory substances such as complement, have evolved in order to facilitate the achievement of this basic mechanism when different viruses are encountered also cannot yet be answered.

The *in vitro* study of viral neutralization represents the "probe" for understanding the *in vivo* mechanism of the humoral defense system. As indicated by Adler *et al.* (1971) and Leddy *et al.* (1977), there now appears to be a "reason" for the evolvement of the complement system. A current problem related to the immune response is the existence of unsuccessful virus–antibody interactions in the form of infectious virus–antibody complexes. This subversion of the immune reaction has resulted in the recognition of a pathological syndrome now classified as immune complex diseases. It is to be hoped that further studies of the mechanism of neutralization may yield a clue to the nature of this unsuccessful attempt on the part of antibody to neutralize the offending virus.

Because of the requirement for very high concentrations of viral particles to initiate infection, little has been done on the characteristics of the neutralization of plant viruses. In one study, Rappaport (1957) described the kinetic aspects of the reaction of TMV with neutralizing antibody. In the major aspects, the reaction resembled that of animal viruses—namely, a single-hit first-order reaction which eventually approached a constant surviving level. In the past few years, cell culture systems have been developed for the cultivation of plant viruses. The use of protoplasts from tobacco and barley plant tissue for replication of such viruses as TMV, cucumber mosaic virus, potato virus X, and brome mosaic virus has been reported (Takebe and Otsuki, 1969; Otsuki and Takebe, 1973; Otsuki *et al.*, 1974; Okuno and Furusawa, 1978). These developments have been reviewed by Takebe (1977). Early and late phases of the replication of plant viruses have been described. It appears likely that in its major aspects this system should resemble the animal virus–animal cell system. Certainly, with respect to penetration and uncoating these are essential events, as, for example, reported by Kurtz-Fritsch and Hirth (1972).

Similar developments now permit studies on the neutralization of insect viruses. Cell culture systems have been developed for replication of insect viruses in which cells from various genera of insects (e.g., *Aedes*, *Drosophila*, *Spodoptera*) have been used. Plaque assays for nuclear polyhedrosis and iridescent viruses have been described (Brown and Faulkner, 1977; Brown *et al.*, 1977). In terms of plating efficiency, Brown *et al.* have shown that the particle-to-plaque ratio is approximately 75, a value which is intermediate with respect to values reported for various animal viruses.

In view of these technological developments, it is anticipated that studies will be undertaken to examine the characteristics of the neutralization of both plant and insect viruses. The feasibility for such studies has been demonstrated in the report of Elliott *et al.* (1977), who examined the serological relationships among several strains of iridescent virus in a cell culture system. Studies on the neutralization of plant and insect viruses should ultimately help to establish whether a fundamental underlying principle pertains to the neutralization of viruses as a whole, or whether the divergence among viruses as to host (i.e., animal, plant, insect, protist) is also reflected in a divergence of neutralization mechanisms.

12. REFERENCES

Ablashi, D. V., Martos, L. M., Gilden, R. V., and Hampar, B., 1969, Preparation of rabbit immune serum with neutralizing activity against a simian cytomegalovirus (SA6), *J. Immunol.* **102**:263.

Adler, F. L., Walker, W. S., and Fishman, M., 1971, Amplification of phage neutralization by complement, antiglobulin, and allotype sera, *Virology* **46**:797.

Almeida, J. D., and Laurence, G. D., 1969, Heated and unheated antiserum on rubella virus; morphological effect, *Am. J. Dis. Child.* **118**:101.

Almeida, J. D., and Waterson, A. P., 1969, The morphology of virus–antibody interaction, *Adv. Virus Res.* **15**:307.

Almeida, J. D., Brown, F., and Waterson, A. P., 1967, The morphologic characteristics of 19 S antibody, *J. Immunol.* **98**:186.

Andersen, H. K., 1971, Serologic differentiation of human cytomegalovirus strains using rabbit hyperimmune sera, *Arch. Gesamte Virusforsch.* **33**:187.

Andersen, H. K., 1972, The influence of complement on cytomegalovirus neutralization by antibodies, *Arch. Gesamte Virusforsch.* **36**:133.

Andrewes, C. H., and Elford, W. J., 1933a, Observations on antiphage sera. I. "The percentage law," *Br. J. Exp. Pathol.* **14**:367.

Andrewes, C. H., and Elford, W. J., 1933b, Observations on antiphage sera. II. Properties of incompletely neutralized phage, *Br. J. Exp. Pathol.* **14**:376.

Arnon, R., 1971, Antibodies to enzymes—A tool in the study of antigenic specificity determinants, *Curr. Top. Microbiol. Immunol.* **54**:47.

Ashe, W. K., and Notkins, A. L., 1966, Neutralization of an infectious herpes simplex virus–antibody complex by anti-γ-globulin, *Proc. Natl. Acad. Sci. USA* **56**:447.

Ashe, W. K., and Notkins, A. L., 1967, Kinetics of sensitization of herpes simplex virus and its relationship to the reduction in the neutralization rate constant, *Virology* **33**:613.

Ashe, W. K., Mage, M., Mage, R., and Notkins, A. L., 1968, Neutralization and sensitization of herpes simplex virus with antibody fragments from rabbits of different allotypes, *J. Immunol.* **101**:500.

Ashe, W. K., Mage, M., and Notkins, A. L., 1969, Kinetics of neutralization of sensitized herpes simplex virus with antibody fragments, *Virology* **37**:290.

Ashe, W. K., Daniels, C. A., Scott, G. S., and Notkins, A. L., 1971, Interaction of rheumatoid factor with infectious herpes simplex virus–antibody complexes, *Science* **172**:176.

Austin, R. M., and Daniels, C. A., 1974, Interaction of staphylococcal protein A with virus–IgG complexes, *J. Immunol.* **113**:1568.

Barlow, J. L., Van Vunakis, H., and Levine, L., 1958, Studies of the inactivation of phage by the properdin system. I. Evidence for complement, properdin and magnesium requirements, *J. Immunol.* **80**:339.

Baughman, R. H., Fenters, J. D., Marquis, G. S., Jr., and Holper, J. C., 1968, Effect of complement and viral filtration on the neutralization of respiratory syncytial virus, *Appl. Microbiol.* **16**:1076.

Béclère, A., Chambon, and Ménard, 1898, Études sur l'immunité vaccinale: L'immunité consécutive à l'inoculation sous-cutanée du vaccin, *Ann. Inst. Pasteur* **12**:837.

Bendinelli, M., Nardini, L., and Campa, M., 1974, Neutralization of Friend leukemia virus by sera of unimmunized animals, *J. Gen. Virol.* **22**:207.

Ben-Yoseph, Y., Geiger, B., and Arnon, R., 1975, Antibody-mediated thermal stabilization of human hexosaminidases, *Immunochemistry* **12**:221.

Berry, D. M., and Almeida, J. D., 1968, The morphological and biological effects of various antisera on avian infectious bronchitis virus, *J. Gen. Virol.* **3**:97.

Bowman, B. U., Jr., and Patnode, R. A., 1963, Infection of protoplasts of *Escherichia coli* by bacteriophage φX174 treated with specific antibody, *Virology* **21**:506.

Bowman, B. U., and Patnode, R. A., 1964, Neutralization of bacteriophage φX174 by specific antiserum, *J. Immunol.* **92**:507.

Bradish, C. J., Farley, J. O., and Ferrier, H. E. N., 1962, Studies on the nature of the neutralization reaction and the competition for neutralizing antibody between components of the virus system of foot-and-mouth disease, *Virology* **18**:378.

Brandtzaeg, P., 1978, Polymeric IgA is complexed with secretory component (SC) on the surface of human intestinal epithelial cells, *Scand. J. Immunol.* **8**:39.

Brown, D. A., Lescott, T., Harrap, K. A., and Kelly, D. C., 1977, The replication and titration of iridescent virus type 22 in *Spodoptera frugiperda* cells, *J. Gen. Virol.* **38**:175.

Brown, F., Cartwright, B., and Newman, J. F. E., 1964, Further studies of the early antibody in the sera of cattle and guinea pigs infected with foot-and-mouth disease virus, *J. Immunol.* **93**:397.

Brown, J. C., and Koshland, M. E., 1975, Activation of antibody Fc function by antigen-induced conformational changes, *Proc. Natl. Acad. Sci. USA* **72**:5111.

Brown, M., and Faulkner, P., 1977, A plaque assay for nuclear polyhedrosis viruses, using a solid overly, *J. Gen. Virol.* **36**:361.

Burnet, F. M., Keogh, E. V., and Lush, D., 1937, The immunological reactions of the filterable viruses, *Aust. J. Exp. Biol. Med. Sci.* **15**:227.

Burns, W. H., and Allison, A. C., 1975, Virus infections and the immune responses they elicit, in: *The Antigens* (M. Sela, ed.), pp. 479–574, Academic Press, New York.

Cann, J. R., and Clark, E. W., 1954, On the kinetics of neutralization of bacteriophage T2 by specific antiserum, *J. Immunol.* **72**:463.

Carthew, P., 1976, The surface nature of a bovine enterovirus, before and after neutralization, *J. Gen. Virol.* **32**:17.

Chesebro, B., Bloth, B., and Svehag, S.-E., 1968, The ultrastructure of normal and pathological IgM immunoglobulins, *J. Exp. Med.* **127**:399.

Cinader, B., ed., 1966, *Antibodies to Biologically Active Molecules*, Pergamon Press, New York.

Cohn, M., 1971, The take-home lesson—1971, *Ann. N.Y. Acad. Sci.* **190**:529.

Copra, J. D., and Kehoe, J. M., 1974, Antibody diversity: Is it all coded for by the germ line genes? *Scand. J. Immunol.* **3**:1.

Cowan, K. M., 1962, Studies on the coliphage neutralizing activity of normal human serum, *J. Immunol.* **88**:476.

Cowan, K. M., 1973, Antibody response to viral antigens, *Adv. Virus Res.* **17**:195.

Cremer, W. E., Riggs, J. L., Fujimoto, F. Y., Hagens, S. J., Ota, M. I., and Lennette, E. H., 1964, Neutralizing activity of fragments obtained by papain digestion of viral antibody, *J. Immunol.* **93**:283.

Cremer, N. E., Riggs, J. L., and Lennette, E. H., 1975, Neutralization kinetics of Western equine encephalitis virus by antibody fragments, *Immunochemistry* **12**:597.

Crothers, D. M., and Metzger, H., 1972, The influence of polyvalency on the binding properties of antibodies, *Immunochemistry* **9**:341.

Cunningham, A. J., 1974, The generation of antibody diversity: Its dependence on antigenic stimulation, *Contemp. Top. Mol. Immunol.* **3**:1.

Cunningham, A. J., and Pilarski, L. M., 1974, Antibody diversity: A case for its generation after antigenic stimulation, *Scand. J. Immunol.* **3**:5.

Dales, S., and Kajioka, R., 1964, The cycle of multiplication of vaccinia virus in Earle's strain L cells, *Virology* **24**:278.

Daniels, C. A., 1975, Mechanisms of viral neutralization, in: *Viral Immunology and Immunopathology* (A. L. Notkins, ed.), pp. 79–97, Academic Press, New York.

Daniels, C. A., Borsos, T., Rapp, H. J., Snyderman, R., and Notkins, A. L., 1970, Neutralization of sensitized virus by purified components of complement, *Proc. Natl. Acad. Sci. USA* **65**:528.

Day, E. D., 1972, *Advanced Immunochemistry*, pp. 273–291, Williams and Wilkins, Baltimore.

Day, L. A., Sturtevant, J. M., and Singer, S. J., 1962, The direct measurement of the rate of a hapten–antibody reaction, *J. Am. Chem. Soc.* **84**:3768.

Day, L. A., Sturtevant, J. M., and Singer, S. J., 1963, The kinetics of the reactions between antibodies to the 2,4 dinitrophenyl group and specific haptens, *Ann. N.Y. Acad. Sci.* **103**:611.

Delbrück, M., 1945, Effects of specific antisera on the growth of bacterial viruses (bacteriophages), *J. Bacteriol.* **50**:137.

Della-Porta, A. J., and Westaway, E. G., 1978, A multi-hit model for the neutralization of animal viruses, *J. Gen. Virol.* **38**:1.

De Sena, J., and Mandel, B., 1976, Studies on the *in vitro* uncoating of poliovirus. I. Characterization of the modifying factor and the modifying reaction, *Virology* **70**:470.

Douglas, S. R., and Smith, W., 1930, A study of vaccinal immunity in rabbits by means of *in vitro* methods, *Br. J. Exp. Pathol.* **11**:96.

Dourmashkin, R. R., and Tyrrell, D. A. J., 1974, Electron microscopic observations on the entry of influenza virus into susceptible cells, *J. Gen. Virol.* **24**:129.

Dozois, T. F., Wagner, J. C., Chemerda, C. M., and Andrew, V. M., 1949, The influence of certain factors on the neutralization of Western equine encephalomyelitis virus, *J. Immunol.* **62**:319.

Drake, W. P., and Mardiney, M. R., Jr., 1975, Complement-mediated alteration of antibody specificity *in vivo, J. Immunol.* **114**:1053.

Dudley, M. A., Henkens, R. W., and Rowlands, D. T., Jr., 1970, Kinetics of neutralization of bacteriophage f2 by rabbit G-antibodies, *Proc. Natl. Acad. Sci. USA* **65**:88.

Dulbecco, R., Vogt, M., and Strickland, A. G. R., 1956, A study of the basic aspects of neutralization of two animal viruses, Western equine encephalitis virus and poliomyelitis virus, *Virology* **2**:162.

Eisen, H. N., and Karush, F., 1949, Interaction of purified antibody with homologous hapten. Antibody valence and binding constant, *J. Am. Chem. Soc.* **71**:363.

Eisen, H. N., and Siskind, G. W., 1964, Variations in affinities of antibodies during the immune response, *Biochemistry* **3**:996.

Elliott, R. M., Lescott, T., and Kelly, D. C., 1977, Serological relationships of an iridescent virus (type 25) recently isolated from *Tipula* sp. with two other iridescent viruses (types 2 and 22), *Virology* **81**:309.

Epstein, S. I., Doty, P., and Boyd, W. C., 1956, A thermodynamic study of hapten–antibody association, *J. Am. Chem. Soc.* **78**:3306.

Erickson, R. P., 1974, Inactivation of trypsin by antibodies of high affinity, *Immunochemistry* **11**:41.

Fazekas de St. Groth, S., 1961, Methods in immunochemistry of viruses. 2. Evaluation of parameters from equilibrium measurements, *Aust. J. Exp. Biol. Med. Sci.* **39**:563.

Fazekas de St. Groth, S., 1962, The neutralization of viruses, *Adv. Virus Res.* **9**:1.

Fazekas de St. Groth, S., and Reid, A. F., 1958, The neutralization of animal viruses. II. A critical comparison of hypotheses, *J. Immunol.* **80**:225.

Fazekas de St. Groth, S., and Webster, R. G., 1961, Methods in immunochemistry of viruses. I. Equilibrium filtration, *Aust. J. Exp. Biol. Med. Sci.* **39**:549.

Fazekas de St. Groth, S., and Webster, R. G., 1963a, The neutralization of animal viruses. III. Equilibrium conditions in the influenza virus–antibody system, *J. Immunol.* **90**:140.

Fazekas de St. Groth, S., and Webster, R. G., 1963b, The neutralization of animal viruses. IV. Parameters of the influenza virus-antibody system, *J. Immunol.* **90**:151.

Fazekas de St. Groth, S., Watson, G. S., and Reid, A. F., 1958, The neutralization of animal viruses. I. A model of virus–antibody interaction, *J. Immunol.* **80**:215.

Feinstein, A., and Munn, E. A., 1966, An electron microscopic study of the interaction of macroglobulin (IgM) antibodies with bacterial flagella and of the binding of complement, *J. Physiol. (London)* **186**:64P.

Feinstein, A., and Rowe, A. J., 1965, Molecular mechanisms of formation of an antigen-antibody complex, *Nature (London)* **205**:147.

Feinstein, R. N., Jaroslow, B. N., Howard, J. B., and Faulhaber, J. T., 1971, Stabilization of mutant catalase by complex formation with antibody to normal catalase, *J. Immunol.* **106**:1316.

Fenwick, M. L., and Cooper, P. D., 1962, Early interactions between poliovirus and ERK cells: Some observations on the nature and significance of the rejected particles, *Virology* **18**:212.

Finkelstein, M. S., and Uhr, J. W., 1966, Antibody formation. V. The avidity of γM and γG guinea pig antibodies to bacteriophage ϕX174, *J. Immunol.* **97**:565.

Foti, A. G., Glovsky, M. M., and Cooper, J. F., 1975, The effect of antibody on human prostatic acid phosphatase activity. I. Temperature and pH stabilization of acid phosphatase enzyme activity by rabbit antibody to acid phosphatase, *Immunochemistry* **12**:131.

Froese, A., 1968, Kinetic and equilibrium studies on 2,4-dinitrophenyl hapten–antibody systems, *Immunochemistry* **5**:253.

Froese, A., and Sehon, A. H., 1965, Kinetic and equilibrium studies of the reaction between anti-*p*-nitrophenyl antibodies and a homologous hapten, *Immunochemistry* **2**:135.

Froese, A., Sehon, A. H., and Eigen, M., 1962, Kinetic studies of protein–dye and antibody–hapten interactions with the temperature-jump method, *Can. J. Chem.* **40**:1786.

Gard, S., 1955, Neutralization of Theiler's virus, *Acta Pathol. Microbiol. Scand.* **37**:21.

Gard, S., 1957, Immuno-inactivation of poliovirus, *Acta. Gesamte Virusforsch.* **7**:449.

Gipson, T. G., Daniels, C. A., and Notkins, A. L., 1974, Interaction of rheumatoid factor with infectious vaccinia virus–antibody complexes, *J. Immunol.* **112**:2087.

Goodman, J. W., and Donch, J. J., 1964, Neutralization of bacteriophage by intact and degraded rabbit antibody, *J. Immunol.* **93**:96.

Goodman, J. W., and Donch, J. J., 1965, Phage-neutralizing activity in light polypeptide chains of rabbit antibody, *Immunochemistry* **2**:351.

Gopalakrishnan, P. V., and Karush, F., 1974*a*, Antibody affinity. VI. Synthesis of bivalent lactosyl haptens and their interaction with anti-lactosyl antibodies, *Immunochemistry* **11**:279.

Gopalakrishnan, P. V., and Karush, F., 1974*b*, Antibody affinity. VII. Multivalent interaction of anti-lactoside antibody. *J. Immunol.* **113**:769.

Gordon, M. H., 1925, Studies of the viruses of vaccinia and variola, *Med. Res. Counc. G.B. Spec. Rep. Ser.*, No. 98.

Graham, B. J., Minamishima, Y., Dreesman, G. R., Haines, H. G., and Benyesh-Melnick, M., 1971, Complement-requiring neutralizing antibodies in hyperimmune sera to human cytomegaloviruses, *J. Immunol.* **107**:1618.

Granoff, A., 1965, The interaction of Newcastle disease virus and neutralizing antibody, *Virology* **25**:38.

Graves, J. H., Cowan, K. M., and Trautman, R., 1964, Characterization of antibodies produced by guinea pigs inoculated with inactivated foot-and-mouth disease antigen, *J. Immunol.* **92**:501.

Green, N. M., 1969, Electron microscopy of the immunoglobulins, *Adv. Immunol.* **11**:1.

Gudnadóttir, M., and Pálsson, P. A., 1965, Host–virus interaction in visna infected sheep, *J. Immunol.* **95**:1116.

Hahon, N., 1969, The kinetics of neutralization of Venezuelan equine encephalomyelitis virus by antiserum and the reversibility of the reaction, *J. Gen. Virol.* **4**:77.

Hahon, N., 1970, Neutralization of residual infectivity of Venezuelan equine encephalomyelitis virus by anti-gamma globulin, *J. Gen. Virol.* **6**:361.

Haimovich, J., and Sela, M., 1966, Inactivation of poly-DL-alanyl bacteriophage T4 with antisera specific toward poly-DL-alanine, *J. Immunol.* **97**:338.

Hajek, P., 1966, Properties of the neutralizing factors against T2 and ϕX174 phages present in normal sera, *Folia Microbiol. (Prague)* **11**:290.

Hajek, P., 1968, Dependence of the neutralizing activity of 19 S and 7 S antibodies on complement in the primary and secondary response in infant rabbits to phage T2, *Folia Microbiol. (Prague)* **13**:557.

Hajek, P., 1969, Neutralization of bacterial viruses by antibodies of young animals. I. Dependence of neutralizing activity of 19 S and 7 S on complement in the course of the primary and secondary response of young rabbits immunized with T2 phage, *Folia Microbiol. (Prague)* **14**:165.

Hajek, P., and Mandel, L., 1966, Antibody response of young animals to bacteriophages of different immunological behaviour: ϕX174 and T2, *Folia Microbiol. (Prague)* **11**:282.

Hale, E. M., Hirata, A. A., Brusenback, R. A., and Overby, L. R., 1969, Antiserum neutralization of bacteriophage Qβ: A mathematical analysis, *J. Immunol.* **102**:206.

Hampar, B., Notkins, A. L., Mage, M., and Keehn, M. A., 1968, Heterogeneity in the properties of 7 S and 19 S rabbit-neutralizing antibodies to herpes simplex virus, *J. Immunol.* **100**:586.

Hardie, G., and van Regenmortel, M. H. V., 1975, Immunochemical studies of tobacco mosaic virus. I. Refutation of the alleged homogeneous binding of purified antibody fragments, *Immunochemistry* **12**:903.

Harris, J. E., Siminovitch, L., McCulloch, E. A., and Cinader, B., 1962, Restoration of heat-labile activity in mouse and human antiserum to *B. megatherium* bacteriophage, *Fed. Proc.* **21**:17.

Hashimoto, N., and Prince, A. M., 1963, Kinetic studies on the neutralization reaction between Japanese encephalitis virus and antiserum, *Virology* **19**:261.

Haukenes, G., 1977, Demonstration of host antigens in the myxovirus membrane: Lysis of virus by antibody and complement, *Acta Pathol. Microbiol. Scand. Sect. B* **85**:125.

Haurowitz, F., 1973, The problem of antibody diversity. Immunodifferentiation versus somatic mutation, *Immunochemistry* **10**:775.

Hawkes, R. A., 1964, Enhancement of the infectivity of arboviruses by specific antisera produced in domestic fowls, *Aust. J. Exp. Biol. Med. Sci.* **42**:465.

Hawkes, R. A., and Lafferty, K. J., 1967, The enhancement of virus infectivity by antibody, *Virology* **33**:250.

Heineman, H. S., 1967, Herpes simplex neutralizing antibody—Quantitation of the complement-dependent fraction in different phases of adult human infection, *J. Immunol.* **99**:214.

Hoffman, L. G., 1976a, Antibodies as allosteric proteins. I. hypothesis, *Immunochemistry* **13**:725.

Hoffman, L. G., 1976b, Antibodies as allosteric proteins. II. Comparison with experiment, *Immunochemistry* **13**:731.

Hoffman, L. G., 1976c, Antibodies as allosteric proteins. III. An alternative model and some predictions, *Immunochemistry* **13**:737.

Hornick, C. L., and Karush, F., 1969, The interaction of hapten-coupled bacteriophage ϕX174 with antihapten antibody, *Isr. J. Med. Sci.* **5**:163.

Hornick, C. L., and Karush, F., 1972, Antibody affinity. III. The role of multivalence, *Immunochemistry* **9**:325.

Huggett, D. O., Rodríguez, J. E., and McKee, A. P., 1972, Infectious antibody–reovirus complexes, *Infect. Immun.* **6**:996.

Hultin, J. V., and McKee, A. P., 1952, Fixation of "neutralized" influenza virus by susceptible cells, *J. Bacteriol.* **63**:437.

Hyllseth, B., and Pettersson, U., 1970, Neutralization of equine arteritis virus: Enhancing effect of guniea pig serum, *Arch. Gesamte Virusforsch.* **32**:337.

Ide, K., and Yoshino, K., 1974, Studies on the neutralization of herpes simplex virus. VII. Reevaluation of the equilibrium theory concerning the unneutralizable persistent fraction, *Jpn. J. Microbiol.* **18**:397.

Ikegami, M., and Francki, I. B., 1973, Presence of antibodies to double-stranded RNA in sera of rabbits immunized with rice dwarf and maize rough dwarf viruses, *Virology* **56**:404.

Iwasaki, T., and Ogura, R., 1968a, Studies on complement-potentiated neutralizing antibodies (C′-PNab) induced in rabbits inoculated with Japanese encephalitis virus (JEV). 1. The nature of C′-PN-ab, *Virology* **34**:46.

Iwasaki, T., and Ogura, R., 1968b, Studies on neutralization of Japanese encephalitis virus (JEV). I. Further neutralization of the resistant fraction by an interaction between antivirus IgG antibody and IgG heterotype or allotype antibody, *Virology* **34**:141.

Jaton, J.-C., Huser, H., Braun, D. G., Givol, D., Pecht, I., and Schlessinger, J., 1975, Conformational changes induced in a homogeneous anti-type III pneumococcal antibody by oligosaccharides of increasing size, *Biochemistry* **14**:5312.

Jerne, N. K., and Avegno, P., 1956, The development of the phage-inactivating properties of serum during the course of specific immunization of an animal; reversible and irreversible inactivation, *J. Immunol.* **76**:200.

Joklik, W. K., 1964, The intracellular fate of rabbitpox virus rendered noninfectious by various reagents, *Virology* **22**:620.

Joklik, W. K., and Darnell, J. E., Jr., 1961, The adsorption and early fate of purified poliovirus in HeLa cells, *Virology* **13**:439.

Kalmanson, G. M., Hershey, A. D., and Bronfenbrenner, J., 1942, Factors influencing the rate of neutralization of bacteriophage by the antibody, *J. Immunol.* **45**:1.

Kärber, G., 1931, Beitrag zur kollektiven Behandlung pharmakologischer Reihenversuche, *Arch. Exp. Pathol. Pharmakol.* **162**:480.

Karl, S. C., and Thormar, H., 1971, Antibodies produced by rabbits immunized with visna virus, *Infect. Immun.* **4**:715.

Karush, F., 1956, The interaction of purified antibody with optically isomeric haptens, *J. Am. Chem. Soc.* **78**:5519.

Karush, F., 1962, Immunologic specificity and molecular structure, *Adv. Immunol.* **2**:1.

Karush, F., 1976, Multivalent binding and functional affinity, in: *Contemporary Topics in Molecular Immunology*, Vol. 5 (H. N. Eisen and R. A. Reisfeld, eds.), pp. 217–228, Plenum Press, New York.

Keller, R., 1965, Reactivation by physical means of antibody-neutralized poliovirus, *J. Immunol.* **94**:143.

Keller, R., 1966, The stability of neutralization of poliovirus by native antibody and enzymatically derived fragments, *J. Immunol.* **96**:96.

Keller, R., 1968, Studies on the mechanism of the enzymatic reactivation of antibody-neutralized poliovirus, *J. Immunol.* **100**:1071.

Keller, R., and Dwyer, J. E., 1968, Neutralization of poliovirus by IgA coproantibodies, *J. Immunol.* **101**:192.

Ketler, A., Hinuma, Y., and Hummeler, K., 1961, Dissociation of infective poliomyelitis virus from neutralizing antibody by fluorocarbon, *J. Immunol.* **86**:22.

Kindt, T. J., 1975, Rabbit immunoglobulin allotypes; structure, immunology, and genetics, *Adv. Immunol.* **21**:35.

Kjellén, L., 1957, Studies on *in vitro* neutralization of adenoviruses, *Arch. Gesamte Virusforsch.* **7**:307.

Kjellén, L., 1962, Studies on the interactions of adenovirus, antibody, and host cells in vitro, *Virology* **18**:448.

Kjellén, L., 1964, Reactions between adenovirus antigens and papain digested rabbit immune globulin. *Arch. Gesamte Virusforsch.* **14**:189.

Kjellén, L., 1965*a*, On the capacity of pepsin-digested antibody to neutralize adenovirus infectivity, *Immunology* **8**:557.

Kjellén, L., 1965*b*, Density gradient centrifugations of adenovirus-antibody complexes, *Arch. Gesamte Virusforsch.* **17**:398.

Kjellén, L., and Pereira, H. G., 1968, Role of adenovirus antigens in the induction of virus neutralizing antibody, *J. Gen. Virol.* **2**:177.

Kjellén, L. E., and Schlesinger, R. W., 1959, Influence of host cell on residual infectivity of neutralized vesicular stomatitis virus, *Virology* **7**:236.

Klinman, N. R., Long, C. A., and Karush, F., 1967, The role of antibody bivalence in the neutralization of bacteriophage, *J. Immunol.* **99**:1128.

Krummel, W. M., and Uhr, J. W. 1969, A mathematical and experimental study of the kinetics of neutralization of bacteriophage ϕX174 by antibodies, *J. Immunol.* **102**:772.

Kulberg, A. J., and Pervikov, Ju. V., 1976, Naturally occurring antiglobulin factors in virus neutralization: Homoreactant as a factor enhancing neutralization of the infectious complex of poliovirus with the Fab' antibody fragment, *Infect. Immun.* **13**:322.

Kurtz-Fritsch, C., and Hirth, L., 1972, Uncoating of two spherical plant viruses, *Virology* **47**:385.

Lafferty, K. J., 1963*a*, The interaction between virus and antibody. I. Kinetic studies, *Virology* **21**:61.

Lafferty, K. J., 1963*b*, The interaction between virus and antibody. II. Mechanism of the reaction, *Virology* **21**:76.

Lafferty, K. J., and Oertelis, S., 1963, The interaction between virus and antibody. III. Examination of virus–antibody complexes with the electron microscope, *Virology* **21**:91.

Lanni, F., and Lanni, Y. T., 1953, Antigenic structure of bacteriophage, *Cold Spring Harbor Symp. Quant. Biol.* **18**:159.

Leddy, J. P., Simons, R. L., and Douglas, R. G., 1977, Effect of selective complement deficiency on the rate of neutralization of enveloped viruses by human sera, *J. Immunol.* **118**:28.

Leerhoy, J., 1968, Rubella virus neutralization in heated sera, *Acta Pathol. Microbiol. Scand.* **73**:275.

Lewenton-Kriss, S., and Mandel, B., 1972, Studies on the nonneutralizable fraction of poliovirus, *Virology* **48**:666.

Leymaster, G. R., and Ward, T. G., 1949, The effect of complement in the neutralization of mumps virus, *J. Immunol.* **61**:95.

Linscott, W. D., and Levinson, W. E., 1969, Complement components required for virus neutralization by early immunoglobulin antibody, *Proc. Natl. Acad. Sci. USA* **64**:520.

Long, P. H., and Olitzky, P. K., 1930, The recovery of vaccine virus after neutralization with immune serum, *J. Exp. Med.* **51**:209.

Macario, A. J. L., and Conway de Macario, E., 1975, Antigen-binding properties of antibody molecules: Time-course dynamics and biological significance, *Curr. Top. Microbiol. Immunol.* **71**:125.

Maess, J., 1971, Komplementabhangige *in vitro*-Neutralisation des equine arteritis virus, *Arch. Gesamte Virusforsch.* **33**:194.

Majer, M., 1972, Virus sensitization, *Curr. Top. Microbiol. Immunol.* **58**:69.

Majer, M., and Link, F., 1970, Studies on the non-neutralizable fraction of vaccinia virus, *Clin. Exp. Immunol.* **7**:283.

Majer, M., and Link, F., 1971, Sensitization of influenza virus A2/Singapore by antineuraminidase, *J. Gen. Virol.* **13**:355.

Majer, M., and Link, F., 1972, Studies on a recombinant influenza A virus by indirect neutralization, *Z. Immunitaetsforsch.* **144**:96.

Mäkelä, O., 1966, Assay of anti-hapten antibody with the aid of hapten-coupled bacteriophage, *Immunology* **10**:81.

Mamet-Bratley, M. D., 1966, Evidence concerning homogeneity of the combining sites of purified antibody, *Immunochemistry* **3**:155.

Mandel, B., 1958, Studies on the interactions of poliomyelitis virus, antibody, and host cells in a tissue culture system, *Virology* **6**:424.

Mandel, B., 1960, Neutralization of viral infectivity: Characterization of the virus–antibody complex, including association, dissociation, and host-cell interaction, *Ann. N.Y. Acad. Sci.* **83**:515.

Mandel, B., 1961, Reversibility of the reaction between poliovirus and neutralizing antibody of rabbit origin, *Virology* **14**:316.

Mandel, B., 1967a, The interaction of neutralized poliovirus with HeLa cells. I. Adsorption, *Virology* **31**:238.

Mandel, B., 1967b, The interaction of neutralized poliovirus with HeLa cells. II. Elution, penetration, uncoating, *Virology* **31**:248.

Mandel, B., 1971a, Methods for the study of virus–antibody complexes, *Methods Virol.* **5**:375.

Mandel, B., 1971b, Characterization of type 1 poliovirus by electrophoretic analysis, *Virology* **44**:554.

Mandel, B., 1976, Neutralization of poliovirus: A hypothesis to explain the mechanism and the one-hit character of the neutralization reaction, *Virology* **69**:500.

Mandel, B., 1978, Neutralization of animal viruses, *Adv. Virus Res.* **23**:205.

Mannweiler, E., 1963, Die Neutralisation von Influenza-virus in der Gewebekultur von Huhnerembryo-nieren-zellen. II. Die unspezifische Neutralisation, *Arch. Gesamte Virusforsch.* **12**:197.

Markenson, J. A., Daniels, C. A., Notkins, A. L., Hoofnagle, J. H., Gerety, J., and Barker, L. F., 1975, The interaction of rheumatoid factor with hepatitis B surface antigen–antibody complexes, *Clin. Exp. Immunol.* **19**:209.

Martos, L. M., Ablashi, D. V., Gilden, R. V., Siguenza, R. F., and Hampar, B., 1970, Preparation of immune rabbit sera with neutralizing activity against human cytomegalovirus and varicella-zoster virus, *J. Gen. Virol.* **7**:169.

McKercher, P. D., and Giordano, A. R., 1967, Foot-and-mouth disease in swine. II. Some physical-chemical characteristics of antibodies produced by chemically-treated and non-treated foot-and-mouth disease virus, *Arch. Gesamte Virusforsch.* **20**:54.

McNeill, T. A., 1968, The neutralization of pox viruses. I. Evidence for antibody interference, *J. Hyg.* **66**:541.

Metzger, H., 1974, Effect of antigen binding on the properties of antibody, *Adv. Immunol.* **18**:169.

Miller, G. W., 1977, Complement-mediated dissociation of antibody from immobilized antigen, *J. Immunol.* **119**:488.

Minamishima, Y., Graham, B. J., and Benyesh-Melnick, M., 1971, Neutralizing antibodies to cytomegaloviruses in normal simian and human sera, *Infect. Immun.* **4**:368.

Monod, J., Wyman, J., and Changeux, J.-P., 1965, On the nature of allosteric transitions: A plausible model, *J. Mol. Biol.* **12**:88.

Morgan, C., and Rose, H. M., 1968, Structure and development of viruses as observed in the electron microscope. VIII. Entry of influenza virus, *J. Virol.* **2**:925.

Morgan, C., Rose, H. M., and Mednis, B., 1968, Electron microscopy of herpes simplex virus. I. Entry, *J. Virol.* **2**:507.

Mueller, J. H., 1931, The effect of alexin in virus–antivirus mixtures. *J. Immunol.* **20**:17.

Muschel, L. H., and Toussaint, A. J., 1962, Studies on the bacteriophage neutralizing activity of serums. II. Comparison of normal and immune phage neutralizing antibodies, *J. Immunol.* **89**:35.

Nagano, Y., and Mutai, M., 1954, Études sérologiques sur le bactériophage. 2. Adsorption du bactériophage neutralisé sur le bactérie hote, *C. R. Acad. Sci. Paris* **148**:766.

Nagano, Y., Takeuti, S., and Iwasa, S., 1952, Études sérologiques de bactériophage. II. Influence de l'immunsérum sur l'adsorption du phage T2 sur la bactérie hôte, *Jpn. J. Exp. Med.* **22**:145.

Neva, F. A., and Weller, T. H., 1964, Rubella interferon and factors influencing the indirect neutralization test for rubella antibody, *J. Immunol.* **93**:466.

Nicklin, M. G., and Stephen, J., 1973, Solubilities of protein-antigen/rabbit-antibody complexes as a measure of serum avidity, *Immunochemistry* **10**:717.

Nisonoff, A., Wissler, F. C., Lipman, L. N., and Woernley, D. L., 1960, Separation of univalent fragments from the bivalent rabbit antibody molecule by reduction of disulfide bonds, *Arch. Biochem. Biophys.* **89**:230.

Notkins, A. L., 1971, Infectious virus–antibody complexes: Interaction with anti-immunoglobulins, complement, and rheumatoid factor, *J. Exp. Med.* **134**:41S.

Notkins, A. L., Mahar, S., Scheele, C., and Goffman, J., 1966, Infectious virus–antibody complex in the blood of chronically infected mice, *J. Exp. Med.* **124**:81.

Notkins, A. L., Mage, M., Ashe, W. K., and Mahar, S., 1968, Neutralization of sensitized lactic dehydrogenase virus by anti-globulin, *J. Immunol.* **100**:314.

Notkins, A. L., Rosenthal, J., and Johnson, B., 1971, Rate zonal centrifugation of herpes simplex virus–antibody complexes, *Virology* **43**:321.

Ogra, P. L., Karzon, D. T., Righthand, F., and MacGillivray, M., 1968, Immunoglobulin response in serum and secretions after immunization with live and inactivated poliovaccine and after natural infection, *New Engl. J. Med.* **279**:893.

Ogra, P. L., Marag, A., and Tiku, M. L., 1975, Humoral immune response to viral infections, in: *Viral Immunology and Immunopathology* (A. L. Notkins, ed.), pp. 57–77, Academic Press, New York.

Okuno, T., and Furusawa, I., 1978, Use of osmotic shock for the inoculation of barley protoplasts with brome mosaic virus, *J. Gen. Virol.* **39**:187.

Oldstone, M. B. A., 1975, Virus neutralization and virus-induced immune complex disease, *Prog. Med. Virol.* **19**:84.

Oldstone, M. B. A., Larson, D. L., and Cooper, N. R., 1972, Virus-antiviral antibody (V-Ab) complexes: Interaction with complement, *Fed. Proc.* **31**:791.

Oldstone, M. B. A., Cooper, N. R., and Larson, D. L., 1974, Formation and biologic role of polyoma virus–antibody complexes: A critical role for complement, *J. Exp. Med.* **140**:549.

Oroszlan, S., and Gilden, R. V., 1970, Immune virolysis: Effect of antibody and complement on C-type RNA virus, *Science* **168**:1478.

Örvell, C., and Norrby, E., 1977, Immunologic properties of purified Sendai virus glycoproteins, *J. Immunol.* **119**:1882.

Osler, A. G., 1976, *Complement—Mechanisms and Functions*, Prentice-Hall, Englewood Cliffs, N.J.

Otsuki, Y., and Takebe, I., 1973, Infection of tobacco mesophyll protoplasts by cucumber mosaic virus, *Virology* **52**:433.

Otsuki, Y., Takebe, I., Honda, Y., Kajita, S., and Matsui, C., 1974, Infection of tobacco mesophyll protoplasts by potato virus X, *J. Gen. Virol.* **22**:375.

Ozaki, Y., 1968, Neutralization kinetics of poliovirus by specific antiserum during the course of immunization of rabbits, *Arch. Gesamte Virusforsch.* **25**:137.

Ozaki, Y., and Kumagai, K., 1969, Studies on the neutralization of Japanese encephalitis virus. II. Variations in reaction properties of virus to antibody during replication in PS cell cultures, *J. Immunol.* **103**:850.

Ozaki, Y., and Tabeyi, K., 1967, Studies on the neutralization of Japanese encephalitis virus. I. Application of kinetic neutralization to the measurement of the neutralizing potency of antiserum, *J. Immunol.* **98**:1218.

Ozaki, Y., Kumagai, K., Kawanishi, M., and Seto, A., 1974, Studies on the neutralization of Japanese encephalitis virus. III. Analysis of the neutralization reaction by anti-rabbit-γ-globulin serum, *Arch. Gesamte Virusforsch.* **45**:7.

Palmer, J. L., Mandy, W. J., and Nisonoff, A., 1962, Heterogeneity of rabbit antibody and its subunits, *Proc. Natl. Acad. Sci. USA* **48**:49.

Parkman, P. D., Mundon, F. K., McCown, J. M., and Buescher, E. L., 1964, Studies of rubella. II. Neutralization of the virus, *J. Immunol.* **93**:608.

Pernis, B., Ghezzi, I., and Turri, M., 1963, Properties of phage-neutralizing antibodies produced by new-born rabbits, *Nature (London)* **197**:807.

Petty, R. E., and Steward, W. M., 1977, The effect of immunological adjuvants on the relative affinity of anti-protein antibodies, *Immunology* **32**:49.

Philipson, L., 1966, Interaction between poliovirus and immunoglobulins. II. Basic aspects of virus–antibody interaction, *Virology* **28**:35.

Philipson, L., and Bennich, H., 1966, Interaction between poliovirus and immunoglobulins. III. The effect of cleavage products of rabbit γ-G globulin on infectivity and distribution of virus in polymer phase systems, *Virology* **29**:330.

Porter, D. D., and Larsen, A. E., 1967, Aleutian disease of mink: Infectious virus–antibody complexes in the serum, *Proc. Soc. Exp. Biol. Med.* **126**:680.

Porter, R. R., 1959, The hydrolysis of rabbit γ-globulin and antibodies with crystalline papain, *Biochem. J.* **73**:119.

Putnam, F. W., Tan, M., Lynn, L. T., Easley, C. W., and Migita, S., 1962, The cleavage of rabbit γ-globulin by papain, *J. Biol. Chem.* **237**:717.

Radwan, A. I., and Burger, D., 1973a, The complement-requiring neutralization of equine arteritis virus by late antisera, *Virology* **51**:71.

Radwan, A. I., and Burger, D., 1973b, The role of sensitizing antibody in the neutralization of equine arteritis virus by complement or anti-IgG serum, *Virology* **53**:366.

Radwan, A. I., Burger, D., and Davis, W. C., 1973, The fate of sensitized equine arteritis virus following neutralization by complement or anti-IgG serum, *Virology* **53**:372.

Rappaport, I., 1957, The kinetics of antibody inactivation of tobacco mosaic virus, *J. Immunol.* **78**:256.

Rappaport, I., 1965, The antigenic structure of tobacco mosaic virus, *Adv. Virus Res.* **11**:223.

Rappaport, I., 1970, An analysis of the inactivation of MS2 bacteriophage with antiserum, *J. Gen. Virol.* **6**:25.

Rawls, W. E., Desmyter, J., and Melnick, J. L., 1967, Rubella virus neutralization by plaque reduction, *Proc. Soc. Exp. Biol. Med.* **124**:167.

Reed, L. J., and Muench, H., 1938, A simple method of estimating fifty per cent endpoints, *Am. J. Hyg.* **27**:493.

Rohrman, G. F., and Krueger, R. G., 1970, Precipitation and neutralization of bacteriophage MS2 by rabbit antibodies, *J. Immunol.* **104**:353.

Rosenstein, R. W., Nisonoff, A., and Uhr, J. W., 1971, Significance of bivalence of antibody in viral neutralization, *J. Exp. Med.* **134**:1431.

Rotman, M. B., and Celada, F., 1968, Antibody-mediated activation of a defective β-D-galactosidase extracted from an *Escherichia coli* mutant, *Proc. Natl. Acad. Sci. USA.* **60**:660.

Rowlands, D. T., Jr., 1967, Precipitation and neutralization of bacteriophage f2 by rabbit antibodies, *J. Immunol.* **98**:958.

Rubin, H., 1957, Interactions between Newcastle disease virus (NDV), antibody and cell, *Virology* **4**:533.

Rubin, H., and Franklin, R. M., 1957, On the mechanism of Newcastle disease virus neutralization by immune serum, *Virology* **3**:84.

Sabin, A. B., 1935a, The mechanism of immunity to filterable viruses. I. Does the virus combine with the protective substance in immune serum in the absence of tissue? *Br. J. Exp. Pathol.* **16**:70.

Sabin, A. B., 1935b, II. Fate of the virus in a system consisting of susceptible tissue, immune serum and virus, and the role of the tissue in the mechanism of immunity, *Br. J. Exp. Pathol.* **16**:84.

Sagik, B. P., 1954, A specific reversible inhibition of bacteriophage T2, *J. Bacteriol.* **68**:430.

Sarvas, H., and Mäkelä, O., 1970, Haptenated bacteriophage in the assay of antibody quantity and affinity: Maturation of an immune response, *Immunochemistry* **7**:933.

Scatchard, G., 1949, The attractions of proteins for small molecules and ions, *Ann. N.Y. Acad. Sci.* **51**:660.

Schluederberg, A., Ajello, C., and Evans, B., 1976, Fate of rubella genome ribonucleic acid after immune and nonimmune virolysis in the presence of ribonuclease, *Infect. Immun.* **14**:1097.

Schrader, J. A., and Muschel, L. H., 1975, Coliphage T2 neutralization by 7 S antibody and C1, *Immunochemistry* **12**:791.

Schultz, E. W., 1928, Studies on the antigenic properties of the ultraviruses. I. Introductory remarks, *J. Immunol.* **15**:229.

Seidman, J. G., Leder, A., Nau, M., Norman, B., and Leder, P., 1978, Antibody diversity, *Science* **202**:11.

Shinkai, K., and Yoshino, K., 1975a, Complement requirement of neutralizing antibodies in different classes of immunoglobulin appearing in rabbits and guinea pigs after primary and booster immunization with herpes simplex virus, *Jpn. J. Microbiol.* **19**:25.

Shinkai, K., and Yoshino, K., 1975b, Neutralizing activities of early and late IgG fragments from rabbits immunized with herpes simplex virus, *Jpn. J. Microbiol.* **19**:211.

Shortridge, K. F., 1972, Adenovirus neutralization—behavior of virion derived capsid components in the production of an in vitro neutralizing antibody, *Microbios* **5**:265.

Shortridge, K. F., and Biddle, F., 1970, The proteins of adenovirus type 5, *Arch. Gesamte Virusforsch.* **29**:1.

Silverstein, S. C., and Marcus, P. I., 1964, Early stages of Newcastle disease virus–HeLa cell interaction: An electron microscopic study, *Virology* **23**:370.

Smith, K. O., Galasso, G., and Sharp, D. G., 1961, Effect of antiserum on adsorption of vaccinia virus to Earle's L cells, *Proc. Soc. Exp. Biol. Med.* **106**:669.

Smith, W., 1930, Specific antibody absorption by the viruses of vaccinia and herpes, *J. Pathol. Bacteriol.* **33**:273.

Smorodintsev, A. A., and Yabrov, A. A., 1963, The mechanism of enhanced activity of anti-influenza virus neutralizing antisera on their interaction with native serum from normal animals, *Acta Virol. Engl. Ed.* **7**:193.

Spielberg, H., 1974, Biological activities of immuno-globulins of different classes and subclasses, *Adv. Immunol.* **19**:259.

Stemke, G. W., 1969, Mechanism of bacteriophage T4 neutralization by rabbit immunoglobulin and its proteolytic digestion fragments, *J. Immunol.* **103**:596.

Stemke, G. W., and Lennox, E. S., 1967, Bacteriophage neutralizing activity of fragments derived from rabbit immunoglobulins by papain digestion, *J. Immunol.* **98**:94.

Sternberg, G. M., 1892, Practical results of bacteriological researches, *Trans. Assoc. Am. Physicians* **7**:68.

Stevens, D. A., Pincus, T., Burroughs, M. A. K., and Hampar, B., 1968, Serologic relationship of a simian herpes virus (SA8) and herpes simplex virus: Heterogeneity in the degree of reciprocal cross-reactivity shown by rabbit 7 S and 19 S antibodies, *J. Immunol.* **101**:979.

Stinski, M. F., and Cunningham, C. H., 1970, Antibody-neutralized avian infectious bronchitis virus in chicken embryo kidney cells: Entry and degradation, *J. Gen. Virol.* **8**:173.

Strunk, R. C., John, T. J., and Sieber, O. F., 1977, Herpes simplex virus infections in guinea pigs deficient in the fourth component of complement, *Infect. Immun.* **15**:165.

Styk, B., 1965, Cofactor and specific antibodies against influenza viruses. XI. Mechanism of the action of antibody cofactor, *Acta Virol. Engl. Ed.* **9**:210.

Styk, B., and Hana, L., 1965a, Cofactor and specific antibodies against influenza viruses. IX. Formation of 19 S and 7 S type influenza antibodies in white mice; the role of "antibody cofactor," *Acta Virol. Engl. Ed.* **9**:109.

Styk, B., and Hana, L., 1965b, Cofactor and specific antibodies against influenza viruses. X. Formation of 19 S and 7 S type influenza antibodies in young and adult rabbits and roosters; the role of antibody cofactor, *Acta Virol. Engl. Ed.* **9**:200.

Styk, B., Rathova, V., and Blaskovic, D., 1958, Thermolability of specific hemagglutination inhibiting antibodies against the FE influenza virus and their reactivation by the addition of fresh serum, *Acta Virol. Engl. Ed.* **2**:179.

Svehag, S.-E., 1963, Reactivation of neutralized virus by fluorocarbon: Mechanism of action and demonstration of reduced reactivability with time of virus–antibody interaction, *Virology* **21**:174.

Svehag, S.-E., 1965a, The dissociability of different poliovirus–antibody complexes as tested by hypertonic salt solutions, *Arch. Gesamte Virusforsch.* **17**:504.

Svehag, S.-E., 1965b, The formation and properties of poliovirus neutralizing antibody. 5. Changes in the quality of 19 S and 7 S rabbit antibodies following immunization, *Acta Pathol. Microbiol. Scand.* **64**:103.

Svehag, S.-E., 1966, Diversity of antibodies formed against viruses, in: *Antibodies to Biologically Active Molecules* (B. Cinader, ed.), pp. 301–348, Pergamon Press, New York.

Svehag, S.-E., 1968, Formation and dissociation of virus–antibody complexes with special reference to the neutralization process, *Prog. Med. Virol.* **10**:1.

Svehag, S.-E., and Mandel, B., 1962, The production and properties of poliovirus neutralizing antibody of rabbit origin, *Virology* **18**:508.

Svehag, S.-E., and Mandel, B., 1964a, The formation and properties of poliovirus-neutralizing antibody. I. 19 S and 7 S antibody formation: Differences in kinetics and antigen dose requirement for induction, *J. Exp. Med.* **119**:1.

Svehag, S.-E., and Mandel, B., 1964b, The formation and properties of poliovirus-neutralizing antibody. II. 19 S and 7 S antibody formation: Differences in antigen dose requirement for sustained synthesis, anamnesis, and sensitivity to X-irradiation, *J. Exp. Med.* **119**:21.

Svehag, S.-E., Chesebro, B., and Bloth, B., 1968, Ultrastructure of IgM immunoglobulins, *Bull. Soc. Chim. Biol.* **50**:1013.

Symington, J., McCann, A. K., and Schlesinger, M. J., 1977, Infectious virus-antibody complexes of sindbis virus, *Infect. Immun.* **15**:720.

Szweczuk, M. R., and Mukkur, T. K. S., 1977, Enthalpy-entropy compensation in dinitrophenyl-anti-dinitrophenyl antibody interaction(s), *Immunology* **32**:11.

Takebe, I., 1977, Protoplasts in the study of plant virus replication, in: *Comprehensive Virology*, Vol. 11 (H. Fraenkel-Conrat and Robert R. Wagner, eds.), Plenum Press, New York.

Takebe, I., and Otsuki, Y., 1969, Infection of tobacco mesophyll protoplasts by tobacco mosaic virus, *Proc. Natl. Acad. Sci. USA* **64**:843.

Taniguchi, S., and Yoshino, K., 1965, Studies on the neutralization of herpes simplex virus. II. Analysis of complement as the antibody-potentiating factor, *Virology* **26**:54.

Thomssen, R., 1963, Ein chromatographisches Verfahren zur Bestimmung typenspezifischer Poliovirus-antikörper mit ^{32}P-markierten Poliovirus, *Z. Naturforsch.* **18B**:798.

Thormar, H., 1963, Neutralization of visna virus by antisera from sheep, *J. Immunol.* **90**:185.

Tiselius, A., and Kabat, E. A., 1939, An electrophoretic study of immune sera and purified antibody preparations, *J. Exp. Med.* **69**:119.

Tolmach, L. J., 1956, Immunological aspects of bacteriophage–host cell interaction, *Fed. Proc.* **15**:619.

Toolan, H. W., 1965, H-1 virus viremia in adult hamster, *Proc. Soc. Exp. Biol. Med.* **119**:715.

Toussaint, A. J., and Muschel, L. H., 1962, Studies on the bacteriophage neutralizing activity of serums. I. An assay procedure for normal antibody and complement, *J. Immunol.* **89**:27.

Trautman, R., 1976, Unified mass-action theory for virus neutralization and radioimmunology, *Scand. J. Immunol.* **5**:609.

Trautman, R., and Harris, W. F., 1977, Modeling and computer simulation approach to the mechanism of foot-and-mouth disease virus neutralization assays, *Scand. J. Immunol.* **6**:831.

Tyrrell, D. A. J., and Horsfall, F. L., Jr., 1953, Neutralization of viruses by homologous immune serum. I. Quantitative studies on factors which affect the neutralization reaction with Newcastle disease, influenza A, and bacterial virus, T3, *J. Exp. Med.* **97**:845.

Uhr, J. W., 1964, The heterogeneity of the immune response, *Science*, **145**:457.

Uhr, J. W., and Finkelstein, M. S., 1963, Antibody formation. IV. Formation of rapidly and slowly sedimenting antibodies and immunological memory to bacteriophage ϕX174, *J. Exp. Med.* **117**:457.

Uhr, J. W., Finkelstein, M. S., and Baumann, J. B., 1962, Antibody formation. III. The primary and secondary response to bacteriophage ϕX174 in guinea pigs, *J. Exp. Med.* **115**:655.

Valentine, R. C., and Green, N. M., 1967, Electron microscopy of an antibody–hapten complex, *J. Mol. Biol.* **27**:615.

van Regenmortel, M. H. V., 1966, Plant virus serology, *Adv. Virus Res.* **12**:207.

Van Vunakis, H., Barlow, J. L., and Levine, L., 1956, Neutralization of bacteriophage by the properdin system, *Proc. Natl. Acad. Sci. USA* **42**:391.

Vogt, A., Kopp, R., Maass, G., and Reich, L., 1964, Poliovirus type 1: Neutralization by papain-digested antibodies, *Science*, **145**:1447.

Wadell, G., 1972, Sensitization and neutralization of adenovirus by specific sera against capsid subunits, *J. Immunol.* **108**:622.

Wallis, C., 1971, The role of antibody, complement, and anti-IgG in the persistent fraction of herpesvirus, in: *Viruses Affecting Man and Animals* (M. Sanders and M. Schaeffer, eds.), pp. 102–123, Warren H. Green, St. Louis.

Wallis, C., and Melnick, J. L., 1967, Virus aggregation as the cause of the nonneutralizable persistent fraction, *J. Virol.* **1**:478.

Wallis, C., and Melnick, J. L., 1970, Herpesvirus neutralization: Induction of the persistent fraction by insufficient antibody, *Virology* **42**:128.

Wallis, C., Shirley, A., and Melnick, J. L., 1973, Total recovery of infectious virus from noninfectious type 1 poliovirus–antibody complex by heating in salts, *Intervirology* **1**:41.

Way, H. J., and Garwes, D. J., 1970, Serum accessory factors in the measurement of arbovirus neutralization reactions, *J. Gen. Virol.* **7**:211.

Werner, T. C., Bunting, J. R., and Cathou, R. E., 1972, The shape of immunoglobulin G molecule in solution, *Proc. Natl. Acad. Sci. USA* **69**:795.

Westaway, E. G., 1965a, The neutralization of arboviruses. I. Neutralization in homologous virus–serum mixtures with two group B arboviruses, *Virology* **26**:517.

Westaway, E. G., 1965b, The neutralization of arboviruses. II. Neutralization in heterologous virus–serum mixtures with four group B arboviruses, *Virology* **26**:528.

Westaway, E. G., 1968, Antibody responses in rabbits to the group B arbovirus Kunjin: Serologic activity of the fractionated immunoglobulins in homologous and heterologous reactions, *J. Immunol.* **100**:569.

Wigzell, H., 1973, Antibody diversity: Is it all coded for by the germ line genes? *Scand. J. Immunol.* **2**:199.

Yguerabide, J., Epstein, H. F., and Stryer, L., 1970, Segmental flexibility in an antibody molecule, *J. Mol. Biol.* **51**:573.

Yoshino, K., and Isono, N., 1978, Studies on the neutralization of herpes simplex virus. IX. Variance in complement requirement among IgG and IgM from early and late sera under different sensitization conditions, *Microbiol. Immunol.* **22**:403.

Yoshino, K., and Taniguchi, S., 1964, The appearance of complement-requiring neutralizing antibodies by immunization and infection with herpes simplex virus, *Virology* **22**:193.

Yoshino, K., and Taniguchi, S., 1965a, Studies on the neutralization of herpes simplex virus. I. Appearance of neutralizing antibodies having different grades of complement requirement, *Virology* **26**:44.

Yoshino, K., and Taniguchi, S., 1965b, Studies on the neutralization of herpes simplex virus. III. Mechanism of the antibody-potentiating action of complement, *Virology* **26**:61.

Zimmerman, S. E., Brown, R. K., Curti, B., and Massey, V., 1971, Immunochemical studies of L-amino acid oxidase, *Biochim. Biophys. Acta* **229**:260.

CHAPTER 3

Humoral Immunity to Viruses

Neil R. Cooper

Department of Molecular Immunology
Scripps Clinic and Research Foundation
La Jolla, California 92037

1. INTRODUCTION

Viruses are the causative agents of a number of acute and chronic infectious diseases and are undoubtedly involved in the pathogenesis of certain chronic debilitating diseases of man. Furthermore, a number of viruses may become latent in cells and reemerge at a later time to produce disease. It is therefore not surprising that vertebrates have evolved a multitude of defense mechanisms, operative at multiple levels, to cope with the omnipresent threat posed by viruses. These defenses range from simple physical barriers to sophisticated, complex systems such as the finely tuned interacting members of the immunological network. Disease may result not only from a failure of primary or secondary defense mechanisms but also in some cases from overzealous efforts of the host to cope with the viruses.

This chapter will focus on humoral defense mechanisms which function to neutralize and inactivate viruses. Specific and nonspecific, antibody- and complement-dependent and -independent mechanisms resident in the plasma will be examined. Although not to be considered here, it is important to emphasize that the humoral systems to be described here do not operate alone *in vivo* but rather function in a coordinated and integrated manner with other immunological and nonimmunological defenses. Particularly relevant are the collaborative interrelationships of the various arms of the immune network, i.e., antibody and the various subsets of B and T cells and macrophages in the induction and control of the immune response to viruses. Also crucial are the roles played by the various populations of lymphocytes and macrophages and other phagocytic cells in eliminating viruses and virus-infected cells. The reader is referred to other articles dealing with these important areas (Oldstone and Lampert, 1979; Oldstone, 1975; Notkins *et al.*, 1970; Wheelock and Toy, 1973; Joseph *et al.*, 1975; Zinkernagel and Welsh, 1976; Katz, 1977; Daniels, 1975).

2. THE COMPLEMENT SYSTEM

2.1. Constituents and Molecular Mechanisms

The complement system consists of at least 20 distinct proteins, which represent a significant proportion of the total plasma proteins as their cumulative concentration exceeds 3 mg/ml (Table 1). Although immunologically non-cross-reactive and distinct from one another in size, structure, and physicochemical parameters, these proteins are capable of interacting following activation of the complement system. Activation triggers a well-defined and orderly sequence of interactions of the complement proteins with each other and with biological membranes. These various reactions generate the numerous and potent biological activities which characterize activation of the complement system, as will be considered in the next section.

The reactions involving the complement factors, most of which are termed "components," can be grouped into several units, each of which involves several of the complement proteins (Fig. 1). There are two activation pathways, the classical pathway and the alternative, or

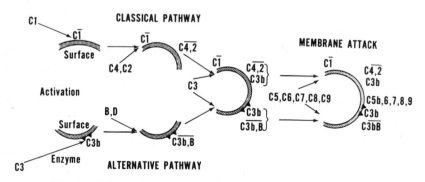

Fig. 1.   Schematic representation of the complement pathways.

TABLE 1

Proteins of the Complement System

	Charge	Molecular weight	Average serum concentration (μg/ml)
Classical pathway			
C1q	γ_2	400,000	70
C1r	β	190,000	34
C1s	α	88,000	31
C4	β_1	206,000	640
C2	β_1	117,000	25
C3	β_1	180,000	1200
Alternative pathway			
Factor B	β	93,000	200
Factor D	α	24,000	2
C3	β_1	180,000	1200
Properdin	γ	180,000	20
Membrane attack pathway			
C5	β_1	180,000	75
C6	β_2	128,000	64
C7	β_2	121,000	54
C8	γ_1	154,000	54
C9	α	79,000	58
Control proteins			
C$\overline{1}$ In	α	105,000	240
AI	α	310,000	50
β1H	β	150,000	470
C3b In	β	80,000	34
S protein	α	71,000	500

properdin, pathway. Either of these may be selectively triggered by several kinds of activators. The two pathways converge at the step involving C3 and thereafter share the remainder of the complement reaction sequence. The latter portion of the reaction sequence is termed the "membrane attack" mechanism because of its ability to lyse or otherwise damage biological membranes. In addition, there are several control proteins which act to modulate and inhibit these steps in the reaction sequence.

The classical complement pathway is generally activated by antigen–antibody complexes in which the antibody is of the IgG or the IgM class. Among immunoglobulins, IgM is the most efficient activator, since a single molecule of IgM in complex with antigen is sufficient to activate the first complement component, C1, while at least two molecules of IgG in close proximity to each other are required for complexes containing IgG. The site of attachment of C1 is in the Fc portion of immunoglobulin molecules. C1 may also be activated in the absence of antibody by a large number of different substances including a polypeptide located on the external surface of retroviruses, C-reactive protein in complex with phosphorylcholine, its natural substrate, polyanions such as DNA or RNA, certain cellular membranes, and lipid A of lipopolysaccharides. The structural or chemical features responsible for C1 binding and activation are not yet known.

The classical complement pathway comprises the reaction steps of C1, C4, and C2. C1 in normal plasma is a trimolecular calcium-dependent complex of three different proteins, C1q, C1r, and C1s. The C1q constituent of C1 bears the site or sites for attachment of C1 to the activator molecule as it is able to bind to activators in the absence of C1r and C1s. C1q is an unusual molecule chemically, and in the electron microscope it resembles a "bouquet of six flowers." Several lines of evidence suggest that the six heads of the molecule, the flowers in the bouquet, are the sites utilized for the attachment of C1q to immunoglobulin molecules and presumably also to other activators, while the C1r and C1s subcomponents are thought to be in close proximity to the clustered stems of the flowers. Following attachment of C1 via C1q to an activator, a series of intramolecular changes in the C1 molecule involving C1q, C1r, and C1s follows. These changes lead to the proteolytic cleavage of the polypeptide chains of C1r. By this process C1r is converted from a zymogen into an enzyme of the serine protease type. The newly activated $\overline{\text{C1r}}$ enzyme (according to accepted convention, a bar over the symbol for a component denotes an activated state, usually an enzyme) activates C1s by proteolytic cleavage. Cleavage of C1s at a single site by the $\overline{\text{C1r}}$ enzyme converts C1s from a zymogen into an active protease, also of the serine esterase type. With the activation of the C1s subcomponent, activation of C1 is completed.

$\overline{\text{C1s}}$ in $\overline{\text{C1}}$ activates the next two reacting molecules in the complement reaction sequence, C4 and C2, by proteolytic cleavage. The cleavage of C4 by $\overline{\text{C1}}$ engenders several sites in the larger fragment, C4b. One of these, a labile binding site, enables C4b, for a brief period of time, to attach to biological membranes. The C4b molecules do not bind to $\overline{\text{C1}}$ or to the antibody molecule but rather attach to the membrane around the $\overline{\text{C1}}$ molecule. Another site in C4b is an acceptor for a fragment of the newly cleaved C2 molecule. The protein–protein complex thus formed, $\overline{\text{C4,2}}$, is another indigenous complement enzyme. $\overline{\text{C4,2}}$ cleaves C3, the complement component in highest concentration in the plasma, into two fragments, each of which has potent biological activity. The smaller fragment, C3a, is released with cleavage and diffuses away from the site of its generation, while the larger fragment, C3b, possesses a short-lived binding site which permits attachment of this molecule to the membrane of the activator in a cluster-type distribution around the $\overline{C4,2}$ enzyme. The binding of C3b molecules in close proximity to the $\overline{C4,2}$ molecules generates yet another enzyme, $\overline{C4,2,3b}$, which has C5 as its substrate. The proteolytic cleavage of C5 by $\overline{C4,2,3b}$ initiates the membrane attack mechanism, as considered below.

The mechanism of initiation of the alternative complement pathway is quite different. There is the initial generation of a low-level C3-cleaving enzyme. This protease appears to be formed by the action of factor $\overline{D}$, a serine protease enzyme normally found in serum, on a loose complex of native C3 with factor B. Some of the C3b generated by the action of this enzyme becomes attached to membranes. The nature of the surface to which these C3b molecules become bound determines whether or not the alternative pathway is activated. On "nonactivators" the control proteins $\beta 1H$ and C3b inactivator degrade the bound C3b and thereby prevent progression of the complement reaction sequence. However, on the surface of particles termed "activators," the C3b which has become bound is not degraded by the control proteins $\beta 1H$ and C3b inactivator. The mechanism of this protection is not presently clear. Bound C3b on the protected surface of the activator interacts with factors B and $\overline{D}$ to generate a protease, $\overline{C3b,Bb}$, which is able to cleave large amounts of C3 into the typical C3a and C3b fragments. $\overline{C3b,Bb}$ is an enzyme analogous in structure and mechanism of action to $\overline{C4,2}$ of the classical pathway. Some of the C3b generated by $\overline{C3b,Bb}$ becomes adherent to the cell surface in the vicinity of the enzyme and forms an additional enzyme, $\overline{C3b_n Bb}$, which has C5 as its substrate.

The cleavage of C5 by the respective C5-cleaving enzymes of either the classical or alternative pathways, $\overline{C4,2}$ or $\overline{C3b,Bb}$, respectively, initiates formation of the membrane attack mechanism. The products of C5 cleavage are C5a, a molecule with potent biological activities as will be considered below, and C5b, the larger fragment. C5b is able to bind C6 and C7 to form a trimolecular complex, C5b,6,7. The C5b–7 complex can bind to lipid containing membranes; in addition, C5b–7 has an acceptor site for C8. With the attachment of C8 a tetramolecular complex, C5b–8, is formed which has the ability to bind several C9 molecules. The complete C5b–9 complex has a molecular weight of approximately 1 million and, in its nascent form, just after activation, is able to damage or lyse many membranes having a lipid bilayer structure.

The remaining proteins of the complement system are involved in regulation and control. They include $\overline{C1}$ inhibitor ($\overline{C1}$ In), a multispecific enzyme inhibitor which is able to block the action of a number of enzymes of the complement, kinin, coagulation, and fibrinolytic systems. Within the complement system $\overline{C1}$ In combines with $\overline{C1r}$ and $\overline{C1s}$ and blocks the actions of these enzymes on C1s, and C4 and C2, respectively. In this manner, $\overline{C1}$ In effectively controls activation of the classical pathway. The protein $\beta 1H$ and the enzyme C3b inactivator are involved in regulation of the critical steps involving C3. The anaphylatoxin inactivator (AI), also known as serum carboxypeptidase type B, is an enzyme which cleaves the C-terminal amino acid arginine from C3a and C5a, thereby inactivating some of the biological properties of these fragments. S protein binds to newly generated C5b–9 complexes in a competitive reaction with lipid membranes and modulates the ability of C5b–9 to produce cytolytic damage.

2.2. Biological Reactions Accompanying Complement Activation

There are three categories of biological activities of the complement system (Table 2). First, complement has the ability to produce a number of ultrastructural changes in lipid-containing membranes which range from the accumulation of complement protein on the surface of the cell, virus, or complex, inducing activation, to overt lysis. Alterations in electrical charge and resistance of membranes with complement deposition have been described. A foaminess or swelling of the bilayer membrane has been observed with activation of the late complement components. The C5b–9 complex also produces characteristic circular

TABLE 2
Biological Consequences of Complement Activation

Alterations in membrane ultrastructure	Biological actions of complement fragments
Accumulation of bulk	Histamine release, anaphylatoxin
Changes in charge	Smooth muscle contraction
Membrane swelling	Chemotaxis
Increased fluidity	Cellular activation
Ultrastructural lesions	Enzyme release
Disruption	C3b- and C4b-dependent cross-linking

lesions with a diameter of approximately 10 nm in lipid bilayers. However, the presence of such lesions is not synonymous with lysis as unlysed membranes bearing these hallmarks of complement action have been described. The most familiar biological action of complement is the ability to produce cytolytic damage, and many kinds of cells including erythrocytes, platelets, bacteria, and viruses possessing a lipid-containing membrane are susceptible to lysis, although with greatly varying efficiency in each instance. The newly formed C5b–9 complex is the lytic agent.

A second category of complement biology consists of the activities of the fragments of complement molecules generated during activation. As a result of the attack by complement enzymes, smaller fragments are generated and released from factor B, C3, and C5 during complement activation. These fragments, as well as fragments from C4 and C2 for which no biological activity has yet been described, may be released from the cleaved protein and diffuse away from the area of complement activation. In this process, they may encounter cells such as neutrophils, mast cells, and basophils which have specific receptors for the complement fragments on their membranes. Interaction of the complement peptides with these cellular receptors can trigger specific responses by the cells. For example, C3a and C5a specifically bind to mast cells and trigger histamine release by the cells. The ability to induce histamine release is termed "anaphylatoxin activity." C5a and the smaller factor B fragment interact with neutrophils to stimulate their directed migration into the area of complement activation, a property termed "chemotaxis." C5a also induces enzyme release and activation of certain cells. A kinin-like activity derived from C2 has been reported.

Certain cells also have receptors for the larger fragments of several of the complement proteins. These receptors are distinct from those utilized by the minor fragments. Also, the sites in the complement molecules interacting with these receptors (stable binding sites) are not the same sites as those utilized by the same activated complement molecules to bind to the surface of a cell undergoing complement attack (labile binding site). Thus the larger fragments of C3 and C4, C3b and C4b, respectively, interact with specific receptors located on the surfaces of neutrophils, B lymphocytes, and other cells. The larger fragment of factor B, Bb, binds to macrophages and monocytes. These interactions may also lead to specific responses by the cells involved.

The third general cateogry of biological activities of the activated complement system is cross-linking of cells by C3b and C4b. The ability to bridge cells is due to the presence of at least two different kinds of binding sites in C3b and C4b molecules, as described in the preceding section. One of these, a labile binding site, mediates the attachment of C3b or C4b to a virus, cell, or immune complex undergoing complement attack, while the other, a stable binding site, is recognized by effector cells having C3b receptors, such as neutrophils and B lymphocytes. In this manner, C4b and C3b mediate the direct approximation of the virus, bacteria, immune complex, or cell bearing the activated complement molecules to the surface of these various types of effector cells. C3b and C4b may be considered opsonins as they facilitate adherence to phagocytic cells such as neutrophils and macrophages. The biological function of the comparable reaction with B lymphocytes has not yet been elucidated.

These various biological activities of the activated complement system are the individual facets of an integrated system that mediates an acute inflammatory reaction which serves to confine an injurious or infectious process to the area of complement activation. For example, complement activation generates C3a and C5a fragments, which induce histamine release from mast cells or basophils. The released histamine in turn produces changes in permeability with edema and smooth muscle contraction. Simultaneously, the C5a fragment and the smaller fragment of factor B trigger the directed movement of leukocytes into the area of complement activation where they become adherent to the specific sites on C3b and C4b. The phagocytic cells attempt to ingest the particles or pathogens to which C3b and C4b are adherent and in this process release enzymes which activate more complement and amplify the process. All of these reactions represent the ingredients of an acute inflammatory reaction serving to localize the complement-activating substance.

Quite distinct from these activities, complement may play a role in the early stages of an immune response, possibly through the recognition site on B lymphocytes for C3b and C4b. This property could be relevant to agents such as retroviruses, which activate complement directly without the participation of antibody. Separate from these considerations, the bridging activities of C3b and C4b may focus a virus bearing C3b and C4b onto the surface of cells with receptors for these proteins, such as B lymphocytes, thus facilitating infection of these cells.

Complement also possesses a physiogenic role *in vivo* of unknown nature as indicated by the very high frequency of autoimmune disease in individuals with congenital absence of C1r, C1s, C2, and C4. The mechanism by which the absence of these components predisposes to such diseases is not clear. It may be, however, that components of the classical pathway are essential for the clearance of certain viruses involved in the pathogenesis of autoimmune diseases like lupus erythematosus. Alternatively, the absence of C2 and C4, which are encoded within the major histocompatibility complex, may reflect an immune response gene defect, and numerous pieces of evidence indicate that genes in the major histocompatibility complex are involved in susceptibility to certain diseases. Recent reviews detailing the reactions and biology of the complement system are found in the following: Schreiber *et al.* (1978) Hugli and Müller-Eberhard (1978), Müller-Eberhard (1975), Lachmann and Rosen (1978), Osler (1976), Reid and Porter (1975), Day and Good (1977), and Cooper and Ziccardi (1976).

3. GENERAL CONSIDERATIONS OF VIRUS STRUCTURE AND INTERACTIONS WITH HUMORAL ELEMENTS

Viruses contain nucleic acid which is enclosed and surrounded by, and in some cases intermingled with, a protein coat termed the "capsid." The nucleic acid together with the protein coat represents the nucleocapsid. The internal core also contains a nucleic acid polymerase and frequently other molecules involved in maintaining structure or assisting in transcription. The capsid consists of repeating arrays of subunits of protein molecules. Many viruses, in addition, contain an outer envelope acquired in budding through cellular membranes. A schematic representation of a moderately complex enveloped virus similar to members of the retrovirus group is depicted in Fig. 2. The envelope, which has a lipid bilayer configuration, is derived from the host-cell membrane and therefore contains lipids and glycolipids in proportions similar to but not identical to those of the cellular membrane from which it originated. In addition, however, the envelope contains multiple copies of protein subunits. These proteins are virtually all specified by the viral genome, although occasionally host-cell proteins may be present. Some of the proteins are hydrophobic membrane (M) proteins not exposed on the viral surface while others, which appear as spikes or knobs in electron micrographs, project from the viral envelope. The projecting proteins are glycosylated, a property which gives such viruses hydrophilic properties. In some virus systems, the external projecting protein may be linked to or associated with a transmembrane protein.

Humoral and cellular defense mechanisms are effective only if directed against the external structural features of viruses. The viral

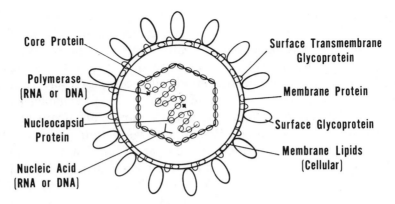

Fig. 2.   Schematic representation of an enveloped virus.

proteins of both enveloped and nonenveloped viruses are antigenic and stimulate antibody production, as well as the formation of various immune lymphocyte populations. The repeating array arrangement of the external proteins of enveloped and nonenveloped viruses probably facilitates recognition by the various humoral and cellular elements of the immune network. Antibody-coated viruses may interact with cellular Fc receptors on phagocytes, lymphocytes, and other cells. As immune complexes, antibody on viral surfaces may activate complement, leading to complement deposition on the viral surface, also facilitating neutralization. In addition, lipid-containing enveloped viruses may be lysed by complement. The same external features are undoubtedly the structures recognized by nonimmune non-antibody-mediated defense systems. These include the complement system, which is directly triggered in the absence of antibody by some viruses like retroviruses, factors such as serum lipoproteins, and potentially other factors which directly interact with some viruses as well as certain types of cells, as, for example, natural killer (NK) cells. This chapter will focus selectively on the role of various humoral elements in neutralizing virions and the various mechanisms by which this is accomplished. The reader is referred to other recent reviews for a discussion of the various cellular and combined humoral–cellular defense mechanisms operative against viruses and virus-infected cells (Fenner *et al.*, 1974; Notkins, 1975; Rawls and Tompkins, 1975; Oldstone and Lampert, 1979).

4. NONIMMUNE NON-COMPLEMENT-RELATED HUMORAL VIRAL NEUTRALIZING FACTORS

Levy *et al.* (1975) described a factor in mouse serum which neutralized the activity of murine xenotropic retroviruses. Ecotropic murine retroviruses were not affected by the factor. Xenotropic and ecotropic retroviruses are both endogenous in murine cells but differ from each other in external antigens and in host-cell range. Xenotropic virus derived from murine cells was inactivated by murine plasma, as was xenotropic virus passed through cells from other species. The factor in murine plasma did not appear to be antibody as it was not precipitated by 50% ammonium sulfate and not removed by antiserum to murine immunoglobulins. Furthermore, it was unaffected by heating to 100°C. Other workers (Fischinger *et al.*, 1976) also confirmed the presence of a nonimmunoglobulin factor in murine plasma which neutralized xenotropic but not ecotropic murine retroviruses or retroviruses from other sources. Subsequently, further characterization (Leong *et al.*, 1977) showed the factor in murine plasma to be unaffected by treatment with proteases including pronase as well as treatment with phospholipase A or carbohydrate-cleaving enzymes. Ultracentrifugal and other studies suggested that the neutralizing factor is associated with mouse serum lipoproteins.

5. ANTIBODY-DEPENDENT VIRAL NEUTRALIZATION

5.1. General Considerations

Extensive clinical and epidemiological studies document the major role of antibody in preventing or terminating viral infection in man. *In vitro* assays have supported and extended these data and amply demonstrated that antibody can reduce, or entirely neutralize, the infectivity of a large number of plant, bacterial, and animal viruses. The attachment of IgG or IgM antibody molecules to the external membrane of viruses does not lead to permanent alterations in viral morphology as shown by the fact that any of several treatments which disrupt the antibody–virus bond restore infectivity (Hummeler and Ketler, 1958; Lafferty, 1963; Granoff, 1965; Keller, 1968).

It is likely that the ability of antibody to neutralize viruses *in vitro* is usually due either to the presence of a blanket of antibody around the virus or to the ability of antibody to reduce the net number of infectious particles through aggregation or to a combination of these two effects as described below. Either of these activities of antibody would retard adsorption and probably also entry of the virus into a potentially susceptible cell. In addition, however, effects of antiviral antibody on subsequent intracellular critical steps in the infectious process have been reported with several viruses, as reviewed by Svehag (1968), Daniels (1975), and Dales (1965). Although not considered here, virus particles coated with antibody would bind to cells possessing Fc receptors such as phagocytes and Fc-receptor-positive lymphocytes. In addition to the above, other reviews of the mechanisms involved in antibody-dependent neutralization are found in articles by Fazekas de St. Groth (1962), Dulbecco *et al.* (1956), Fenner *et al.* (1974), and Silverstein (1970).

5.2. Neutralization by Envelopment

As the external surface of viruses consists of repeating subunits, each of which may function as at least a monovalent and more likely a polyvalent antigen, each virion is able to bind multiple antibody molecules. The contribution of antibody protein to the viral surface may be considerable as convincingly demonstrated by electron microscopic studies of virus–antibody mixtures. Berry and Almeida (1968) showed that antibody enveloped avian infectious bronchitis virus (AIBV), a coronavirus, with a halo of protein up to 300 Å thick. Virus incubated with serum containing only antibody was significantly neutralized.

5.3. Neutralization by Aggregation

Antibody molecules are multivalent, and therefore it is not surprising that they can cross-link viral particles into clumps. Aggregation, by reducing the net number of infectious viral units, can produce neutralization. Hummeler *et al.* (1962) employed electron microscopy to show that antibody clumped polio virus while Almeida *et al.* (1963) used the same technique to demonstrate that antibody to polyoma virus selectively agglutinated polyoma virus particles in mixtures of polyoma and wart virus, a structurally similar virus. Electron microscopy was also used to show antibody-dependent aggregation of influenza virus (Lafferty and Oertelis, 1963), foot and mouth virus (Almeida *et al.*, 1967), and rubella virus (Best *et al.*, 1967). Wallis and Melnick (1971) used filtration through membranes of different pore sizes to show that antibody obtained late after immunization aggregated herpes simplex virus.

Employing a different approach, Oldstone *et al.* (1974) analyzed differentially labeled polyoma virus particles and antibody by rate zonal sucrose density gradient ultracentrifugation and showed that as few as two antibody molecules per virion aggregated the viral particles. Slightly greater degrees of sensitization with antibody (20 molecules per virion) produced marked viral neutralization. Gradient sedimentation has also been used to document aggregation of a number of other viruses by antibody, including herpes simplex virus (Notkins *et al.*, 1971), retroviruses (Orozlan and Gilden, 1970), and lymphocytic choriomeningitis virus (Welsh *et al.*, 1976*b*).

Although antibody can clearly aggregate virus, this is not an inevitable consequence of the addition of antibody to virus. The degree of aggregation is modulated, as in all immune reactions, by steric and physical considerations related to the density and distribution of antigenic sites, concentration of reactants, and the type and affinity of antibody. In addition, as the antigens are located on a particle, aggregation is influenced by the relationship of the antigenic sites to the surface topography. Antibody directed against antigens located on the envelope of a virus having prominent projections would probably not agglutinate viral particles. One would not anticipate agglutination where there existed a considerable excess of virus over antibody because of shear forces and insufficient contacts for the formation of stable aggregates. At the opposite extreme, agglutination would be precluded if the viral particles were saturated with antibody, leaving no sites available for bridging. These various considerations have been well addressed from both theoretical and experimental standpoints by Lafferty and Oertelis (1963) and Almeida and Waterson (1969).

6. GENERAL FEATURES OF ANTIBODY- AND COMPLEMENT-DEPENDENT VIRAL NEUTRALIZATION

6.1. Historical Considerations and Overview

Perhaps the first report of the ability of complement, or alexin, as it was earlier called, to enhance antibody-dependent neutralization of a virus is that of Gordon (1925), who found that heating reduced the neutralizing activity of immune sera directed against vaccinia. The addition of fresh sera containing complement increased the neutralization a hundredfold. Since that time there have been many studies showing that complement either enhances or, in some cases, is necessary for antibody-dependent neutralization of a number of viruses. Among these are various members of the following genera or species: alphavirus (Dozois *et al.*, 1949; Whitman, 1947), arbovirus group B (Sabin, 1950; Ozaki and Tabeyi, 1967; Westaway, 1965), coliphages (Toussaint and Muschel, 1962; Adler *et al.*, 1971), herpesvirus (Yoshino and Taniguchi, 1965; Taniguchi and Yoshino, 1965; Hampar *et al.*, 1968;

Heineman, 1969), paramyxoviruses (Leymaster and Ward, 1949; Neva and Weller, 1964; Parkman *et al.*, 1964; Rawls *et al.*, 1967; Wedgwood *et al.*, 1956), poxviruses (McCarthy and Germer, 1952), and retroviruses (Mueller, 1931).

The mechanisms involved were not analyzed in these studies, although several did show that the effect was related to complement, as then understood. In a few cases, participation of C1, C4, C2, and C3 and/or properdin was assessed employing older methods based on the use of sera depleted of individual complement components, termed "R reagents." Although these reagents are known to be deficient in more than one complement component, the general conclusions regarding complement participation obtained with R reagents remain valid.

A number of mechanisms have been identified by which complement can enhance the neutralizing activity of antibody. As considered in detail in later sections, complement can augment neutralization of some antibody-coated viruses by contributing an additional envelope of protein to the surface of the virus which interferes with attachment and/or penetration. In some cases complement can aggregate viruses. These complement-dependent effects do not require lysis; in fact, it is likely that many viruses which undergo complement-dependent lysis are neutralized before completion of the lytic process. Complement can lyse a number of enveloped viruses. Various *in vitro* studies suggest that antibody-initiated complement-dependent mechanisms are primarily involved early in the course of a viral disease when lesser amounts of antibody are present which often have a lower binding affinity than antibody developed later in the disease.

Complement can also directly neutralize some viruses without the participation of antibody. These nonimmune processes, which are highly efficient in undiluted serum, can also be divided into nonlytic and lytic mechanisms. Complement may well serve as a first line of defense against viruses which are directly inactivated by complement and prevent infection by such viruses.

6.2. The Complement-Fixation Test

The complement-fixation test is frequently used in laboratory immunology, particularly as a retrospective diagnostic tool in viral infections. In the test, the patient's convalescent serum, possibly containing antibody, is heated to inactivate complement in the sample. Dilutions are then prepared and incubated with a source of viral antigens, thus forming immune complexes. Next, a source of complement, generally guinea pig serum, is added to the samples. Immune complexes, where present, activate ("consume" or "fix") the complement. Red cells coated with anti-red-cell antibody are subsequently added to detect and quantitate the complement activity remaining in the samples. Reduced lysis of the sensitized red cells indicates that the complement has been consumed and therefore that the sample contained antiviral antibody.

The complement fixation assay as usually performed generally detects antibody to the most immunogenic viral antigens. With a number of viruses (e.g., influenza), the antigen involved in the complement-fixation test is the nucleocapsid antigen. It should be appreciated that antibody to internal antigens, although present, does not inactivate viruses *in vivo* either alone or in conjunction with complement. Other antibodies to surface viral structures, which are capable of neutralizing the virus *in vivo* and *in vitro*, also develop, but their contribution to the complement-fixation assay is small. Thus the complement-fixation test itself does not provide a measure of the presence of neutralizing antibody.

6.3. Host-Cell Modification of Viruses

The surface properties of an enveloped virus are altered by the cell in which it is grown. These host-cell modifications are often due to the assimilation of cellular lipids, glycolipids, and carbohydrates and possibly occasionally proteins into the viral envelope (Klenk *et al.*, 1972; Laver and Webster, 1966; Rott *et al.*, 1966; Simpson and Hauser, 1966). Enveloped viruses may be inactivated by antibody to various incorporated antigenic moieties of the membrane of the host cell of derivation (Laver and Webster, 1966; Rott *et al.*, 1966). Complement may also potentiate that inactivation (Welsh, 1977). Viral inactivation and viral lysis by antibody to cells have been demonstrated in several instances and inferred in others (Welsh, 1977; Berry and Almeida, 1968; Haukenes, 1977; Apostolov and Sawa, 1976). Welsh (1977) found that lymphocytic choriomeningitis virus (LCMV) was inactivated by fresh but not heated normal human serum after passage through L929 cells, a mouse cell line, but not after passage through three other cell lines from various species. The neutralizing activity of normal human serum for L929-cell-derived LCMV was eliminated by adsorbing the serum with L929 cells; furthermore, it was shown that antibody with specificity for L929 cells bound to the LCMV derived from these cells but not to LCMV grown in BHK cells. The use of complement-depleted and -reconstituted sera established that LCMV (L929 cells) was inactivated via the classical complement pathway. Welsh (1977) concluded that natural antibody in human serum to the cells of origin of the virus activated the classical complement pathway leading to inactivation of the virus. Natural antibodies are often heat labile and of low titer, and reactive against lipid moieties (Wilson and Miles, 1975), properties which render them difficult to detect.

The cell through which viruses are passed may also change the susceptibility of the viruses to nonimmune complement-dependent inactivation. Theoretically, host-cell lipids, glycolipids, carbohydrates, or possibly proteins present in the viral envelope may have the ability to directly trigger the classical or alternative pathway. There is ample precedent for substances able to directly activate the classical complement pathway in the absence of antibody. Such substances include proteins, such as p15E of retroviruses, lipids like lipid A of lipopolysaccharide, some lipid bilayer membranes, and cholesterol, nucleic acids, and certain simple chemicals like sodium urate crystals. The alternative pathway is usually initiated without the participation of antibody by many substances, including complex carbohydrates. In this context it would not be surprising to find that viruses derived from certain cells directly activate the classical or alternative pathways due to acquisition from the cells of substances which possess complement-activating ability. Although few examples have thus far been reported, Welsh (1977) observed that Newcastle disease virus (NDV) grown in chick embryo cells was inactivated by human serum while NDV passed through HeLa cells was resistant to inactivation. No evidence for antibody involvement was obtained. Thiry *et al.* (1978) also found marked differences in susceptibility of VSV to inactivation and lysis by human serum depending on the cell in which the virus had been grown in another apparent antibody-independent reaction. The studies of Bendinelli *et al.* (1974) may represent another example.

6.4. Factors Involved in Susceptibility to Lysis

Complement-dependent damage to viruses bearing a lipid envelope may occur, as noted before. The structural alterations resulting from the actions of the complement system on lipid bilayer membranes range from relatively minor degrees of damage to complete loss of viral integrity. Such changes include complement-dependent alterations in permeability allowing probable osmotic lysis or, alternatively, influx of plasma proteins and nucleases into the virus (Welsh *et al.*, 1976*b*; Schluederberg *et al.*, 1976). More extensive changes include varying degrees of disruption of the envelope to complete separation of the residual envelope fragments from the nucleic acid (Welsh *et al.*, 1976*b*). the released nucleic acid may retain integrity as a dense core or may be partially or completely degraded, depending on the sensitivity of the capsid proteins and the nucleic acid to plasma enzymes and nucleases.

Although not yet extensively examined, it is unlikely that serum-derived accessory factors, in addition to complement, are needed to lyse enveloped viruses. An example of an accessory factor of this type is lysozyme, needed for lysis of gram-negative bacteria after complement action. It is also quite probable that complement-dependent viral lysis is a one-hit phenomenon, as is complement-mediated lysis of erythrocytes and nucleated cells. With these cells one lesion or successful complement attack site per cell is sufficient for lysis.

The action of antibody and complement on an enveloped virus would not, however, be expected to invariably lead to lysis. There are several reasons for a potential failure of complement to lyse cells and presumably also enveloped viruses. For example, complement may not be activated at all or may only be minimally activated by the viral antigen-antibody complex. Some antibodies are not able to activate complement. The antigenic sites on some viruses may be situated too far apart for binding of two or more IgG molecules in close proximity, which is a requirement for C1 binding and activation. Also, although difficult to define in quantitative terms, the stimulus to activation, i.e., the relative concentration of antibody bound to viral antigens, may not be sufficiently great for the complement reaction to overcome the inhibitory effects of the various complement control proteins, including $\overline{\text{C1}}$ In, C3b In, β1H, and S protein. Failure to activate complement obviously would also occur with an antibody directed against internal viral constituents.

For lysis to occur, the attack mechanism must be activated by a C5-cleaving enzyme. Generally this occurs through the action of the C5 convertases of the classical or alternative pathway, $\overline{\text{C4,2,3}}$ or $\overline{\text{C3b}_n\text{Bb}}$, respectively, situated on or near the lipid bilayer. In addition, the ability of the newly cleaved C5b to adhere to a membrane is a very transient property and lost within a fraction of a second. Failure of the nascent C5b to achieve binding to a lipid bilayer within its very short half-life of <0.1 sec would preclude initiation of a lytic C5b–9 complex on the membrane. It is not difficult to conceive of formation of the $\overline{C4,2,3}$ or $\overline{C3b_nB}$ enzymes on the ends of the surface projections of an enveloped virus due to initiation of complement action by antibody directed against antigenic sites on the protruding protein. C5b generated at such a site may well lose its ability to bind to a lipid membrane before it has time to diffuse the necessary distance to achieve binding. It is quite likely that this represents the reason for the failure of chicken antibody to AIBV to initiate complement-dependent lysis of the virus despite dramatic evidence of complement activation and binding to the virus (Berry and Almeida, 1968). Chicken antibody reacted solely with the virus projections of this coronavirus. In contrast, rabbit antibody as well as antibody against the cell of origin, which efficiently initiated lytic complement action, reacted not only with the surface projections but also with antigens located between the projections on the envelope.

Although studies have not yet been performed with viruses, it is likely that lipid composition will also prove important in determining susceptibility to lysis. Inoue *et al.* (1971) examined antibody- and complement-dependent release of internally trapped markers from synthetic lipid vesicles (liposomes) prepared with antigen and various combinations of phospholipids, cholesterol, and charged amphiphiles. Liposomes prepared with lecithin were more readily lysed than those containing sphingomyelin while liposomes with an equimolor combination of both were the most sensitive. Alving *et al.* (1974) confirmed these findings with other immune systems and further found that phospholipids with longer-chain fatty acids generated liposomes which were less sensitive to antibody- and complement-mediated lysis. An influence of fatty acid chain length was also found by Akiyama and Inoue (1977) in their studies of bacteria resistant to antibody- and complement-dependent lysis. These authors felt that the presence of more longer-chain saturated fatty acids in the membrane of the resistant bacteria rendered the membranes more rigid, which had the effect of decreasing susceptibility to antibody- and complement-mediated lysis. Interestingly, resistant strains could be generated from susceptible strains by growth in media containing antibody and complement.

Chemical composition of membrane lipids was also implicated in the resistance of mutant mycoplasma strains to lysis by antibody and complement (Dahl *et al.*, 1977). In addition to composition, membrane thickness and relative fluidity have been implicated (Mayer, 1976).

7. ANTIBODY- AND COMPLEMENT-DEPENDENT VIRAL NEUTRALIZATION: NONLYTIC MECHANISMS

7.1. Envelopment with Complement Proteins

Complement activation by an immune complex located on a surface, as, for example, a viral envelope, is characterized by the deposition of complement proteins near the activating complex, as described earlier. Studies with numerous cells and other complexes indicate that large numbers of molecules of complement components, in particular C1q, C4b, and C3b, may become bound to the surface during complement deposition. In their electron microscopic studies Berry and Almeida (1968) observed and described this accumulation of complement on the envelope of antibody-sensitized AIBV as a halo of protein enveloping the virus. Whereas antibody alone produced a halo of 30 nm in diameter, this was increased up to 70 nm in the presence of an intact complement source. The protein halo was most clearly visualized when avian complement was used, as this source of complement is not lytic to AIBV. It is not surprising that a blanket of complement protein can interfere with attachment and/or penetration of potentially susceptible cells by the virus and be manifested as a reduction in infectivity. Where antibody alone neutralized 2.5 of 6.2 log units of virus, the addition of nonlytic avian complement reduced infectivity by an additional 2.2 log units.

Another virus neutralized by antibody and complement without lysis is herpes simplex virus (HSV). Daniels *et al.* (1969) found that C1 and high concentrations of C4 were sufficient to neutralize HSV in the presence of IgM antibody. On using low concentrations of C4, neutralization occurred on addition of functionally purified C2 and C3 to the mixture. Subsequent extensive studies showed that the later-reacting components, C5 to C9, and thus lysis, were not necessary for neutralization (Daniels *et al.*, 1970). Yoshino and Taniguchi (1969) reached a similar conclusion in their briefly described studies. Daniels *et al.* (1969) postulated that complement neutralized HSV by covering the viral surface with additional protein. Wallis and Melnick (1971), however, challenged this interpretation on the basis of their data derived from filtration of complement-related HSV–antibody complexes through membranes of varying pore sizes. They found that HSV–antibody complexes passed through 0.45-μm filters but after complement addition failed to traverse 0.45- or 0.8-μm membranes and two-thirds of the virus failed to pass through a 3-μm filter. They interpreted these data as indicating that complement neutralized HSV by aggregating the virions. While these data are certainly compatible with this interpretation, later studies of Notkins *et al.* (1971) employing sucrose density gradient ultracentrifugation indicated that complement does not aggregate antibody-sensitized HSV. The impaired ability of antibody- and complement-coated HSV to pass through the filters employed by Wallis and Melnick (1971) may be a consequence of the accumulation of complement protein on the viral envelope.

7.2. Aggregation by Complement Proteins

The studies of Oldstone *et al.* (1974) provide the first direct demonstration of complement-dependent cross-linking of virions. While the sedimentation rate of radiolabeled polyoma virus was increased from 240 S to 260 S on addition of 2.18 molecules of IgG anti-polyoma antibody per virion, the sedimentation rate was further increased to approximately 450 S on addition of serum. The addition of serum led to neutralization of the virus (Table 3). Comparative experiments with polyoma virus surface labeled with ^{125}I and internally labeled with [^{3}H]thymidine showed that serum was not lytic as it did not release labeled DNA and the external and internal labels cosedimented. Studies with isolated complement components revealed that purified C1q alone cross-linked and also neutralized polyoma virus sensitized with the same limited amounts of antibody (Fig. 3, Table 3). These properties

TABLE 3

Complement Requirements for Neutralization of Polyoma Virus

Reagents added to polyoma virus–antibody	Percent neutralization
None	0
Rabbit serum	73
C6-deficient rabbit serum	65
Human serum	80
Human C1q	60
Human C1	0
Human C1, C4	0
Human C1, C4, C2	0
Human C1, C4, C2, C3	84

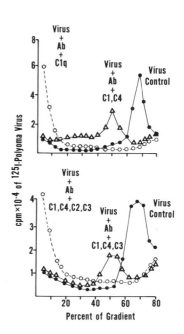

Fig. 3. Complement-dependent aggregation of polyoma virus. Externally labeled polyoma virus was incubated with antibody and various combinations of purified complement components. The mixtures were subjected to sucrose density gradient ultracentrifugation. The direction of sedimentation is to the left. Aggregation by C1q but not by C1 is apparent (upper panel). Aggregation by the C1, C4, C2, C3 mixture but not by the C1, C4, C3 mixture indicates that activation of C3 is necessary for cross-linking (lower panel).

were not, however, retained by C1, indicating that C1r and C1s apparently rendered some of the binding sites of C1q unavailable for agglutination of the virus particles. No agglutination or neutralization occurred when even very large amounts of C4 were included in the virus–antibody–C1 mixture, and the subsequent addition of C2 was also without effect. Dramatic aggregation and also neutralization reoccurred, however, on adding C3 (Fig. 3, Table 3). The cross-linking was apparently a property of C3b since comparable antibody–C1, C4, C3 mixtures lacking C2, which is essential for C3 cleavage, were unable to aggregate the virus. The ability of C3b to cross-link virions was unexpected as C3b does not generally mediate agglutination reactions. The reaction could occur, however, if polyoma virions possess C3b receptors. Under these conditions C3b attached to one virion by its labile binding site could attach to the postulated C3b receptor on another virion by its stable binding site, thus producing viral aggregation. Preliminary evidence tends to support the presence of a C3b receptor on polyoma virions. Although C3b receptors have been reported on a number of cells including B lymphocytes, macrophages, and neutrophils, they have not previously been reported to occur on viruses.

Externally labeled LCMV was found by Welsh et al. (1976b) to sediment very rapidly in sucrose density gradient studies after incubation with antibody and complement. The rapidly sedimenting complexes represent envelopes, as experiments with internally labeled LCMV showed the RNA at the top of the same gradients. These findings may provide another example of complement-dependent aggregation, in this instance of viral envelopes.

7.3. Uncertain Mechanisms

Linscott and Levinson (1969) observed that NDV was neutralized by early IgM antibody and complement. Their observation that rabbit serum genetically lacking C6 effectively neutralized NDV indicated that lysis was not necessary for neutralization. Studies with purified complement components established that the addition of C1, C4, C2, and C3 to a mixture of NDV and antibody was sufficient for neutralization. It is probable, as postulated by Linscott and Levinson (1969), that neutralization with completion of the C3 step results from envelopment of the virus with complement protein. Later studies (Apostolov and Sawa, 1976) showed that NDV is susceptible to lysis by complement, although neutralization by early-reacting components does not require lysis. Thus this virus, like the virus described below and potentially other viruses, can be neutralized prior to lysis.

Radwan and Burger (1973) observed that equine arteritis virus (EAV)–antibody complexes were neutralized by fresh complement at 2°C without lysis, as labeled RNA was not released from the virus. In further studies Radwan and Crawford (1974) observed that C1, C4, C2, and C3 alone effectively neutralized EAV sensitized with high antibody concentrations. The addition of C5, C6, C7, C8, and C9 did not further potentiate neutralization, although it did induce lysis. Some neutralization was also observed at the C1,4 step when very high concentrations of C4 were added. When limited antibody concentrations were employed, the neutralization observed on addition of C1, C4, C2, and C3 was slightly increased by the addition of C5–C9. Although the mechanism of the nonlytic neutralization was not defined, it is probable that it is due to envelopment by complement protein.

Vesicular stomatitis virus (VSV) and vaccinia virus are also neutralized in the absence of lysis by antibody and complement, as shown by Leddy *et al.* (1977). These viruses were found to be neutralized by antibody and complement sources containing C1, C4, C2, and C3 but lacking C5 or other components reacting later in the sequence. Leddy *et al.* (1977) also observed some neutralization of both antibody-sensitized viruses by sera lacking C2 or C3, but the rates of neutralization were slower than obtained with sera containing these components. The mechanism underlying this neutralization was not explored but most likely is the consequence of the accumulation of complement protein, especially C3, on the viral surface and resulting interference with attachment and infection of potentially susceptible cells.

8. ANTIBODY- AND COMPLEMENT-DEPENDENT VIRAL NEUTRALIZATION: LYTIC MECHANISMS

8.1. Methods Employed to Demonstrate Viral Lysis

Several methods have been used to demonstrate complement-dependent lysis of enveloped viruses. These include electron microscopy, as most clearly demonstrated in the pioneering studies of Almeida and her co-workers (Berry and Almeida, 1968; Almeida and Waterson, 1969). Employing negatively stained preparations of a coronavirus, AIBV, they observed marked changes in morphology with the lytic action of complement. These ultrastructural alterations included increased radiolucency with stain penetration, increased size of the virus with apparent flattening, and the presence of numerous circular lesions with a diameter of approximately 10 nm. These lesions were morphologically indistinguishable from those shown earlier by Borsos *et al.* (1964) to be characteristic of the action of complement on antibody-sensitized red cells. Humphrey *et al.* (1967) showed that these lesions were due to the action of complement on the lipid of the erythrocyte membrane. The lesions were thought to be the actual lytic "holes," a conclusion now known to be incorrect, although they do represent C5b–9-dependent alterations in the ultrastructure of the lipid bilayer membrane. They are not, however, the functional holes in the membrane, for a number of reasons including the fact that various cells and membranes can sustain such lesions without undergoing lysis. Berry and Almeida (1968) interpreted their electron micrographs of AIBV as indicating viral lysis, primarily on the basis of the presence of the lesions. Later knowledge and comparison of electron microscopic and other techniques to demonstrate lysis indicate that the other morphological changes they observed and not primarily the presence of the lesions alone indicate viral lysis. Changes of this type showing lysis of a murine leukemia virus (MuLV) in the presence of antibody and complement are illustrated in Fig. 4. Electron microscopy has now been used to show that a number of other viruses are lysed by antibody and complement, as detailed below and in Table 4. In the case of certain viruses, in particular rubella (Almeida and Laurence, 1969), additional changes, in particular destruction of the envelope and the presence of free nucleocapsids, have been observed. In another study, Welsh *et al.* (1976*b*) electron microscopically examined thin sections of LCMV acted on by antibody and complement (Fig. 5). Antibody alone increased the width of the surface projections of the virus while the

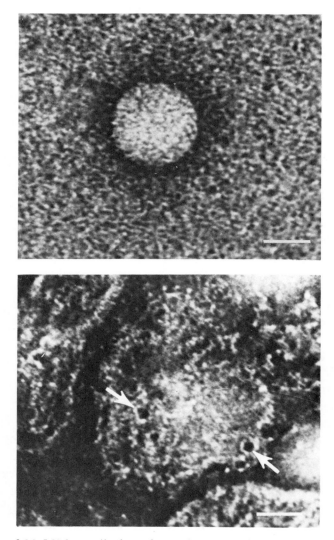

Fig. 4.   Lysis of MuLV by antibody and complement as demonstrated by electron microscopic examination of a negatively stained preparation. Top, virus control; bottom, antibody and complement added.

TABLE 4

Antibody- and Complement-Mediated Lysis of Enveloped Viruses

Virus	Classification	Method of showing lysis	Specificity of			Reference
			Source of Ab	Ab	Source of C	
AKR-MuLV	Retrovirus	[³H]Uridine release	Rat, guinea pig	Viral	Guinea pig	Orozlan and Gilden (1970)
Avian infectious bronchitis	Coronavirus	Electron microscopy	Rabbit	Viral, cellular	Rabbit, guinea pig	Berry and Almeida (1968)
Equine arteritis		[³H]Uridine release	Horse, guinea pig	Viral	Horse, guinea pig	Radwan et al. (1973), Radwan and Crawford (1974)
Influenza	Myxovirus	Electron microscopy	[a]	[a]	[a]	Almeida and Waterson (1969)
Lymphocytic chorio-meningitis	Arenavirus	Electron microscopy, [³H]-RNA release	Guinea pig	Viral	Rabbit, guinea pig	Welsh et al. (1976b)
Moloney MuLV	Retrovirus	Electron microscopy	Rat	Viral	Human	Oldstone (1975), Cooper and Oldstone (unpublished)
Newcastle disease	Paramyxovirus	Electron microscopy	Human	Cellular	Human	Apostolov and Sawa (1976)
Rauscher MuLV	Retrovirus	RDDP release	Human	Viral	Guinea pig	Welsh et al. (1976a)
Rubella	Paramyxovirus	Electron microscopy	Rabbit, human	Viral	Human	Almeida and Laurence (1969)
		Electron microscopy, [³H]-RNA release	Human	Viral	Guinea pig, human	Schluederberg et al. (1976)
Sendai	Paramyxovirus	Electron microscopy	Rabbit	Cellular	Guinea pig	Haukenes (1977)
		Electron microscopy	Human	Cellular	Human	Apostolov and Sawa (1976)
Sindbis	Alphavirus	[³H]-RNA release	Rabbit	Viral	Guinea pig	Stollar (1975)

[a] Exact findings were not described.

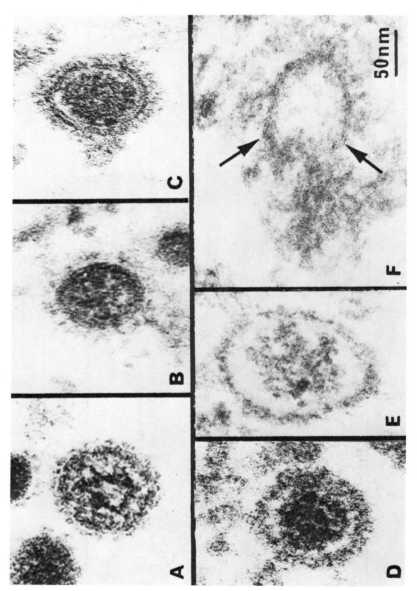

Fig. 5. Lysis of LCMV by antibody and complement as demonstrated by electron microscopic examination of thin sections. A: LCMV exposed to normal control serum. B: LCMV exposed to heated guinea pig serum containing antibody to LCMV. C–F: LCMV exposed to guinea pig serum containing antibody and complement. From Welsh et al. (1976b).

addition of complement produced a diversity of changes which apparently represent a continuum. Minimal changes were the deposition of electron-dense material on the envelope, probably consisting of complement protein. This was accompanied by thickening of the envelope with loss of the typical lipid bilayer appearance, membrane swelling, and progressive separation of the envelope from the electron-dense core. Disintegration of the RNA cores as evidenced by loss of radiodensity followed, and ultimately there were large physical breaks in the envelope and expulsion of the degenerating cores.

Another technique widely used to document viral lysis is a demonstration of release of internal viral constituents such as nucleic acid, antigens, or enzymes. Orozlan and Gilden (1970), in the first study of this type, employed sucrose density gradient ultracentrifugation to show that [^{3}H]uridine-labeled RNA and the internal group-specific antigen (p30) of AKR leukemia virus were released from the virus by antibody and complement. Both the RNA and internal p30 antigen were at the top of the gradient while untreated virus and antibody-sensitized virus sedimented well into such gradients. Furthermore, the released labeled RNA at the top of the gradient was RNase sensitive. Sucrose density gradient ultracentrifugation of virus–antibody–complement mixtures has since been extensively used to prove lysis of a number of viruses, as detailed below and in Table 4.

In a related approach Radwan et al. (1973) exposed RNA-labeled EAV to antibody and complement and then quantitated RNase-sensitive labeled RNA in the supernatant fluid. In a similar approach Stollar (1975) incubated RNA-labeled Sindbis virus with antibody and complement, then directly added RNase followed by trichloroacetic acid. Acid-soluble radioactivity was taken as the measure of lysis.

Release of the enzyme, RNA-dependent DNA polymerase (RDDP), has been widely used to demonstrate and quantitate complement-dependent, Ab-independent lysis of retroviruses (Welsh et al., 1975). RDDP enzyme activity is not present unless released from the virus by antibody and complement or detergent.

8.2. Viruses Lysed by Antibody and Complement

Using the various approaches described above, antibody- and complement-dependent lysis of a number of enveloped viruses has been demonstrated (Table 4). These include AKR-MuLV (Orozlan and Gilden, 1970), AIBV (Berry and Almeida, 1968), EAV (Radwan et al., 1973; Radwan and Crawford, 1974), influenza virus (Almeida and

Waterson, 1969; Haukenes, 1977), LCM (Welsh *et al.*, 1976*b*), Moloney-MuLV (Oldstone *et al.*, 1974; Cooper and Oldstone, unpublished), NDV (Apostolov and Sawa, 1976), Rauscher MuLV (Welsh *et al.*, 1976*a*), rubella virus (Almeida and Laurence, 1969; Schluederberg *et al.*, 1976), Sendai virus (Haukenes, 1977; Apostolov and Sawa, 1976), and Sindbis virus (Stollar, 1975).

9. NONIMMUNE COMPLEMENT-DEPENDENT VIRAL INACTIVATION

9.1. The Properdin System

Ginsberg and Horsfall (1949) reported that NDV, influenza A and B viruses, and mumps virus (grown in chicken eggs) were neutralized by normal, nonimmune serum. Heated sera (56°C, 30 min) did not neutralize, indicating not only that the property in serum was heat labile but also that it was not classical heat-stable neutralizing antibody. Adsorption and depletion studies suggested the factor(s) in serum was similar to but also different from complement. Howitt (1950) also observed that normal human and other sera inactivated NDV, although her studies did not permit a differentiation of the factor(s) in serum from complement. Bang *et al.* (1950), however, showed that removal of complement activity by adsorption of human serum with an immune precipitate at 4°C did not impair the ability of the same normal, nonimmune human serum to neutralize NDV.

Some of these properties were similar to those of the properdin system, first described by Pillemer *et al.* (1954) as a nonimmune, nonspecific serum system similar to but also different from complement. The system was characterized as a natural defense mechanism operative in lysis of certain abnormal erythrocytes, gram-negative bacteria, and protozoa. Wedgwood *et al.* (1956) further explored the relationship of the properdin system to the serum factors involved in neutralization of NDV. These studies indicated a requirement for the protein termed "properdin," the four then-described complement proteins, C1, C2, C3, and C4, and magnesium but not calcium. No antibody requirement was evident. These studies implicated the properdin system in the neutralization of viruses.

The concept of the properdin system as a separate and distinct natural immune system was challenged by Nelson (1958), who cited experiments indicating that the properdin system was entirely explained by natural antibody acting in conjunction with C1, C2, C3, and C4.

Interest in the properdin system as a distinct system subsided after Nelson's publication (1958) and other studies about that time which also implicated antibody (Osler and Sandberg, 1973; Götze and Müller-Eberhard, 1976). Developments within the last few years from several laboratories (Gewurz *et al.*, 1968; Sandberg *et al.*, 1970; Frank *et al.*, 1971; Marcus *et al.*, 1971; Götze and Müller-Eberhard, 1971) have verified the existence of the properdin system as a system of natural immmunity.

More recently, Welsh (1977) confirmed that NDV grown in chicken cells (see Section 6.3) was inactivated by normal, nonimmune human serum. Antibody was apparently not involved, as agammaglobulinemic human serum and serum previously adsorbed with the cell of origin were effective in neutralizing NDV. The alternative complement pathway was able to inactivate NDV in the absence of the classical pathway as C4-depleted human serum inactivated NDV, furnishing a confirmation of the participation of the alternative pathway (Wedgwood *et al.*, 1956) in the neutralization of NDV. Interestingly, Welsh observed (1977) that NDV could also be neutralized by the classical pathway as factor-B-depleted normal human-serum-inactivated NDV. Thus NDV can trigger either the alternative or the classical complement pathways in the absence of antibody, with resulting neutralization of the virus. It was not determined whether neutralization resulted from lysis or occurred prior to completion of the complement reaction.

The repeating glycosylated projecting membrane proteins which are characteristic of the external surface structure of many viruses would appear to be good candidates for direct alternative pathway activators. In addition, a number of viruses in conjunction with antibody selectively activate the alternative pathway as they bud from cells with cytolytic consequences to the host cell (Perrin *et al.*, 1976). It is therefore anticipated that other viruses will be found with additional study which directly activate the properdin or alternative pathway in the absence of antibody.

9.2. Nonlytic Mechanisms: Vesicular Stomatitis Virus

VSV was reported to be neutralized by normal serum from several species, including sera genetically deficient in late-reacting complement components (Oldstone, 1975; Welsh, 1977). This observation was confirmed and the detailed mechanism of the reactions examined by Mills and Cooper (1978*b*). Normal, nonimmune human sera were found to neutralize up to 5 logs/ml of VSV derived from hamster, mouse, or human cell lines when mixed in equal volume with the virus (Table 5). Human sera congenitally deficient in or immunochemically depleted of components reacted after C3 were able to neutralize VSV, as were sera lacking factor B (Table 5); however, sera devoid of C2 or C4 were ineffective. These observations indicated that nonimmune neutralization, like immune neutralization of VSV examined earlier by Leddy *et al.* (1977), proceeds through the classical complement pathway and occurs with completion of the C3 step. Several experimental approaches indicated that antibody was not required for this reaction. These included, first, the lack of significant neutralizing activity after heating, as would be expected with classical heat-stable neutralizing activity. Second, human IgG, IgA, and IgM were tested in concentrations that encompassed and exceeded normal serum concentrations and found to be unable to neutralize VSV or to enhance VSV neutralization by human serum. IgG also did not sensitize VSV for neutralization by human serum. Third, adsorption of normal serum with normal cells or VSV carrier cells expressing VSV antigens did not change the neutralizing activity. Fourth, immunoglobulin-free C1q and C1 bound to VSV and to the purified external glycoprotein of VSV (G protein).

Despite the ability of VSV to bind C1, it was unable to activate C1, and mixtures of purified C1, C4, C2, and C3 at serum concentrations did not neutralize VSV. These findings suggested that serum contained another factor(s) which was involved in VSV neutralization

TABLE 5
Human Complement Requirements for VSV Neutralization

Serum	C activity (% normal)	Log_{10}/ml titer change
NHS	100	−4.9
C1q depleted	0	−0.3
C1q depleted + C1q[a]	75	−2.0
C2 deficient	0	−0.6
C2 deficient + C2	100	−4.9
C4 depleted + C1q[a]	0	−0.6
Factor B depleted + C1q	61	−2.4
Factor B depleted + C1q + B[a]	nd	−3.4
C5 deficient	0	−3.8
C6 depleted + C1q[a]	0	−2.0
C7 depleted + C1q[a]	0	−2.4
C8 depleted + C1q[a]	0	−2.5

[a] Immunochemically depleted sera are also generally deficient in C1q, which must therefore be added back.

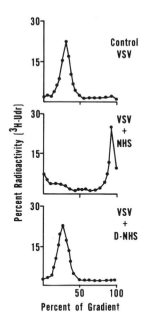

Fig. 6. Effect of human serum and delipidated human serum on VSV. VSV was incubated alone (control), with normal human serum (NHS), or with delipidated serum (D-NHS) and subjected to sucrose density gradient ultracentrifugation. The direction of sedimentation is to the left. Flotation of VSV by normal serum but not by delipidated serum is apparent.

in addition to C1, C4, C2, and C3, In beginning a search for the accessory factor in human serum, Mills and Cooper (1978a; Mills and Cooper, manuscript in preparation) observed that the density of VSV was dramatically reduced from 1.19 g/ml to < 1.065 g/ml after incubation in either fresh or heated normal human serum but was unchanged after comparable incubations in delipidated serum (Fig. 6). Studies with serum lipoproteins indicated that very-low-density lipoproteins (VLDL) but not chylomicrons, low-density-lipoproteins, or high-density-lipoproteins had the ability to attach to VSV and strikingly change its density (Fig. 7). Present experiments are directed toward determining whether the VSV–VLDL complex, which is the normal state of VSV in the presence of serum, has enhanced ability to bind and activate C1. There may be a relationship between these interactions of VSV and serum lipoproteins and the studies of Leong et al. (1977), which indicated that serum lipoproteins have the ability to neutralize xenotropic MuLV.

9.3. Lytic Mechanisms: Retroviruses

The first demonstration of viral lysis in the absence of demonstrable antibody comes from the studies of Welsh et al. (1975). Welsh and

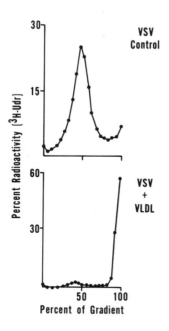

Fig. 7. Effect of VLDL on VSV. VSV was incubated alone or with VLDL and was subjected to sucrose density gradient ultracentrifugation. The direction of sedimentation is to the left. Flotation of VSV by VLDL is apparent.

co-workers observed that fresh normal human serum inactivated 2.5×10^5 plaque-forming units (PFU) of Moloney leukemia virus (M-MuLV) as tested in an XC cell plaque reduction assay. Inactivation was accompanied by viral lysis as radiolabeled RNA and the internal enzyme, RDDP, were released from virus preparations by normal human serum (Fig. 8, Table 6). Further study (Jensen *et al.*, 1976); Welsh *et al.*, 1976*a*; Gallagher *et al.*, 1978; Sherwin *et al.*, 1978; Bartholomew *et al.*, 1978; Thiry *et al.*, 1978) showed that a large number of retroviruses from avian, feline, murine, rat, and simian sources were inactivated by human serum as tested in either plaque or focus reduction assays (Table 7). Lysis was demonstrated by either sucrose density gradient or reverse transcriptase assays in most instances. The phenomenon was not an artifact of tissue culture as avian myeloblastosis virus isolated from chicken plasma and Moloney MuLV obtained directly from mouse plasma were also inactivated by human serum. Furthermore, Moloney MuLV harvested from cells grown in heated human serum was susceptible to lysis by human serum. Lytic susceptibility was not appreciably influenced by growing the same virus in different cells or by growing different viruses in the same cell.

Six lines of evidence indicate that antibody is not involved in this reaction. First, the reaction occurred with antigenically unrelated viruses grown in many kinds of cells, and all of the more than 50

TABLE 6

Human Complement Requirements for Lysis of MuLV

	pmol of [³H]-TMP polymerized		
	a[a]	b[a]	c[a]
Normal human serum	2.17	1.55	0.78
C2-deficient serum	0.10		
C4-depleted serum	0.02		
C8-deficient serum	0.17		
Factor-B-depleted human serum		0.83	
Factor-D-depleted human serum			0.26
Control (detergent)	3.37		
Heated human serum	0.04		

[a]a, b, and c represent separate experiments.

normal human sera tested to date were able to lyse retroviruses. Similar amounts of antibodies to a number of different kinds of viruses and/or different cells would obviously be highly unlikely. Second, heated human sera did not inactivate retroviruses, a classical test for neutralizing antibody. Third, normal human sera did not deposit immunoglob-

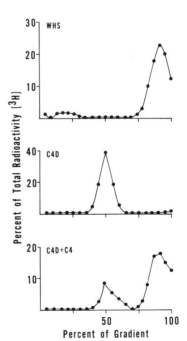

Fig. 8. Nonimmune complement-dependent lysis of a retrovirus. Rat leukemia virus containing RNA was incubated in normal serum (WHS) (top panel), C4-depleted human serum (C4D) (middle panel), and C4D reconstituted with C4 (bottom panel). The mixtures were subjected to equilibrium sucrose density gradient ultracentrifugation. Release of RNA or lysis by human serum and reconstituted human serum is apparent. The density of the virus treated with C4D is 1.15 g/ml, identical to that of untreated virus. Sedimentation is to the left. From Cooper *et al.* (1976).

TABLE 7
Retroviruses Inactivated by Primate Sera

	Virus	Viral source	Complement source	Assay system for lysis	Neutralization assay system	Reference
Avian	Avian myeloblastosis	Chicken serum	Human	RDDP release	—	Welsh et al. (1976a)
	Avian sarcoma B77	Chicken embryo fibroblasts	Human	—	Focus reduction	Welsh et al. (1976a)
Feline	Feline leukemia virus–Theilen	Feline fibroblasts	Human, gibbon	RDDP release	—	Welsh et al. (1976a); Gallagher et al. (1978)
	Moloney sarcoma (RD114) pseudotype	Baboon fibroblasts, human lymphoblasts	Human	RDDP release	Focus reduction	Welsh et al. (1976a)
Murine	AKR-MuLV	3T3 mouse cells	Human	RDDP release	Plaque reduction	Welsh et al. (1976a); Cooper et al. (1976); Sherwin et al. (1978)
	Endogenous N-tropic virus from BALBC	3T3 mouse cells	Human, chimpanzee, gibbon, baboon, rhesus, African green, squirrel, and spider monkeys	RDDP release	—	
	Friend MuLV	STV mouse	Human	RDDP release	—	Welsh et al. (1976a)
	Moloney MuLV	Murine fibroblasts	Human	RDDP release; [^{3}H]-RNA release; C5b–9 formation	Plaque reduction	Welsh et al. (1976a); Jensen et al. (1976); Bartholomew et al. (1978)
		Murine lymphoblasts	Human	RDDP release	—	Welsh et al. (1976a)
		Murine plasma	Human	—	Plaque reduction	Welsh et al. (1975)
	Moloney sarcoma	Norwegian rat kidney	Human	—	Focus reduction	Welsh et al. (1976a)
	Rauscher MuLV	JLSV-9 cells, rhesus monkey kidney, murine fibroblasts	Human, chimpanzee, gibbon, baboon, rhesus, African green, squirrel, and spider monkeys	RDDP release	Plaque reduction	Welsh et al. (1976a); Gallagher et al. (1978); Sherwin et al. (1978)
	Wild mouse	Wild mouse 1504 cells	Human	RDDP release	—	Welsh et al. (1976a)

	Virus	Cells	Species			Reference
Primate	Baboon endogenous virus M7	Bat lung fibroblasts	Human, gibbon	RDDP release	—	Gallagher et al. (1978)
	Baboon endogenous virus M28	Human rhabdomyosarcoma cell line	Human, gibbon, chimpanzee, rhesus, African green, squirrel, and spider monkeys	RDDP release	—	Sherwin et al. (1978)
	Gibbon ape leukemia virus	Bat lung fibroblasts	Human, gibbon	RDDP release	—	Gallagher et al. (1978)
	Human virus HL23	Bat lung fibroblasts	Human, gibbon	RDDP release	—	Gallagher et al. (1978)
	Mason-Pfizer monkey virus	Human rhabdomyosarcoma cell line	Human, gibbon, chimpanzee, rhesus, African green, squirrel, and spider monkeys	RDDP release	—	Sherwin et al. (1978)
	Moloney sarcoma (gibbon ape leukemia) pseudotype	Baboon fibroblasts, human fibroblasts, normal rat kidney cells	Human	—	Focus reduction	Welsh et al. (1976a)
	Moloney sarcoma (simian sarcoma) pseudotype	Baboon fibroblasts	Human	RDDP release	Focus reduction	Welsh et al. (1976a)
	Wooly monkey type C virus	Bat lung fibroblasts, human rhabdomyosarcoma cell line	Human, gibbon	RDDP release	—	Sherwin et al. (1978)
	Vesicular stomatitis virus (baboon C virus)	Dog thymus cells	Human	RNA release	Plaque reduction	Thiry et al. (1978)
Rat	Rat leukemia virus	Rat embryo fibroblasts	Human	RDDP release [^{3}H]-RNA release electron microscopy	—	Welsh et al. (1976a) Cooper et al. (1976) Bartholomew et al. (1978)

ulin on cells expressing retroviruses as detectable with fluoresceinated anti-human IgG, IgA, or IgM, as would be the case if antibody were present. Fourth, agammaglobulinemic human sera having no detectable IgA or IgM and less than 1% of normal IgG levels mediated retroviral lysis. Also, cord sera were able to mediate the reaction. Fifth, fresh human sera retained ability to lyse retroviruses after two adsorptions with cells expressing retroviruses. Sixth, although normal human serum was not able to sensitize retroviruses for lysis by guniea pig complement, serum from a volunteer immunized with Rauscher leukemia virus (R-MuLV) and containing antibody to the virus was able to sensitize the virus for lysis by guinea pig complement. Therefore, if antibody had been present in human serum, it could have been detected by this test.

The complement requirement for the lysis of retroviruses by human serum was apparent from the findings that human sera genetically deficient in C2 or C8 immunochemically depleted of C4 failed to mediate release of RDDP from AKR, Moloney, Rauscher, or xenotropic MuLV or rat leukemia virus (Table 6) (Welsh et al., 1976a; Cooper et al., 1976). Sera immunochemically depleted of C4 (by passage through an anti-C4 immunoadsorbent) also failed to support lysis, and lytic ability was restored on reconstituting the serum with physiological levels of C4 (Fig. 8). In contrast, sera immunochemically depleted of factor B of the alternative pathway, which were intact in regard to the classical pathway, were active in lysing retroviruses, although at reduced levels compared to sera with both pathways intact (Table 6). These studies indicate, first, that completion of the complement sequence is required. Second, the absolute requirements for C2 and C4 but not for factors B and D indicate exclusive mediation of the lytic reaction by the classical pathway. Third, the 15–54% reduction in lytic activity on removal of factor B or D indicates that the alternative pathway can significantly augment lysis initiated by the classical pathway, most likely reflecting participation of the C3b-dependent feedback mechanism triggered with deposition of C3b on the viral envelope. Consistent with the complement requirements, deposition of complement proteins on the viral envelope was demonstrated by sucrose density gradient ultracentrifugal studies (Cooper et al., 1976) and these observations were recently confirmed (Bartholomew et al., 1978).

The lack of antibody involvement together with classical pathway mediation indicated that retroviruses directly activate the classical pathway at the C1 stage. Direct binding of C1q to the viral envelope was demonstrated by several assays, including sucrose density gradient ultracentrifugation (Fig. 9). Retroviruses were also shown to directly

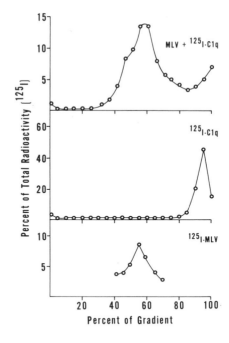

Fig. 9. Rate zonal sucrose density gradient ultracentrifugation of an MuLV–Clq mixture (top panel), ^{125}I-Clq alone (middle panel), and ^{125}I-MuLV alone (bottom panel). Clq incubated with MuLV (top panel) sediments at the same rate as ^{125}I-MuLV alone (bottom panel), documenting direct binding of Clq to MuLV. From Cooper *et al.* (1976).

activate C1 assembled from highly purified Clq, Clr, and Cls (Fig. 10). Activation was assessed by showing specific cleavage of the single polypeptide chain of proenzyme Cls contained within the C1 macromolecule into the 59,000- and 28,000-dalton subunits of activated C1s. This type of cleavage occurs in all C1 activation reactions (Cooper and Ziccardi, 1977). Controls revealed no activation of Clr–Cls complexes on omission of Clq, which not only shows that Clq is required but also eliminates a contaminating enzyme in the viral preparations as responsible for C1 activation.

Therefore, when retroviruses are incubated with human serum, the Clq subunit of C1 specifically recognizes a feature of the retroviral envelope and becomes firmly bound to the viral surface. Activation of C1 follows and in turn activation of the classical pathway with accompanying deposition of complement proteins on the viral envelope and lysis on completion of the reaction sequence. Antibody does not participate in this reaction. Thus, in this system, Clq subserves the recognition function normally associated with the antibody molecule.

Bartholomew *et al.* (1978) isolated the receptor on the viral envelope for C1 and identified it as an external polypeptide with an isoelectric point of 7.5 and a molecular weight of approximately 15,000. Because of these properties, the peptide was referred to as p15E.

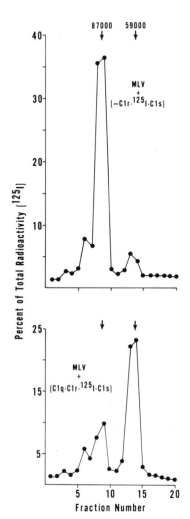

Fig. 10. Demonstration of activation of C1 by MuLV. C1 was reconstituted from a mixture of highly purified C1q, proenzyme C1r, and ^{125}I-proenzyme C1s and incubated with 30 μg of Moloney MuLV (M-MuLV). The mixtures were then reduced and subjected to polyacrylamide gel electrophoresis in the presence of sodium dodecylsulfate, after which the gels were sectioned and radioactivity was measured. C1s in precursor form either in C1 or alone is an 87,000-dalton single polypeptide chain. Activation of C1s is accomplished by cleavage into fragments of 59,000 and 28,000 daltons. Activation of C1 by M-MuLV is demonstrated in the lower panel by cleavage of C1s in C1 into a 59,000-dalton fragment (and also a 28,000-dalton fragment which is unlabeled). In the absence of C1q, as shown in the upper panel, C1s was not activated. Activation of C1 also did not occur on omission of M-MuLV.

Jensen, Robey, and Van de Woude (personal communication) have recently found that Fab antibody directed against the p60 precursor protein of the p30, p15, and p12 proteins of the M1 Moloney sarcoma virus blocked human-complement-mediated lysis of retroviruses. Fab anti-p30 or anti-gp 69–71, however, did not inhibit viral lysis. These workers, therefore, suggested that the p15C or p12 protein may also be C1 receptors.

One striking feature of complement-dependent lysis of retroviruses is the inability of normal sera from most nonprimate species to mediate the reaction whereas normal sera from humans, gibbons, monkeys, baboons, and apes were very active in this regard (Table 8). In attempting to find an explanation for this species specificity, Bartholomew and Esser (1978) found that human C1q and guinea pig C1q bound to retroviruses, but only human C1 and not guinea pig C1 was activated by retroviruses. Hybrid molecules containing various combinations of human and guinea pig C1q, C1r, and C1s were employed to probe the species restriction. The presence of human C1s in the C1 molecule was required for activation, a finding which suggests that human C1s shows some type of recognition for retroviral determinants. The biological relevance of the ability of primate sera to inactivate retroviruses and the failure of most nonprimate species to do so is presently unclear. Nevertheless, the infrequency with which retroviruses are isolated from man in contrast to the frequent presence of such viruses in some nonprimate species raises the possibility that the human complement system functions as a natural defense mechanism *in vivo* in limiting horizontal infection by retroviruses and preventing expression of such viruses by cells which may have been infected or which bear retroviral genomes. The striking absence of antibodies in humans handling large quantities of retroviruses could be interpreted as indicating that the such viruses are cleared prior to the initiation of an immune response, especially as

TABLE 8

**Complement Species Requirements for
Direct Lysis of Retroviruses[a]**

Serum source	Lytic activity
Cat	+
Chicken	0
Cow	0
Dog	0
Goat	0
Guinea pig	0
Mouse	0
Pig	0
Primate	
Baboon	+
Gibbon	+
Green monkey	+
Human	+
Rhesus	+
Rabbit	0, +
Rat	0
Sheep	0

[a] From Welsh *et al.* (1976a), Jensen *et al.* (1976), Gallagher *et al.* (1978), and Sherwin *et al.* (1978).

parenteral immunization of humans with such viruses induces an immune response (Table 4) (Hersch *et al.*, 1974). However, some primates do become infected with retroviruses (Todaro *et al.*, 1976; Kawakami *et al.*, 1972; Heberling *et al.*, 1977; Gallo *et al.*, 1978). Also, many animals exposed to viremic animals develop antibody to retroviral antigens (Gallagher *et al.*, 1978; Kawakami *et al.*, 1972; Charman *et al.*, 1975; Aoki *et al.*, 1976), most likely indicating infectious transmission. Furthermore, sera from the same species which can become infected by retroviruses have the ability to lyse the same viruses (Sherwin *et al.*, 1978; Gallagher *et al.*, 1978). These findings obviously raise questions about the relevance and potency of this system *in vivo* which cannot be presently answered. Little is presently known about transmission of retroviruses between primate species, in particular length of contact, the route by which horizontal infection occurs, and viral dose. Nothing is known of the complement system of animals prior to and during exposure. It should also be noted that serum from the viremic gibbon examined by Gallagher *et al.* (1978) had no ability to lyse retroviruses. Further study is clearly needed to determine the role and potency of the complement system *in vivo* in preventing infection with retroviruses. Particularly relevant would be sequential examinations of the complement system, levels of viremia, and clinical course of primates exposed to graded doses of nonparenterally administered retroviruses.

There have been very few other reports of lysis or presumed lysis of other viruses by nonimmune mechanisms. Schluederberg *et al.* (1976) reported that some unheated normal, nonimmune human sera lysed rubella virus. Antibody to rubella virus was not detected in sera with this activity by hemagglutination-inhibition tests, and all of these individuals subsequently acquired antibody after vaccination or illness. The mechanism of neutralization was by lysis as RNA was released. Thiry *et al.* (1978) observed lysis, assayed by RNA release and neutralization, of VSV grown in certain cells by human serum.

10. CONCLUSIONS

This chapter has selectively focused on the various humoral defense systems which serve to prevent or limit viral infection by directly neutralizing viral infectivity. Particular emphasis has been placed on the specific mechanisms by which antibody alone, antibody and the complement system, and the complement system alone inactivate a number of different viruses.

Antibody alone can neutralize many viruses nondestructively in a number of different ways, which can be grouped into two categories. First, antibody binding to the virus contributes a coat of protein to the viral surface which may interfere with attachment or penetration and thus infection of a potentially susceptible cell. Second, as antibody molecules are bivalent molecules and virions are multivalent antigens, antibody may aggregate virions with a resulting reduction in the net number of infectious particles. Antibody alone would be expected to be important *in vivo*, when relatively large amounts of avid antibody are present, as, for example, late in an infection or on reinfection.

The complement system is often considered as a major mediator of the biological effects of immune complexes. The ability of the immune complexes formed between antibody and viruses to activate complement and the resulting amplification of viral neutralization are not surprising. Complement can potentiate antibody-initiated neutralization by three mechanisms. First, it may neutralize by contributing complement protein to the viral surface with resulting impairment of ability of the virus to attack and/or penetrate a normally susceptible cell. Second, complement neutralizes at least one virus by inducing agglutination, leading to a reduction in the number of infectious particles. As the above two effects are not accomplished by lysis, they do not result in irreversible structural damage to the virus. Third, and most familiar, complement can lyse many viruses, leading to irreversible structural damage. The lytic effects of complement are restricted to viruses surrounded by lipid-containing membranes. Complement-dependent potentiation of the effects of antibody would be anticipated to be most important *in vivo* early in the course of an infection when limited amounts of antibody of relatively low affinity are present.

Several viruses have been found to be neutralized by complement in the complete absence of antibody. In these instances a surface viral structure interacts with the first complement component, leading to its triggering and accompanying activation of the complement system. Complement may neutralize such viruses by contributing additional protein to the viral surface and thus preventing cellular infection by the virus. Lipid-containing viruses which directly activate complement may be lysed and thus inactivated. The ability of complement to efficiently inactivate certain viruses in the absence of antibody suggests the possibility that it may function in this manner *in vivo* as a first line of defense in the nonimmune animal and prevent infection on initial contact. Retroviruses are directly lysed by normal, nonimmune primate complement sources whereas the serum of most nonprimates does not have this property. This observation, together with the rare finding of retroviruses in primates in contrast to their frequent presence and association with malignancies in many nonprimates whose complement sources lack the ability to inactivate such viruses, provides support for the concept that complement functions to prevent infection of man by such viruses. Further study is needed to determine whether the complement system functions in this manner *in vivo*.

ACKNOWLEDGMENTS

This is Publication No. 1665 from the Immunology Departments of the Research Institute of Scripps Clinic. This work was supported by USPHS Grants AI 07007 and CA 14692 and by Biomedical Research Support Grant 1 S07 RR 05514 from the National Institutes of Health. I wish to thank my collaborators in a number of the studies presented here—Fred Jensen, David Larson, Bonnie Mills, Michael B. A. Oldstone, and Raymond M. Welsh, Jr.—and particularly to acknowledge continuing collaborations with Fred Jensen and Michael B. A. Oldstone.

11. REFERENCES

Adler, F. L., Walker, W. S., and Fishman, M., 1971, Amplification of phage neutralization by complement, antiglobulin and anti-allotype sera, *Virology* **46**:797.

Akiyama, Y., and Inoue, K., 1977, Isolation and properties of complement-resistant strains of *Escherichia coli* K-12, *Infect. Immun.* **18**:446.

Almeida, J. D., and Laurence, G. D., 1969, Heated and unheated antiserum on rubella virus, *Am. J. Dis. Child.* **118**:101.

Almeida, J. D., and Waterson, A. P., 1969, The morphology of virus–antibody interaction, *Adv. Virus Res.* **15**:307.

Almeida, J., Cinader, B., and Howatson, A., 1963, The structure of antigen–antibody complexes: A study of electron microscopy, *J. Exp. Med.* **118**:327.

Almeida, J. D., Brown, F., and Waterson, A. P., 1967, The morphologic characteristics of 19 S antibody, *J. Immunol.* **98**:186.

Alving, C. R., Joseph, K. C., and Wistar, R., 1974, Influence of membrane composition on the interaction of a human monoclonal "anti-Forssman" immunoglobulin with liposomes, *Biochemistry* **13**:4818.

Aoki, T., Liu, M., Walling, M. J., Bushar, G. S., Brandchaft, P. B., and Kawakami, T. G., 1976, Specificity of naturally occurring antibody in normal gibbon serum, *Science* **191**:1180.

Apostolov, K., and Sawa, M. I., 1976, Enhancement of haemolysis of Newcastle disease virus (NDV) after pre-treatment with heterophile antibody and complement, *J. Gen. Virol.* **33**:459.

Bang, F. B., Foard, M., and Karzon, D. T., 1950, The determination and significance of substances neutralizing Newcastle virus in human serum, *Bull. Johns Hopkins Hosp.* **87**:130.

Bartholomew, R. M., and Esser, A. F., 1978, Differences in activation of human and guinea pig complement by retroviruses, *J. Immunol.* **121**:1748.

Bartholomew, R. M., Esser, A. F., and Müller-Eberhard, H. J., 1978, Lysis of on-cornaviruses by human serum: Isolation of the viral complement (C1) receptor and identification as p15E, *J. Exp. Med.* **147**:844.

Bendinelli, M., Nardini, L., and Campa, M., 1974, Neutralization of Friend leukemia virus by sera of unimmunized animals, *J. Gen. Virol.* **22**:207.

Berry, D. M., and Almeida, J. D., 1968, The morphological and biological effects of various antisera on avian infectious bronchitis virus, *J. Gen. Virol.* **3**:97.

Best, J. M., Banatvala, J. E., Almeida, J. D., and Waterson, A. P., 1967, Morphological characteristics of rubella virus, *Lancet* **2**:237.

Borsos, T., Dourmashkin, R. R., and Humphrey, J. H., 1964, Lesions in erythrocyte membranes caused by immune haemolysis, *Nature (London)* **202**:251.

Charman, H. P., Kim, N., White, M., Marquardt, H., Gilden, R. V., and Kawakami, T., 1975, Natural and experimentally induced antibodies to defined mammalian type-C virus proteins in primates, *J. Natl. Cancer Inst.* **55**:1419.

Cooper, N. R., and Ziccardi, R. J., 1976, The nature and reactions of complement enzymes, in: *Proteolysis and Physiological Regulation*, Vol. 11 (D. W. Ribbons and K. Brew, eds.), p. 167, Academic Press, New York.

Cooper, N. R., and Ziccardi, R. J., 1977, Reconstitution of C1 in native, proenzyme form and its use in a quantitative C1 activation test, *J. Immunol.* **119**:1664.

Cooper, N. R., Jensen, F. C., Welsh, Jr., R. M., and Oldstone, M. B. A., 1976, Lysis of RNA tumor viruses by human serum: Direct antibody independent triggering of the classical complement pathway, *J. Exp. Med.* **144**:970.

Dahl, J. S., Hellewell, S. B., and Levine, R. P., 1977, A mycoplasma mutant resistant to lysis by C: Variations in membrane composition and altered response to the terminal C complex, *J. Immunol.* **119**:1419.

Dales, S., 1965, Penetration of animal viruses into cells, *Prog. Med. Virol.* **7**:1.

Daniels, C. A., 1975, Mechanism of virus neutralization, in: *Viral Immunology and Immunopathology* (A. L. Notkins, ed.), p. 79, Academic Press, New York.

Daniels, C. A., Borsos, T., Snyderman, R., and Notkins, A. L., 1969, Neutralization of sensitized virus by the fourth component of complement, *Science* **165**:508.

Daniels, C. A., Borsos, T., Rapp, H. J., Snyderman, R., and Notkins, A. L., 1970, Neutralization of sensitized virus by purified components of complement, *Proc. Natl. Acad. Sci. USA* **65**:528.

Day, N. K., and Good, R. A., eds., 1977, *Biological Amplification Systems in Immunology* (*Comprehensive Immunology*, Vol. 2), Plenum Press, New York.

Dozois, T. F., Wagner, J. C., Chemerda, C. M., and Andrew, V. M., 1949, The influence of certain serum factors of the neutralization of western equine encephalomyelitis virus, *J. Immunol.* **62**:319.

Dulbecco, R., Vogt, M., and Strickland, A. G. R., 1956, A study of the basic aspects of neutralization of two animal viruses, western equine encephalitis virus and poliomyelitis virus, *Virology* **2**:162.

Fazekas de St. Groth, S., 1962, The neutralization of viruses, *Adv. Virus Res.* **9**:1.

Fenner, F., McAuslan, B. R., Mims, C. A., Sambrook, J., and White, D. O., 1974, *The Biology of Animal Viruses*, 2nd ed., Academic Press, New York.

Fischinger, P. J., Ihle, J. N., Bolognesi, D. P., and Schäfer, W., 1976, Inactivation of murine xenotropic oncornavirus by normal mouse sera is not immunoglobulin-mediated, *Virology* **71**:346.

Frank, M. M., May, J., Gaither, T., and Ellman, L., 1971, *In vitro* studies of complement function in sera of C4-deficient guinea pigs, *J. Exp. Med.* **134**:176.

Gallagher, R. E., Schrecker, A. W., Walter, C. A., and Gallo, R. C., 1978, Oncornavirus lytic activity in the serum of gibbon apes, *J. Natl. Cancer Inst.* **60**:677.

Gallo, R. C., Gallagher, R. E., Wong-Staal, F., Aoki, T., Markham, P. D., Schetters, H., Ruscetti, F., Valerio, M., Walling, M. J., O'Keeffe, R. T., Saxinger, W. C., Smith, R. G., Gillespie, D. H., and Reitz, M. S., Jr., 1978, Isolation and tissue distribution of type-C virus and viral components from a gibbon ape (*Hylobates lar*) with lymphocytic leukemia, *Virology* **84**:359.

Gewurz, H., Shin, H. S., and Mergenhagen, S. E., 1968, Interactions of the complement system with endotoxic lipopolysaccharide: Consumption of each of the six terminal complement compounds, *J. Exp. Med.* **128**:1049.

Ginsberg, H. S., and Horsfall, F. L., 1949, A labile component of normal serum which combines with various viruses: Neutralization of infectivity and inhibition of hemagglutination by the component, *J. Exp. Med.* **90**:475.

Gordon, M. H., 1925, Studies of the viruses of vaccinia and variola, *Spec. Rep. Ser. Med. Res. Counc. G. B.*, No. 98.

Götze, O., and Müller-Eberhard, H. J., 1971, The C3-activator system: An alternate pathway of complement activation, *J. Exp. Med.* **134**:90s.

Götze, O., and Müller-Eberhard, H. J., 1976, The alternative pathway of complement activation, *Adv. Immunol.* **24**:1.

Granoff, A., 1965, The interaction of Newcastle disease virus and neutralizing antibody, *Virology* **25**:38.

Hampar, B., Notkins, A. L., Mage, M., and Keehn, M. A., 1968, Heterogeneity in the properties of 7 S and 19 S rabbit-neutralizing antibodies to herpes simplex virus, *J. Immunol.* **100**:586.

Haukenes, G., 1977, Demonstration of host antigens in the myxovirus membrane: Lysis of virus by antibody and complement, *Acta Pathol. Microbiol. Scand. Sect. B* **85**:125.

Heberling, R. L., Barker, S. T., Kalter, S. S., Smith, G. C., and Helmke, R. J., 1977, Oncornavirus: Isolation from a squirrel monkey (*Saimiri sciureus*) lung culture, *Science* **195**:289.

Heineman, H. S., 1969, Herpes simplex neutralizing antibody—Quantitation of the complement dependent fraction in different phases of adult human infection, *J. Immunol.* **99**:214.

Hersch, E. M., Hanna, M. G., Jr., Gutterman, J. V., Mavligit, G., Yurconic, M., Jr., and Gschwind, C. R., 1974, Human immune response to active immunization with Rauscher leukemia virus. II. Humoral immunity, *J. Natl. Cancer Inst.* **53**:327.

Howitt, B. F., 1950, A nonspecific heat-labile factor in the serum neutralization test for Newcastle disease virus, *J. Immunol.* **64**:73.

Hugli, T. E., and Müller-Eberhard, H. J., 1978, Anaphylatoxins: C3a and C5a, *Adv. Immunol.* **26**:1.

Hummeler, K., and Ketler, A., 1958, Dissociation of poliomyelitis virus from neutralizing antibody, *Virology* **6**:297.

Hummeler, K., Anderson, T. F., and Brown, R. A., 1962, Identification of poliovirus particles of different antigenicity by specific agglutination as seen in the electron microscope, *Virology* **16**:84.

Humphrey, J. H., Dourmashkin, R. R., and Payne, S. N., 1967, The nature of lesions in cell membranes produced by action of C′ and antibody, in: *Immunopathology, V International Symposium* (P. A. Miescher and P. Grabar, eds.), p. 209, Grune and Stratton, New York.

Inoue, K., Kataoka, T., and Kinsky, S. C., 1971, Comparative responses of liposomes prepared with different ceramide antigens to antibody and complement, *Biochemistry* **10**:2574.

Jensen, F. C., Welsh, R. M., Cooper, N. R., and Oldstone, M. B. A., 1976, Lysis of oncornaviruses by human serum, *Comp. Leuk. Res. Bibl. Haematol.* **43**:438.

Joseph, B. S., Lampert, P. W., and Oldstone, M. B. A., 1975, Replication and persistence of measles virus in defined subpopulations of human leukocytes, *J. Virol.* **16**:1638.

Katz, D. H., 1977, *Lymphocyte Differentiation, Recognition and Regulation*, Academic Press, New York.

Kawakami, T. G., Huff, S. D., Buckley, P. M., Dungworth, D. L., Snyder, S. P., and Gilden, R. V., 1972, C-type virus associated with gibbon lymphosarcoma, *Nature (London) New Biol.* **235**:170.

Keller, R., 1968, Studies on the mechanism of the enzymatic reactivation of antibody-neutralized poliovirus, *J. Immunol.* **100**:1071.

Klenk, H.-D., Rott, R., and Becht, H., 1972, On the structure of the influenza virus envelope, *Virology* **47**:579.

Lachmann, P. J., and Rosen, F. S., 1978, Genetic defects of complement in man, in: *Springer Seminars in Immunopathology*, Vol. 1 (P. A. Miescher and H. J. Müller-Eberhard, eds.), p. 339, Springer-Verlag, New York.

Lafferty, K. J., 1963, The interaction between virus and antibody. II. Mechanism of the reaction, *Virology* **21**:76.

Lafferty, K. J., and Oertelis, S., 1963, The interaction between virus and antibody. III. Examination of virus–antibody complexes with the electron microscope, *Virology* **21**:91.

Laver, W. G., and Webster, R. G., 1966, The structure of influenza viruses. IV. Chemical studies of the host antigen, *Virology* **30**:104.

Leddy, J. P., Simons, R. L., and Douglas, R. G., 1977, Effect of selective complement deficiency on the rate of neutralization of enveloped viruses by human sera, *J. Immunol.* **118**:28.

Leong, J. C., Kane, J. P., Oleszko, O., and Levy, J. A., 1977, Antigen-specific nonimmunoglobulin factor that neutralizes xenotropic virus is associated with mouse serum lipoproteins, *Proc. Natl. Acad. Sci. USA* **74**:276.

Levy, J. A., Ihle, J. N., Oleszko, O., and Barnes, R. D., 1975, Virus-specific neutralization by a soluble non-immunoglobulin factor found naturally in normal mouse sera, *Proc. Natl. Acad. Sci. USA* **72**:5071.

Leymaster, G. R., and Ward, T. G., 1949, The effect of complement in the neutralization of mumps virus, *J. Immunol.* **61**:95.

Linscott, W. D., and Levinson, W. E., 1969, Complement components required for virus neutralization by early immunoglobulin antibody, *Proc. Natl. Acad. Sci. USA* **64**:520.

Marcus, R. L., Shin, H. S., and Mayer, M. M., 1971, An alternate complement pathway: C-3 cleaving activity, not due to $\overline{C4,2a}$, on endotoxic lipopolysaccharide after treatment with guinea pig serum; relation to properdin, *Proc. Natl. Acad. Sci. USA* **68**:1351.

Mayer, M., 1976, *The Nature and Significance of Complement Activation* (W. Pollack, ed.), Ortho Research Institute, International Symposium, Raritan, N.J.

McCarthy, K., and Germer, W. D., 1952, Two heat-labile factors in normal sera which neutralize variola virus, *Br. J. Exp. Pathol.* **33**:529.

Mills, B. J., and Cooper, N. R., 1978a, Analysis of the mechanism of VSV inactivation by human serum, *J. Immunol.* **120**:1786.

Mills, B. J., and Cooper, N. R., 1978b, Antibody-independent neutralization of vesicular stomatitis virus by human complement. I. Complement requirements, *J. Immunol.* **121**:1549.

Mueller, J. H., 1931, The effect of alexin in virus–antivirus mixtures, *J. Immunol.* **20**:17.

Müller-Eberhard, H. J., 1975, Complement, *Annu. Rev. Biochem.* **44**:697.

Nelson, R. A., 1958, An alternative mechanism for the properdin system, *J. Exp. Med.* **108**:515.

Neva, F. A., and Weller, T. H., 1964, Rubella, interferon and factors influencing the indirect neutralization test for rubella antibody, *J. Immunol.* **93**:466.

Notkins, A., 1975, *Viral Immunology and Immunopathology*, Academic Press, New York.

Notkins, A. L., Mergenhagen, S. E., and Howard, R. J., 1970, Effect of virus infections on the function of the immune system, *Annu. Rev. Microbiol.* **24**:525.

Notkins, A. L., Rosenthal, J., and Johnson, B., 1971, Rate-zonal centrifugation of herpes simplex virus–antibody complexes, *Virology* **43**:321.

Oldstone, M. B. A., 1975, Virus neutralization and virus-induced immune complex disease. Virus-antibody union resulting in immunoprotection or immunologic injury– two sides of the same coin, *Prog. Med. Virol.* **19**:84.

Oldstone, M. B. A., and Lampert, P. W., 1979, Antibody-mediated complement-dependent lysis of virus infected cells, in: *Springer Seminars in Immunopathology* (P. A. Miescher and H. J. Müller-Eberhard, eds.), Springer-Verlag, New York, in press.

Oldstone, M. B. A., Cooper, N. R., and Larson, D. L., 1974, Formation and biologic role of polyoma virus–antibody complexes, *J. Exp. Med.* **140**:549.

Orozlan, S., and Gilden, R. V., 1970, Immune virolysis: Effect of antibody and complement on C-type RNA virus, *Science* **168**:1478.

Osler, A. G., 1976, *Foundations of Immunology Series*, Prentice-Hall, Englewood Cliffs, N.J.

Osler, A. G., and Sandberg, A. L., 1973, Alternate complement pathways, *Prog. Allergy* **17**:51.

Ozaki, Y., and Tabeyi, K., 1967, Studies on the neutralization of Japanese encephalitis virus. I. Application of kinetic neutralization to the measurement of the neutralizing potency of antiserum, *J. Immunol.* **98**:1218.

Parkman, P. D., Mundon, F. K., McCowan, J. M., and Buescher, E. L., 1964, Studies of rubella. II. Neutralization of the virus, *J. Immunol.* **93**:608.

Perrin, L. H., Joseph, B. S., Cooper, N. R., and Oldstone, M. B. A., 1976, Mechanism of injury of virus infected cells by antiviral antibody and complement: Participation of IgG, Fab'2 and the alternative complement pathway, *J. Exp. Med.* **143**:1027.

Pillemer, L., Blum, L., Lepow, I. H., Ross, O. A., Todd, E. W., and Wardlaw, A. C., 1954, The properdin system and immunity. I. Demonstration and isolation of a new serum protein, properdin, and its role in immune phenomena, *Science* **120**:279.

Radwan, A. I., and Burger, D., 1973, The complement-requiring neutralization of equine arteritis virus by late antisera, *Virology* **51**:71.

Radwan, A. I., and Crawford, T. B., 1974, The mechanisms of neutralization of sensitized equine arteritis virus by complement components, *J. Gen. Virol.* **25**:229.

Radwan, A. I., Burger, D., and Davis, W. C., 1973, The fate of sensitized equine arteritis virus following neutralization by complement or anti-IgG serum, *Virology* **53**:372.

Rawls, W., and Tompkins, W., 1975, Destruction of virus infected cells by antibody and complement, in: *Viral Immunology and Immunopathology* (A. Notkins, ed.), p. 99, Academic Press, New York.

Rawls, W. E., Desmyter, J., and Melnick, J. L., 1967, Rubella virus neutralization by plaque reduction, *Proc. Soc. Exp. Biol. Med.* **124**:167.

Reid, K. B. M., and Porter, R. R., 1975, The structure and mechanism of activation of the first component of complement, in: *Contemporary Topics in Molecular Immunology*, Vol. 4 (F. P. Inman and W. J. Mandy, eds.), p. 1, Plenum Press, New York.

Rott, R., Drzeniek, R., Saber, M. S., and Reichert, E., 1966, Blood group substances, Forssman and mononucleosis antigens in lipid-containing RNA viruses, *Arch. Gesamte Virusforsch.* **19**:273.

Sabin, A., 1950, The dengue group of viruses and its family relationships, *Bacteriol. Rev.* **14**:225.

Sandberg, A. L., Osler, A. G., Shin, H. S., and Oliveira, B., 1970, The biologic activities of guinea pig antibodies. II. Modes of complement interaction with $\gamma 1$ and $\gamma 2$ immunoglobulins, *J. Immunol.* **104**:329.

Schluederberg, A., Ajello, C., and Evans, B., 1976, Fate of rubella genome ribonucleic acid after immune and nonimmune virolysis in the presence of ribonuclease, *Infect. Immun.* **14**:1097.

Schreiber, R. D., Pangburn, M. K., Lasavre, P. H., and Müller-Eberhard, H. J., 1978, Initiation of the alternative pathway of complement: Recognition of activators by bound C3b and assembly of the entire pathway from six isolated proteins, *J. Exp. Med.* **75**:3948.

Sherwin, S. A., Benveniste, R. E., and Todaro, G. J., 1978, Complement-mediated lysis of type-C virus: Effect of primate and human sera on various retroviruses, *Int. J. Cancer* **21**:6.

Silverstein, S., 1970, Macrophages and viral immunity, *Semin. Hematol.* **7**:185.

Simpson, R. W., and Hauser, R. E., 1966, Influence of lipids on the viral phenotype. I. Interactions of myxoviruses and their lipid constituents with phospholipases, *Virology* **30**:684.

Stollar, V., 1975, Immune lysis of Sindbis virus, *Virology* **66**:620.

Svehag, S.-E., 1968, Formation and dissociation of virus–antibody complexes with special reference to the neutralization process, *Prog. Med. Virol.* **10**:1.

Taniguchi, S., and Yoshino, K., 1965, Studies on the neutralization of herpes simplex virus. II. Analysis of complement as the antibody-potentiating factor, *Virology* **26**:54.

Thiry, L., Clerc, J. C.-L., Content, J., and Tack, L., 1978, Factors which influence inactivation of vesicular stomatitis virus by fresh human serum, *Virology* **87**:384.

Todaro, G. J., Sherr, C. J., and Benveniste, R. E., 1976, Baboons and their close relatives are unusual among primates in their ability to release nondefective endogenous type C viruses, *Virology* **72**:278.

Toussaint, A. J., and Muschel, L. H., 1962, Studies on the bacteriophage neutralizing activity of serums. I. An assay procedure for normal antibody and complement, *J. Immunol.* **89**:27.

Wallis, C., and Melnick, J. L., 1971, Herpesvirus neutralization: The role of complement, *J. Immunol.* **107**:1235.

Wedgwood, R. J., Ginsberg, H. S., and Pillemer, L., 1956, The properdin system and immunity. VI. The inactivation of Newcastle disease virus by the properdin system, *J. Exp. Med.* **104**:107.

Welsh, R. M., Jr., 1977, Host cell modification of lymphocytic choriomeningitis virus and Newcastle disease virus altering viral inactivation by human complement, *J. Immunol.* **118**:348.

Welsh, R. M., Jr., Cooper, N. R., Jensen, F. C., and Oldstone, M. B. A., 1975, Human serum lyses RNA tumour viruses, *Nature (London)* **257**:612.

Welsh, R. M., Cooper, N. R., Jensen, F. C., and Oldstone, M. B. A., 1976a, Inactivation and lysis of oncornaviruses by human serum, *Virology* **74**:432.

Welsh, R. M., Jr., Lampert, P. W., Burner, P. A., and Oldstone, M. B. A., 1976b, Antibody-complement interactions with purified lymphocytic choriomeningitis virus, *Virology* **73**:59.

Westaway, E. G., 1965, The neutralization of arboviruses. I. Neutralization in homologous virus-serum mixtures with two group B arboviruses, *Virology* **26**:517.

Wheelock, E. F., and Toy, S. T., 1973, Participation of lymphocytes in viral infections, *Adv. Immunol.* **16**:123.

Whitman, L., 1947, The neutralization of western equine encephalomyelitis virus by human convalescent serum: The influence of heat labile substances in serum on the neutralization index, *J. Immunol.* **56**:97.

Wilson, G. S., and Miles, A., 1975, *Principles of Bacteriology and Immunity*, Vol. II, p. 1438, Williams and Wilkins, Baltimore.

Yoshino, K., and Taniguchi, S., 1965, Studies on the neutralization of herpes simplex virus. I. Appearance of neutralizing antibodies having different grades of complement requirement, *Virology* **26**:44.

Yoshino, K., and Taniguchi, S., 1969, Effect of complement upon viral neutralization, *J. Immunol.* **102**:1341.

Zinkernagel, R. M., and Welsh, R. M., 1976, H-2 compatibility requirement for virus-specific T cell-mediated effector functions *in vivo*. I. Specificity of T cells conferring antiviral protection against lymphocytic choriomeningitis virus is associated with H-2K and H-2D, *J. Immunol.* **117**:1495.

CHAPTER 4

Cellular Immune Response to Viruses and the Biological Role of Polymorphic Major Transplantation Antigens

R. M. Zinkernagel

Department of Immunopathology
Scripps Clinic and Research Foundation
La Jolla, California 92037

1. INTRODUCTION

The various categories of infectious agents that confront higher vertebrate hosts are quite different with respect to acuteness and rapidity of the disease process they incite. Consequently, the evolutionary or selective pressure that ultimately determines whether the relationship between parasite and host becomes symbiotic or parasitic is also decisive in shaping a particular part of the host physiology specifically for that function. Since most parasites have an enormously faster generation cycle than the vertebrate host, the parasites' adaptive capacity is much the greater of the two. The ultimate equilibrium of the host–parasite relationship and their relative capacity to adapt mutually

Abbreviations used in this chapter: *Ir* genes, immune response genes; *MHC*, major histocompatibility complex; T cells, thymus-derived lymphocytes; self-H, major transplantation antigen; X, foreign antigenic determinant; HLA, human histocompatibility antigen; LCM, lymphocytic choriomeningitis; Ig, immunoglobulin; ADCC, antibody-dependent cell-mediated cytotoxicity; NK, natural killer; SV40, simian virus 40; MSV, murine sarcoma virus; *ts*, temperature sensitive; VSV, vesicular stomatitis virus.

are obviously determined by both parties. What establishes this balance is poorly understood, but, viewed teleologically, survival of both parasite and host seems to keep the relationship in check. Within the vertebrate host whose reactive systems are called into play by such infections, immune responses by antibodies and cells (reviewed in Notkins, 1975, Bloom and Rager-Zisman, 1975; Blanden *et al.*, 1976*b*), nonspecific resistance by macrophages (Lindenmann *et al.*, 1978; Cheers and McKenzie, 1978) or other cells, past and present experience with infection, as well as concurrent infections all play some part.

Jenner (1978) proved unequivocally that infecting a human with cowpox virus produced only mild disease and prevented later infection by lethal smallpox virus; however, the biological events that produced this immunity were only imagined. Nevertheless, inquiry into the human reaction to virus infection motivated considerable experimentation by those who were to become immunologists and, unquestionably, laid much of the basis for the development of immunology into a distinct field of research.

The path of this research has recently yielded the unexpected information that the major histocompatibility gene complex (*MHC*) is the primary group of genes that control cellular immune responsiveness and specificity (reviewed in Paul and Benacerraf, 1977; Munro and Bright, 1976). Originally, the *MHC* genes were assigned the relatively obscure role of producing antigens that became the targets of rejection of foreign, grafted material or of tumor cells (reviewed in Klein, 1975; Shreffler and David, 1975). Instead, MHC antigens—the molecular products of *MHC* genes—are now being viewed tentatively as the central hinges on which all cell-mediated immune responses turn in mice (Katz *et al.*, 1973*a,b*; Zinkernagel and Doherty, 1974; Miller *et al.*, 1975; Zinkernagel, 1978) and also in humans (Goulmy *et al.*, 1976; McMichael *et al.*, 1977; Dickmeiss *et al.*, 1977; Bergholtz and Thorsby, 1977).

Most of the research that traces the intertwining story of MHC antigens and immune responses to viruses involves the use of mice. The *MHC* of mice has been designated *H-2* and is subdivided into several component parts. Those subdivisions that are most relevant to this discussion are *H-2K* and *H-2D*, whose products participate in the murine immune response to viruses (reviewed in Shreffler and David, 1975; Klein, 1975) and which code for major transplantation antigens that are involved in graft rejection. Less importantly for our purposes is the *H-2I* region, the products of which mediate protection against intracellular bacterial infections and regulate certain cellular immune responsiveness assessed by antibody production.

2. CELLULAR IMMUNITY AND THE MAJOR HISTOCOMPATIBILITY GENE COMPLEX

MHC antigens, as they participate in graft rejection, seem only to harm the host and often function to negate otherwise curative organ transplants in humans. Because such antigens appear in all higher vertebrates, one must believe that they have a biological function that is important in survival. Many attempts have been made to formulate one general concept to explain this biological role. Mitchison (1954) hypothesized that the delayed-type hypersensitivity reaction against chemicals or tuberculin might well be a cellular reaction exclusively against the antigen on cell surfaces and thus parallel the graft rejection. Later, fostered by Thomas' speculation (1959) on immune surveillance, Lawrence (1959) devised the self plus X hypothesis. He theorized that intracellular infection could alter self antigens, rendering them functionally comparable to foreign histocompatibility antigens that could, thereby, trigger an autoaggressive response.

Shortly thereafter it was discovered that susceptibility to tumor induction is linked to major transplantation antigens (Sjögren and Ringertz, 1961; Lilly et al., 1964). Bryere and Williams (1964) and Svet-Moldavsky and Hamburg (1964) explained that the rejection of syngeneic virus-infected cell or tissue grafts resembles that of allograft rejection. At about the same time, Levine et al. (1963) and McDevitt and Sela (1965) came to believe that antibody responses are regulated by immune response (*Ir*) genes, which later were mapped to the *MHC* (McDevitt and Chinitz, 1969).

During the 1960s it also became clear that various classes of lymphocytes underwent complex interactions during an immune response. Thus selected populations of T cells heightened immune responses (helper T cells), diminished or banished the responses (suppressor T cells), or killed immunologically unacceptable cells (cytotoxic T cells) (reviewed in Gershon, 1974; Cantor and Boyse, 1977; Cerottini and Brunner, 1974; Katz, 1977). An important rule that governed such lymphocyte interactions was discovered by Kindred and Shreffler (1972) and later elaborated by Katz, Hamaoka, Benacerraf, and co-workers. They found that T-helper cells usually support B cells in producing antibody only when both cell types share the same major murine histocompatibility locus (*H-2*) (Katz et al. 1973a; Katz and Benacerraf, 1975; Erb and Feldman, 1975). Independently, Shevach and Rosenthal (1973) found that the proliferation of T cells, in response to a given antigen, is not only related to (or dependent on) that inciting antigen but also dependent on the T cell and the antigen carrier macrophage sharing the same *MHC* (Shevach and Rosenthal, 1973; Rosenthal and Shevach, 1973). Both T-cell–B-cell interactions and T-cell–macrophage interactions were later shown to be specific for the cells' surface antigenic determinants, coded in the *I* gene region of the *MHC* or the equivalent thereof (Katz and Benacerraf, 1975). Since both of these T-cell functions were known to be under the control of *Ir* genes, and both mapped to the same subregions of the *MHC*, these distinct phenomena appeared to be interdependent (Katz *et al.*, 1973*b*; Rosenthal and Shevach, 1973). The last addition to this sequence of experiments linking T-cell-mediated immunity and major transplantation antigens derives from studies of the T-cell-mediated immune response to virus. The general rule emerging is that T cells generated to kill virus-infected target cells can do so only when the viral antigens appear on cells whose *H-2* matches the *H-2* type of the T-cell donor. That is, once invaded by virus, the host's infected cells are killed by T lymphocytes in an immune response that is *H-2* restricted in mice (Zinkernagel and Doherty, 1974, 1975; Doherty and Zinkernagel, 1974, 1975). This is true for all murine virus-specific cytotoxic T cells examined: e.g., mouse pox virus (Blanden *et al.*, 1975), vaccinia virus (Koszinowski and Ertl, 1975), Sendai virus (Doherty and Zinkernagel, 1976, Koszinowski *et al.*, 1976; Schrader and Edelman, 1977), influenza virus (Doherty *et al.*, 1977; Ennis *et al.*, 1977; Braciale, 1977), rabies virus (Wiktor *et al.*, 1977), SV40 (Trinchieri *et al.*, 1976; Pfizenmaier *et al.*, 1977), Friend leukemia virus (Blank *et al.*, 1976), murine sarcoma virus (Gomard *et al.*, 1976), vesicular stomatitis virus (VSV) (Zinkernagel *et al.*, 1977*d*), Coxsackie virus (Wong *et al.*, 1977), herpesvirus (Pfizenmaier *et al.*, 1977), and many more. Independently Shearer found that the specific reaction to trinitrophenyl (TNP) by cytotoxic T cells is similarly restricted (Shearer, 1974; Shearer *et al.*, 1975, 1976). Subsequently, the same restriction was found for cytotoxic T cells directed against weak transplantation antigens instead of viral antigens (Bevan, 1975; Simpson and Gordon, 1977; von Boehmer, 1977).

In mice, all T-cell functions that have been tested so far are *H-2* restricted; that is, T cells that act as helpers, that proliferate after exposure to antigen on macrophages, that lyse target cells, or that are responsible for delayed-type hypersensitivity express two specificities. These T cells are specific (1) for self-MHC structures and (2) for foreign antigens X. This dual specificity appears to be universal in higher vertebrates. For example, and not surprisingly, virus-specific cytotoxicity in rats is strain restricted and probably restricted by the rat *MHC* (*Ag-B*) (Zinkernagel *et al.*, 1977*b*; Marshak *et al.*, 1977). Furthermore, strong evidence exists that the *MHC* restriction is also operative in chickens (Toivanen *et al.*, 1974*a,b*; Wainberg *et al.*, 1974). In humans, whose *MHC* is denoted *HLA*, the first indication that the *HLA* restriction may govern T cells has been found for cytotoxic lymphocytes against cells bearing the male H-Y antigen (Goulmy *et al.*, 1976), and more recently evidence has emerged that influenza-virus-specific cytotoxic T cells (McMichael *et al.*, 1977; Dickmeiss *et al.*, 1977) or T cells from humans proliferating when exposed to PPD (Bergholtz and Thorsby, 1977) are *HLA* restricted.

The main characteristics of the *MHC* restriction of T cells that perform critical biological function of many immune responses are outlined in the following paragraphs.

2.1. Dual Specificity

T cells express specificity for a foreign antigenic determinant X and for an *MHC*-coded self-major transplantation antigen (self-H). Several hypotheses have been formulated to explain this finding. Possibly effector T cells possess two recognition sites, anti-X and anti-self-H. Or T cells express a single recognition site for a neoantigenic determinant formed by a complex of X plus self-H antigens (Zinkernagel and Doherty, 1974; Schrader *et al.*, 1975; Doherty *et al.*, 1976*a,b*; Janeway *et al.*, 1976; Paul and Benacerraf, 1977; Langman, 1978; Cohn and Epstein, 1978). Although the dual recognition version seems more probable at this moment, the single T-cell receptor model is not formally dismissed.

The restriction specificity anti-self-H is for distinct gene products of the *MHC* and correlates more or less with the T-cell effector function. Most lytic (cytotoxic) T cells are generally restricted to interacting with the *K* or *D* gene region products of *H-2* or the *A* or *B* products of *HLA* (Alter *et al.*, 1973; Nabholz *et al.*, 1974; Blanden *et al.*, 1975; Shearer *et al.*, 1975; Zinkernagel and Doherty, 1975; Bach *et al.*, 1976). Most nonlytic T cells that are involved in T-cell–B-cell interactions, in delayed-type hypersensitivity, in proliferative response to soluble antigens, and in the activation of macrophages are restricted to interactions with H-2I or HLA-D (Katz and Benacerraf, 1975, Miller *et al.*, 1975, 1976; Schwartz and Paul, 1976).

2.2. Clonality of Anti-X and Anti-Self-H Specificity

Many experiments document the clonal quality of dual specificity, i.e., a single T cell expresses only one anti-X and one anti-self-H specificity. Cytotoxic T cells specific for vaccinia virus do not kill cells infected with lymphocytic choriomeningitis virus (LCMV) or Sendai virus, and *vice versa* (Doherty *et al.*, 1967*a*). Similarly, in the viral immune reactions by inbred mice, the T cells' anti-self-H specificity is stringent for a particular *H-2* type.

2.3. Differentiation of Restriction Specificities in the Thymus

The anti-self-H restriction specificity of T cells is not determined genetically by the T cells' genome but is acquired or selected during the period when T cells mature in the thymus (Bevan, 1977; Zinkernagel *et al.*, 1978*a,b,c*). For example, lymphohemopoietic stem cells originating from heterozygote ($H-2^k \times H-2^b$) F_1 hybrid mice but removed from their natural host and displaced to mature in the thymus of $H-2^k$ type mouse express restriction specificity for $H-2^k$ but not $H-2^b$. The radioresistant portion of the thymus plays a crucial role in this selection (Zinkernagel *et al.*, 1978*a,b*).

2.4. Restriction Specificity of Effector T Cells

The restriction specificity of effector T cells is selected according to the *MHC*-coded-self available in the thymus. Whether all thymically selected restriction specificities are expressed by immunocompetent T cells depends on several factors that are not fully understood as yet. It appears that lymphohemopoietic cells possessing the same MHC as the thymus are essential to induce full T-cell maturation and to present antigen appropriately to T cells (Zinkernagel, 1978).

2.5. Regulation of Immune Responsiveness

Effector T-cell activity is regulated by immune response (*Ir*) genes (reviewed by Benacerraf and McDevitt, 1972; Benacerraf and Katz, 1975; Benacerraf and Germain, 1978). *Ir* genes empowered to control effector T cells have the following general characteristics: (1) They map within the *MHC* (McDevitt and Chinitz, 1969). (2) They seem to be located in or close to the *MHC* subregion that codes restriction specificity: *K* or *D* subregions code *Ir* genes regulating lytic T cells (Bubbers *et al.*, 1977, 1978; Gomard *et al.*, 1977; Doherty *et al.*, 1978; Zinkernagel *et al.*, 1978*d*); *I* subregions code *Ir* genes controlling nonlytic

T cells (McDevitt *et al.*, 1972; Shevach and Rosenthal, 1973; Miller *et al.*, 1975, 1976). (3) Unresponsiveness is dominant. Therefore, T cells from an F_1 (responder × nonresponder) donor cooperate only with B cells (Katz *et al.*, 1973*b*) or macrophages (Shevach and Rosenthal, 1973) of responder *H-2* types or lyse infected target cells of responder *H-2* types (Zinkernagel et al. 1978*d*). (4) Responsiveness or *Ir* phenotype is determined not by the genotype of the T cell but by the genotype of the thymic environment that selects that cell's restriction specificity (von Boehmer *et al.*, 1978; Billings *et al.*, 1978; Zinkernagel *et al.*, 1978*e*; Zinkernagel, 1978). Therefore, selection of the restriction specificity anti-self-H and determination of the *Ir* phenotype seem to be intimately linked.

3. ANTIGENS INVOLVED IN IMMUNE RECOGNITION: VIRAL ANTIGENS AND SELF ANTIGENS CODED BY THE MAJOR HISTOCOMPATIBILITY GENE COMPLEX

3.1. Major Transplantation Antigens and Their Possible Function

T cells play a major role in early host defense against acute virus infections. These T cells kill infected cells only if two conditions are fulfilled; the target cell to be lysed must be infected with the virus that incited T-cell formation and must express the same self-K or self-D as the donor of the cytotoxic T cells. The antiviral effect of T cells *in vivo* probably occurs through T-cell-mediated destruction of freshly infected cells during the eclipse phase of the infectious cycle (Blanden *et al.*, 1975; Zinkernagel, 1977). In fact, viral antigens have been detected on cell surfaces well before viral progeny assemble (Ada *et al.*, 1976; Koszinowski *et al.*, 1977; Schrader and Edelman, 1977; Hapel *et al.*, 1978), and virus-specific cytotoxic T cells have been shown to reduce drastically production of infectious virus if mixed with acutely vaccinia-infected target cells *in vitro* during but not after the eclipse phase (Zinkernagel and Althage, 1977). Since viruses as a class of infectious agents may infect all kinds of host cells, any self marker that might be involved in cell lysis would have to be expressed on all cells, even though different species of virus preferentially infect distinct cell types or organs. The serologically defined major transplantation agencies or the *K*, *D* (or *A*, *B* in humans) products seem to fulfill the requirements excellently; they are (1) ubiquitous and are (2) receptors for lytic signals that are delivered in an immunologically specific fashion.

In contrast to viruses, intracellular bacteria or fungi do not undergo an eclipse phase (and therefore cell lysis cannot eliminate the parasites), nor can they infect all cells. Since these parasites must be phagocytosed to become intracellular, their antigens probably associate only with cell membranes of phagocytes. Therefore, such parasites are best handled by intracellular digestion as documented by the classical studies of Mackaness (1964, 1969). The self cell-surface marker involved should (1) be expressed on phagocytic cells, e.g., macrophages, and (2) function as receptors for *nonlytic* but digestive enzyme activating signals. The *I*-region-coded antigens expressed on certain macrophages seem to comply with this requirement. Similarly, *I* structures on B cells may serve as receptors for B-cell-specific differentiation signals. That is, T cells may operate in an antigen-specific way to trigger B cells so that they begin synthesizing immunoglobulin (Ig) or switch from IgM to IgG production. Therefore, major transplantation antigens may be viewed as an array of receptors for cell-specific differentiation or lytic signals that are triggered by antigen-specific T cells (Zinkernagel *et al.*, 1977c; Zinkernagel, 1977).

3.2. Experimental Virus Infection

Many reviews describe model infections in mice (Blanden, 1974; Doherty *et al.* 1976a; Zinkernagel and Doherty, 1977; Koszinowski *et al.*, 1976; Schrader *et al.*, 1976). Viruses that infect mice systematically grow for the first few days in primary target organs, e.g., skin. These viruses then spread via lymph nodes to secondary lymphoid organs, e.g., spleen, and other secondary target organs, e.g., liver and skin. After some 2–4 days, virus titers start to decrease in blood and organs, and cell-mediated immunity usually begins (Fenner, 1968, Blanden, 1974). The T-cell activity measured *in vitro* by ^{51}Cr release (Cerottini and Brunner, 1974) reflects accurately the time when test animals acquire cellular protection or develop delayed-type hypersensitivity *in vivo* (for reviews, see Doherty and Zinkernagel, 1974; Blanden, 1974; Zinkernagel and Doherty, 1977). The present analysis of T-cell function disregards many other specific and nonspecific immune mechanisms that accompany infection such as antibodies (Notkins, 1975), antibody-dependent cell-mediated cytotoxicity (ADCC) (Perlmann *et al.*, 1972), activated macrophages (Mackaness, 1964, 1969; Blanden, 1974), lymphokines as exemplified by interferon (Notkins, 1975; Bloom and Rager-Zisman, 1975), natural killer (NK) cell activity (Herberman *et al.*, 1977; Welsh and Zinkernagel, 1977; Welsh, 1978), and so on.

However, these mechanisms should be kept in mind, because virus-specific cytotoxic T cells may well be most efficient in controlling early virus spread, whereas these other mechanisms may substitute for T cells to some extent or may protect against reinfection. Also, all viruses do not cause animals to generate detectable levels of cytotoxic T cells for reasons that are not understood (Röllinghoff *et al.*, 1977).

Tumor-virus-specific cytotoxic T cells are induced *in vivo* by injecting mice either with virus (Leclerc *et al.*, 1972, 1973; de Landazuri and Herberman, 1972; Herberman *et al.*, 1973; Gomard *et al.*, 1976, 1977; Plata *et al.*, 1974, 1975, 1976) or with virus-expressing tumor cells (Schrader and Edelman, 1977; Blank *et al.*, 1976; Bubbers *et al.*, 1977, 1978). The kinetics of resulting T-cell expression are prolonged compared with those of acute virus infections of mice and are usually substantially weaker. Peaks of such activity are reached by about 10–14 days after infection (Leclerc *et al.*, 1973; Lavrin *et al.*, 1973). Because of the relatively low activity, secondary *in vitro* mixed lymphocyte stimulation was introduced as a supplementary method of detection and resulted in selection of very highly active tumor-specific cytotoxic T cell (Plata *et al.*, 1975, 1976).

The effector lymphocytes involved in tumor elimination *in vivo* and *in vitro* may belong to more than one class of lymphocytes (Herberman *et al.*, 1973; Leclerc *et al.*, 1973; Plata *et al.*, 1974). At least some effector lymphocytes are T cells since they are sensitive to anti-T-cell serum plus complement treatment but not to anti-immunoglobulin treatment, as shown for Moloney sarcoma virus (MSV) (Herberman *et al.*, 1973; Leclerc *et al.*, 1973), for Friend leukemia virus (Blank *et al.*, 1976), for SV40 (Trinchieri *et al.*, 1976; Pfizenmaier *et al.*, 1977), and for mammary tumor virus (Stutman *et al.*, 1977). These T cells are virus specific, and, when tested in the short-term ^{51}Cr release assay, their killing is usually *MHC* restricted to *D* or *K* at least in the systems tested—MSV (Plata *et al.*, 1975, 1976; Gomard *et al.*, 1976, 1977), Friend leukemia virus (Blank *et al.*, 1976; Bubbers *et al.*, 1978), SV40 (Trinchieri *et al.*, 1976), and mammary tumor virus (Stutman *et al.*, 1977).

3.3. Virally Induced Target Antigens

Virus-induced cell-surface antigens have been studied for many years, and the antigens of certain viruses (e.g., influenza virus and VSV) expressed on cell surfaces or found only in or under the membrane have been analyzed quite thoroughly. Applying this

knowledge to answer some of the questions about the specificity of
antiviral cytotoxic T lymphocytes is a slow process. Efforts have been
made to (1) analyze minimal viral requirements for target antigen
induction (Ada *et al.*, 1976; Jackson *et al.*, 1976; Koszinowski *et al.*,
1977; Sugamura *et al.*, 1977, 1978; Hapel *et al.*, 1978). (2) use mutant
viruses that have defined defects in expressing certain viral antigens
(Hale *et al.*, 1978; Zinkernagel *et al.*, 1978*f*), (3) block killing of
infected cells with specific antisera, and (4) assess cross-reactivities
between unrelated or closely related but serologically distinct viruses by
directly testing cytotoxic cross-reactivity (Doherty *et al.*, 1976*a*; Ennis
et al., 1977; Braciale, 1977; Gomard *et al.*, 1977; Zinkernagel *et al.*,
1977*d*, 1978*f*) or by selectively restimulating simple subspecificities
with serologically or genetically defined recombinant viruses (Ennis *et
al.*, 1977; Zweerink *et al.*, 1977).

3.3.1. Minimal Requirements for Target-Cell Induction

How much of the virus replication cycle must occur in a cell so
that the virally induced antigens recognizable by cytotoxic T lymphocytes appear on target cells? For some viruses no replication at all is
necessary, for example, for Sendai virus, a parainfluenza virus with a
great capacity to fuse with cell membranes (Schrader *et al.*, 1976; Gething *et al.*, 1978; Sugamura *et al.*, 1977, 1978). Ultraviolet-light-inacti-
vated Sendai virus does not generate infectious progeny but still can
render target cells susceptible to virus-specific lysis (Schrader and
Edelman, 1977; Koszinowski *et al.*, 1977). Mere adsorption of Sendai
by the cell is not sufficient, but fusion is mandatory for inactivated
Sendai virus to render targets susceptible to lysis (Gething *et al.*, 1978;
Sugamura *et al.*, 1977, 1978). Thus proper insertion of the hemagglu-
tinins into the cell membrane by fusion is crucial.

These results show clearly that, for certain viruses at least, the relevant antigen determinant (1) is present in or on a viral particle and (2)
can be inserted from "without"; actual infection is not needed to induce
expression of viral antigen from "within" the cell (Koszinowski *et al.*,
1977; Schrader *et al.*, 1976). This renders the explanation unlikely that
the antigens recognized by T cells are generated by glycosyltranferases
or other cell enzyme systems that modify viral antigens during synthesis
in the cell or, alternatively, that viral infection alters these enzymes
specifically so as to change the glycosylation pattern of the host cells'
surface antigen (Rothenberg, 1976; Blanden *et al.*, 1976*a*).

In accord with evidence from Sendai virus experiments, Ada and co-workers demonstrated that target antigen induction occurred within 30 min or so after vaccinia infection and did not need active DNA synthesis (Ada *et al.*, 1976; Jackson *et al.*, 1976). Also, Koszinowski and Ertl (1976) used specific antisera against early or late vaccinia-induced cell-surface antigens or against vaccinia virus to show that only antisera to viral antigens induced soon after infection but none of the other antisera could block T-cell cytotoxicity. This evidence somewhat conflicts with data from Hapel *et al.* (1978), who extended the observation of Ada *et al.* by showing that merely fusing a large amount of viral envelope was quite sufficient to render cells susceptible to lysis and that no virally induced protein synthesis, not even of the early type, was necessary.

These experiments could not be repeated with VSV (Zinkernagel *et al.*, 1978*f*) or LCMV even when very high multiplicities of infection were used. The simplest explanation for this failure is that neither of these viruses fuses to any detectable degree with the cell membrane, and therefore, to appear on the cell surface, viral antigens must be induced from "within" the cells. This notion is supported by the fact that interference with the replication of VSV inhibits the appearance of appropriate target antigens (Zinkernagel *et al.*, 1977*d*). Thus, infecting virus can either imprint the cell surface directly with antigens or induce them very early during infection. Either circumstance would render the host cells susceptible to immunological attack before viral progeny assemble (Ada *et al.*, 1976; Kees and Blanden, 1976; Zinkernagel and Althage, 1977) during the so-called eclipse phase of viral infection. This has been formally proven experimentally *in vitro* with vaccinia virus. Vaccinia virus progeny appeared about 3–4 hr after infection of L-cell fibroblasts. If these targets were exposed to cytotoxic T cells during the eclipse phase, lysis was great and production of viral progeny was low. In contrast, if these targets were overlaid with the T cells starting at 4 hr after infection, cytolysis was still extensive, but the number of generated or released viral progeny equaled that of infected cells not combined with T cells (Zinkernagel and Althage, 1977). This sequence clearly suggests that the antiviral activity of cytotoxic T cells *in vivo* is probably mediated via target-cell killing during the virus's eclipse phase, as discussed earlier.

3.3.2. Virus Mutants

A different approach for analyzing virally induced target antigens is to use temperature-sensitive (*ts*) mutant viruses that either fail to express certain viral antigens or express a mutant variant of a normal antigen.

Recently, Hale *et al.* (1978) and we (Zinkernagel *et al.*, 1978*f*) used VSV-Indiana *ts* mutants to study the nature of viral target antigens. VSV codes for three major viral proteins, the nucleocapsid, the matrix protein, and the glycoprotein; the last is the only one of the three expressed on the cell surface. Two groups of *ts* mutants are of particular interest. Among the first group, *tsM301* (Hale *et al.*, 1978) and *tsG31*) (Pringle, 1970) fail at the nonpermissive temperature of 31–33°C to express the matrix protein but do express both nucleocapsid antigen and the glycoprotein. Cells infected with these mutants at the nonpermissive temperature were lysed by VSV-Indiana-immune T cells, although to a slightly lesser extent than when infected at the permissive temperature. Whether this difference, which was obvious at lower multiplicities of infection with *tsG31*, is due to less efficient adsorption and infection at the lower temperature or reflects faulty or absent matrix protein underneath the cell membrane that prevents optimal distribution of the glycoprotein is unresolved.

The second group of mutants, *tsM501* and *ts045*, fails to develop mature glycoprotein on the cell membrane at the nonpermissive temperature but expresses the matrix protein and nucleocapside antigens (Lafay, 1974; Perlman and Huang, 1974; Knipe *et al.*, 1977). Target cells infected with these mutants at moderately low multiplicities of infections (20–3 : 1) and at nonpermissive temperature were not lysed by virus-specific T cells. Under these conditions, these target cells were also quite resistant to lysis by anti-VSV antibodies plus complement. Additional analyses of the mutant *tl17* (Zavada, 1972), which possesses a mutant glycoprotein, was unrevealing since VSV-Indiana wild-type immune T cells lysed the targets infected with *tl17* as well as wild-type VSV-infected targets (Zinkernagel *et al.*, 1978*f*). Nevertheless, these combined results support but do not prove unequivocally that the glycoprotein is a major target antigen for VSV specific cytotoxic T cells.

3.3.3.   Comparison of Serological and Cytotoxic T-Cell Specificity

The nature of the viral antigen recognized by virus-specific cytotoxic T cells is poorly understood. In many ways these lymphocytes seem to be comparable in specificities to serological specificities. However, since quantification of specificity or cross-reactivity is difficult because of the technical limitations of cytotoxicity assays, most of the results must be interpreted with great reservation. The following methods have been used to analyze T-cell specificity. T cells were tested for cross-protection *in vivo*, for specificity in cytotoxicity assays *in vitro*, or during restimulation in mixed lymphocyte cultures.

It has been known for some time that ectromelia-virus-immune T cells do not protect from LCMV infection (Mims and Blanden, 1972). Experiments with cytotoxic virus-specific effector T cells demonstrated the great degree of specificity attained during ectromelia and LCMV infections (Doherty *et al.*, 1976a). These results also apply to Sendai virus (Doherty and Zinkernagel, 1976).

To analyze antigenic specificity in more detail, influenza viruses were used, and the outcome of this research revealed that the cytotoxic T cells generated *in vivo* and *in vitro* were T cells which were specific for hemagglutinin antigens or for the shared matrix protein (Doherty *et al.*, 1977; Braciale, 1977; Ennis *et al.*, 1977).

More recent experiments with the two serologically different VSV strains, Indiana and New Jersey, revealed that virus-specific cytotoxic T cells generated in these infections are generally comparable in specificities to the serological classifications (Zinkernagel *et al.* 1978*f*; Rosenthal *et al.*, unpublished). An as yet unexplained asymmetry of specificity was observed, the degree of which appeared to depend on the *H-2* type of the mice studied. For example, *H-2^b* VSV-Indiana-immune T cells lysed Indiana-infected targets but also to a substantial extent New Jersey–infected targets. This cross-reactivity was smaller in cells from *H-2^d* type mice. New Jersey–immune *H-2^b* or *H-2^d* murine cells lysed New Jersey–infected targets much better than Indiana-infected targets. The reasons for these asymmetries are not understood and contrast with the fact that these two strains do not cross-react in terms of virus neutralization (Cartwright and Brown, 1972) or antibody-plus-complement-mediated lysis (Zinkernagel *et al.*, 1978*f*).

Buchmeier and Oldstone (1978) studied T-cell specificity and found no cross-reactivity between cytotoxic T cells generated during LCMV or Pichinde virus infections; the latter is an arenavirus which does not cross-react serologically with LCMV in terms of neutralization or complement fixation (reviewed in Hotchin, 1971; Lehmann-Grube, 1972).

Taken together, the evidence accumulated so far suggests that virus-specific, cytotoxic T lymphocytes express a specificity spectrum that is not too different from the familiar serological one, but that general patterns of specificity and cross-reactivity are difficult to assess until more sensitive techniques become available.

3.3.4. Antibody Blocking

Blocking of the activity of virus-specific cytotoxic T cells with antiviral antibodies initially seemed to be difficult to detect, or nonexistent, in the poxvirus (Gardner *et al.*, 1974*a,b*; Blanden *et al.*, 1976*b*) and influenza virus models (Braciale, 1977) and LCMV (Doherty *et al.*, 1976*a*). Yet such blocking was observed in several more recent experiments with antisera of variably well-defined specificity for vaccinia (Koszinowski and Ertl, 1975) and for VSV (Zinernagel *et al.*, 1977*d*; Hale *et al.*, 1978). Blocking of VSV-specific cytotoxicity was mediated strongly by an antiglycoprotein antiserum. Although steric hindrance may explain the data, the composite findings are also compatible with the evidence from the mutant virus studies that the viral glycoprotein is crucially involved in defining an antigenic entity recognized by T cells.

3.4. Evidence for the Interaction of Self and Viral Antigens

The single T-cell receptor model implies very strongly that viral antigens and self-H interact; within a dual recognition model such interactions may not be mandatory. One possibility of mutual interaction is that viral infection influences expression of self-H. That virus infection may influence expression of major transplantation antigens has been documented for vesicular stomatitis virus (VSV) (Hecht and Summers, 1972, 1976) and vaccinia virus (Koszinowski and Ertl, 1975; Ertl and Koszinowski, 1976). The effect of vaccinia or VSV in decreasing the number of H-2 antigens expressed on cells' surfaces appears to be caused by the effect this virus has on host-cell protein synthesis (Hecht and Summers, 1972). For vaccinia virus infections, Ertl and Koszinowski (1976) demonstrated that the alteration of protein synthesis could account for the decrease of expressed *MHC* products; they eliminated H-2 antigens by enzymatic treatment and then infected the cells with vaccinia virus to show that within a few hours the H-2 antigens were again detectable on uninfected but not infected targets. It is by no means clear whether this metabolic effect is the only mechanism influencing the expression of H-2 antigens after virus infection. Quite interestingly, budding VSV incorporates H-2 antigens into its viral envelope (Hecht and Summers, 1976), and Friend leukemia viruses seem to pack selected H-2 molecules into the budding form (Bubbers *et al.*, 1977, 1978).

A more complex mechanism by which virus may influence *MHC* gene expression has been proposed in several hypotheses. Garrido, Festenstein, and co-workers proposed that *H-2* restriction of virus-specific cytotoxic T lymphocytes could be explained by a regulatory mechanism as originally described by Bodmer (1973). *H-2* restrictions have been interpreted to indicate that virus infection may disturb regulation of MHC antigen expression and cause repression or derepression of similar types but antigenically different gene products. Garrido *et al.* (1976*a,b*, 1977) found that vaccinia-virus-infected target cells lost or expressed new antigenic determinants which could react with allo-antisera. For example, vaccinia-virus-infected but no uninfected (*H-2ᵈ*) tumor cells reacted *in vitro* with anti-H-2D.32 (private specificity of Dᵏ); in contrast, lymphosarcoma cells (Gardner *H-2ᵏ*) infected with vaccinia virus *in vivo* did not react with an anti-Kᵏ-specific antiserum, whereas the uninfected tumor cells did do so. More recently these results were confirmed using different antisera by differential absorption or alloreactive T cells as method of detection (Matossian-Rogers *et al.*, 1977). By using the latter approach, we (Zinkernagel *et al.*, 1977*a*) could not detect changes in the *MHC* phenotype of infected target cells. Alloreactive T cells against *H-2ᵏ*, *H-2ᵇ*, *H-2ᵈ* target cells infected with pox, LCM, VSV, or Sendai virus were screened for lost or unexpected new alloantigenic determinants without success.

Evidence for direct interaction of self-H and viral antigen has been sought extensively. Lilly, Bubbers, and Blank, using the T-cell immune response to leukemia induced by Friend leukemia virus as model, made the stunning observation that cytotoxic activity generated *in vivo* was restricted preferentially only to *K* or *D*. For example, *H-2ᵇ* mice generated only *Dᵇ*-restricted Friend-virus-specific cytotoxic T cells as shown by Gomard *et al.* (1977) or by blocking cytotoxicity with anti-D vs. anti-K antiserum (Bubber *et al.*, 1977). When Friend virus isolated and purified from the sera of infected mice was disrupted and tested for content of *MHC* products, Bubbers *et al.* (1977, 1978) found antigenic material within the virus preparation that could absorb anti-K or anti-D antisera of the host *H-2* type. The *MHC* products so incorporated into the intact virion are not accessible to antibodies (Bubbers *et al.*, 1978). Interestingly, this absorptive capacity was specific for Dᵇ for virus grown in *H-2ᵇ* mice but not for Kᵇ. Absorption was equally specific for Kᵏ in *H-2ᵏ* mice, but not for Dᵏ or Kᵈ or for Dᵈ. These findings strikingly paralleled the specificity expressed by cytotoxic T cells generated *in vivo* for Dᵇ and of the absence of *H-2ᵈ* restricted cytotoxic T cells in *H-2ᵈ* mice (Gomard *et al.*, 1977). The authors conclude that self K or D antigens had formed a complex with the viral antigens. To this complex the cytotoxic T-cell response was directed. The fact that D^b and K^k but none of the other four D or K markers simultaneously disappeared from the cell surface when capping was induced by anti-Friend virus antibodies (Bubbers *et al.*, 1978) was also interpreted as an indication that self K or D selectively complexed with viral antigens. The fact that these associations were so selective seems to rule out any possibility that contaminating antibodies were responsible for the results, unless such an unorthodox contingency as *MHC* restriction of antibody specificity is postulated. Similarly, Schrader *et al.* (1975) had reported earlier that capping of H-2 antigens on Rauscher-virus-infected EL4 lymphoma cells entailed cocapping of the viral antigen glycoprotein, gp70. Both antisera—anti-H-2 and anti-gp70—particularly the former, had been characterized (Henning *et al.*, 1976) to exclude as well as possible that contaminating antibodies against endogenous virus (Klein, 1975) might be responsible for the phenomenon. This in itself is a very difficult task, and some possible criticisms remain. Furthermore, interpretation of cocapping studies has become even more difficult since Singer and his co-workers (Bourgignon *et al.*, 1978) described that cell-surface antigens on independent structures can cocap simply because the irrelevant antigens were anchored to the myosin-active microtubular cell skeleton and apparently moved passively along with the actively capping structures.

Several attempts to demonstrate coprecipitation of viral antigens with MHC determinants seem to have produced some evidence that probably noncovalent complexes between X and self-H may form in cell membranes and withstand the usual solubilization procedures. Callahan and Allison (1978) have documented coprecipitation of a tumor-associated antigen and *H-2 K* or *D* products, whereas Zarling *et al.* (1978) have similar results using a MSV tumor-cell line. At this time, no comparable evidence has been produced for acute viruses.

4. *MHC* RESTRICTION AND IMMUNE RESPONSIVENESS

Inbred mice vary according to strain with respect to their capacity to respond to foreign antigens by making antibodies or T cells. The genes relevant to this regulation map to the *MHC*. Since the immune response against intracellular infectious agents is of paramount importance to higher vertebrates' survival, regulation of this responsiveness must have been critical in shaping the immune system and the phenotypic variants of responsiveness encountered today. The degree to which we can unravel the background and mechanisms involved in regulating immune responses will relate directly to how well we ultimately understand susceptibility to disease, which is linked repeatedly to the *MHC* of humans.

4.1. Immune Response (*Ir*) Genes

Two basic models have been proposed to explain how T cells interact with infected or altered cells. Either T cells possess two receptor sites, located on one or two molecules, specific for self-H and X or, alternatively, T cells have one single receptor site specific for a neonantigenic determinant resulting from a complex formed between self-H and X.

Whatever the correct hypothesis, the finding that both restriction specificity and *Ir* phenotype are determined by the MHC of the environment in which T cells mature—that is, the thymus—rather than by the MHC of the T cell itself cannot be chance and fits both models (Doherty and Zinkernagel, 1975; Zinkernagel, 1978; Miller *et al.*, 1976; Schwartz, 1978; von Boehmer *et al.*, 1978, Langman, 1978; Cohn and Epstein, 1978).

The state of the art concerning control of immune responsiveness by *H-2*-linked *Ir* genes relative to antibody responses has been reviewed extensively (Benacerraf and Katz, 1975; Benacerraf and McDevitt, 1972) and was brought up to date in a recent review by Benacerraf and Germain (1978). These *Ir* genes have the following characteristics: (1) they regulate antibody production (Levine *et al.*, 1963; McDevitt and Sela, 1965), and they are probably expressed mainly at the level of T-helper cells which influence B cells (Katz *et al.* 1973b; Rosenthal *et al.*, 1977); (2) they function in an antigen-dose-dependent way; (3) they map to *H-2* in mice (McDevitt and Chinitz, 1969), mainly to *I-A* (McDevitt *et al.*, 1972), but complementing genes may map to *I-C* (Dorf and Benacerraf, 1975).

Not until several years later was *Ir* gene regulation over the expression of cytotoxic T cells found in responses to hapten (Shearer and Schmitt-Verhulst, 1977) or minor transplantation antigen (Simpson and Gordon, 1977; von Boehmer *et al.*, 1978) or in the virus models (Doherty *et al.*, 1978; Zinkernagel *et al.*, 1978d,e) and mapped to the *H-2 K*, *D* regions.

4.2. *Ir* Genes Regulating Responsiveness of Virus-Specific Cytotoxic T Cells Mapping to *K, D* and "Dominance" of Low Responsiveness

Ir genes regulating responsiveness of virus-specific cytotoxic T cells are virus specific and *H-2* allele specific, and map to the *K* or *D* region. Therefore, the *restricting* element (*I-A* product for helper T cells; *K, D* for cytotoxic T cells) and the *Ir* genes that regulate responses restricted to the same (type of) restricting self-marker apparently map to the same *H-2* region. As will be analyzed subsequently, this relationship cannot be coincidental. All inbred mice tested so far are phenotypically high responders to vaccinia virus, a nonbudding DNA virus, and to Sendai virus and LCMV, both budding RNA viruses. However, when one assays virus-immune lymphocytes from inbred mice on infected target cells that are compatible only at *K* or *D*, the *K*- or *D*-restricted responses vary quantitatively. For example, $H\text{-}2^k$ mice generate high cytotoxic activity to K^k plus vaccinia virus but virtually no response to D^k plus vaccinia. Since all mouse strains representing some 30–40 haplotypes respond well to, at least, either virus plus K or virus plus D, conventional T-cell help seems to be operative. Thus the observed *Ir* gene effects are exerted at the level of cytotoxic T-cell responsiveness, unless one invokes T-helper cell defects which are specific for the idiotype of the receptor for self-K or D or for altered self. This possibility, which has some precedence (Ward *et al.*, 1977), cannot be formally excluded but seems unlikely.

The crucial experimental data from which these notions are derived are as follows. Low response is virus-specific since one particular D^k allele allows high response to LCMV but low response to vaccinia virus, or K^k is associated with low response to LCMV but high response to vaccinia virus. Two general forms of *Ir* regulations are apparent: (1) The *K*-region allele determines the responder phenotype of virus-specific T cells that are restricted to D, e.g., B10.A (2R) mice ($K^k I^k D^b$) are low responders whereas B10.BYR ($K^q I^k D^b$) mice are high responders to D^b plus vaccinia. Therefore, the *Ir* gene maps to the left of the recombination event separating $I\text{-}A^k$ from K^q. (2) Response to D^k plus vaccinia is low, independent of the alleles in *K* or *I* (*k,b,d,q,s*) or the non-*H-2* background genes (as tested in AKR, B10, C3H, BALB mice).

The dominance of low responsiveness is documented by the finding that the F_1 hybrid of a [C57BL/6 mouse (K^b high responder to D^b vaccinia) $\times$ C3H mouse (K^k nonresponder to D^b vaccinia)] is a low responder for D^b plus vaccinia and that a heterozygote formed between D^k and any other D or K alleles is a low responder to D^k plus vaccinia.

How can these findings be explained?

1. *Complex formation.* The cause of dominant D^k low response to vaccinia could be that D^k plus vaccinia markers do not form *immunogenic complexes*. This explanation would fit a single-recognition-site theory but might in rare cases also influence immunogenicity in a dual recognition concept (Blanden *et al.*, 1977). Although no data presently support this notion, related experiments are in progress. Whether the precedent set by Friend leukemia virus is generally applicable is unclear. Bubbers and Lilly (Bubbers *et al.*, 1977, 1978) showed that budding Friend virus incorporated D^b specificities but not K^b or $H-2^d$, findings which correlate with the fact that responsiveness in this model is apparently only for D^b plus virus. Similar formation of a complex does not readily explain the K-regulated responsiveness to D^b plus vaccinia. Therefore, the failure to form complexes may not apply to all instances of *Ir*-controlled low responses to virus (Rosenthal *et al.*, 1977).

2. *Tolerance.* Can these low responses be explained in a two-recognition-model conveying that *mimicking* or *tolerance* (Snell, 1968) regulates responsiveness? If D^k mimics vaccinia and therefore causes a low response, it is difficult to understand why the response to K^k plus vaccinia is high in $H-2^k$ mice. However, tolerance may partially govern the K^k-regulated low response to D^b. Thus K^k may mimic vaccinia with respect to certain antigenic specificities of vaccinia; therefore, K^k diminishes the numbers of clones available with receptors for vaccinia. On this basis, the rules of genetic exclusion discussed in the next paragraph may become limiting. An objection to the concept that K^k mimics D^b plus vaccinia is that the expected cross-reactivity of K^k with vaccinia plus D^b was not found when vaccinia-immune $H-2^b$ lymphocytes were tested on $H-2^k$ targets or when anti-K^k-alloreactive T cells were tested on vaccinia-infected $H-2^b$ targets (Zinkernagel *et al.*, 1977*a*). Also, serological testing has yielded no such evidence. A different mode of tolerance may prevail within the single-recognition-site theory (Schwartz, 1978); accordingly, the neoantigenic determinant formed by K^k and other cell-membrane antigens may mimic and therefore tolerize for D^b plus vaccinia. If this were ture, K^k on different non-$H-2$ backgrounds should influence D^b-restricted responsiveness to vaccinia differentially; this has not been tested formally as yet.

3. *Genetic exclusion models.* Langman (1978) and Cohn and Epstein (1978) proposed that *Ir* phenomena that govern *MHC-*

restricted T cells can be explained as follows: If by random or driven somatic mutation the germ line gene coding anti-D^k usually gives rise to the high-affinity antivaccinia receptor(s), then selection to express anti-D^k as anti-self-H specificity would preclude this cell from expressing antivaccinia as its anti-X specificity. In contrast, the anti-K^d germ line gene does not give rise to antivaccinia; therefore, T cells restricted to K^d can express an antivaccinia specificity derived from the anti-D^k germ line gene. Which specificity is expressed depends on the size of the germ line gene pool, on how specific T-cell receptors for X are, and/or on how specific the *Ir* effect is. Available data are fragmentary and difficult to interpret as yet. This model does not readily explain why two unrelated viruses (e.g., vaccinia and Sendai) should be associated with similar nonresponder *K* or *D* alleles, nor does it explain why for many oligoamino acid antigens only few murine *H-2* haplotypes are responders.

A symmetrical but different model was more recently proposed by von Boehmer *et al.* (1978). The assumptions are as mentioned, but their proposition is that a T cell is going to mature and acquire self-restricted immunocompetence only if it expresses two identical anti-self-H receptors. One of the receptors is then preserved as anti-self-H; the other is free to mutate as Jerne (1971) predicted. Accordingly, T cells expressing anti-D^k are driven to proliferate on contacting D^k in the thymus. During proliferation, mutations occur and change the receptor specificity anti-X from anti-D^k to anti-"different from D^k." The latter T cells would then be allowed to leave the thymus and constitute the pool of immunocompetent T cells. If by such somatic mutation, driven by D^k, a receptor for antivaccinia is not generated readily, D^k-restricted T cells would not respond to vaccinia. In contrast, K^d-restricted T cells could readily derive from anti-K^d an antivaccinia receptor and, therefore, respond to this virus. Immunological tolerance induced by *MHC* products may modify the ground rules of these two models slightly.

A third possible model is based on experimental evidence that variable region genes coding for the anti-X binding site on B cells and on T cells may be basically the same (reviewed in Ramseier *et al.*, 1977; Binz and Wigzell, 1977; Rajewsky and Eichmann, 1977). Then the restriction specificity anti-self-H would have to be conferred by other than *V* genes and the germ line genes coding for anti-self-H type receptors (and not *V*-gene-coded receptors) are alloreactive. Regulation by the *MHC* of anti-X responsiveness may then be a matter of tolerance or of an *ad hoc* rule that certain anti-self-H receptors do not, or cannot, associate with certain anti-X receptors. Whichever of these ideas or even an additional model may be correct, all incorporate genetic mechanisms that may explain the association of disease susceptibility with the *MHC*. Furthermore, the polymorphism of MHC products, discussed in the next section, fits into all propositions as an excellent way to improve and maximize immune responsiveness and therefore the survival of both the species as a whole and of the individual in particular.

5. POLYMORPHISM OF *MHC* PRODUCTS AND *MHC*-LINKED SUSCEPTIBILITY TO DISEASE

Polymorphism of a genetically determined trait is so called because of the fact that, for example, the *MHC* codes for an apparently small number of cell-surface structures, which, however, differ markedly from individual to individual (Snell, 1968; Bodmer, 1972; Burnet, 1973; Klein, 1975). It is not known whether the polymorphism of H-2 or HLA antigens is allelic, i.e., the germ line contains one particular gene to code a single selection from all the possible alleles, or is regulatory (Bodmer, 1973; Martin, 1975), i.e., the germ line of each individual contains genes for all possible structures but only one of the gene products is actually expressed under strict regulation. The striking point is that major transplantation antigens coded by the *MHC* that regulates T-cell-mediated immunity, as well as immunoglobulin (Ig) allotypes involved in regulation of responsiveness of antibodies, are both extremely polymorphic (in fact, the most polymorphic systems known).

The findings that the *MHC* has such a profound regulatory role in immune responsiveness and that T cells express restriction specificity suggest a direct relationship among the polymorphism of *MHC*, the immune response, and host survival in the face of infectious disease. The apparently great selective pressure exerted by infectious agents, particularly viruses, may in fact have helped to shape this polymorphism of the *MHC*.

Our assumption is that the main task of immunity is to protect the host from infectious agents. Intracellular parasites (viruses and intracellular bacteria such as *Listeria* and BCG) are kept in check mainly by T lymphocytes, whereas extracellular parasites are eliminated predominately by antibodies and other neutralizing factors in association with complement and phagocytes (Notkins, 1975; Bloom and Rager-Zisman, 1975; Blanden, 1974; Blanden *et al.*, 1976*b*). T cells may protect the host from virus by destroying acutely infected cells during the eclipse phase of virus infection; it is obvious that other immune effector mechanisms such as antibodies and macrophages are involved in antiviral protection as well. In contrast, facultative intracellular bacteria and fungi are not controlled by lytic T cells but rather by nonlytic T cells, which activate macrophages to increased bactericidal capacity (Mackaness, 1964, 1969; Blanden and Langman, 1972; Lane and Unanue, 1972). Thus *immune protection* against viruses is mediated, at least partially, via *host-cell destruction*. The clinical outcome of an infection is determined by the cell-destroying (cytopathic) capacity of the virus and the competing cell destruction by T cells seeking to prevent the virus from spreading. This sequence immediately implies that the balance of beneficial *vs.* harmful effects of cellular immunity depends on such factors as, on the one side, cytopathogenicity of the virus, rapidity of spread, organ and/or cell tropism, and antigenicity of the virus or parasite, and, on the other side, immunocompetence and immune response phenotype of the host.

Two virus infections, which represent extremes, illustrate these concepts. Poxvirus in humans (ectromelia in mice) is a highly cytopathogenic virus. Cell-mediated immunity is essential to overcome its infection, as documented by the fact that T-cell-deficient children often develop general vaccinosis on pox vaccination and that T-cell deficient mice infected with mouse pox rapidly die (Blanden, 1974). Hepatitis virus in humans and LCMV in mice provoke the other extreme of response to infection. The viruses are *not* very cytopathic and immunodeficient hosts do not die of the virus infection. Therefore, the immunocompetent virus-infected hosts' tissue damage seems to be caused by the T-cell response of the host rather than by the virus *per se* (reviewed in Hotchin, 1971; Cole and Nathanson, 1975; Doherty and Zinkernagel, 1974). From the standpoint of cell-mediated immunity, then, the arbiters in permitting intracellular parasites to cause disease can be viewed as (1) a balance of destructive effects of the immune response and (2) the predisposition to high vs. low responsiveness, which is strongly influenced by *H-2*-linked *Ir* genes.

As mentioned, *Ir* genes that control the expression of virus-specific cytotoxic T cells have the following characteristics. First, they are virus specific and *K* or *D* allele specific. Second, they map to either *K* or *D*, i.e., to the same *MHC* regions as the restricting self-H markers (and not to *H-2I*, as do *Ir* genes controlling antibody, T-cell proliferative, or delayed hypersensitivity responses). Third, nonresponsivesness has dominant character.

These findings offer an obvious teleological explanation for *MHC* polymorphism and gene duplication within the *MHC* (Snell, 1968; Bodmer, 1973; Burnet, 1973; McDevitt and Bodmer, 1974; Klein, 1975; Shreffler and David, 1975; Doherty and Zinkernagel, 1975). If mice possessed only one lytic *MHC* restriction structure, e.g., D type, not only the individual but also the entire species would be in jeopardy from, say, poxvirus infection. The high response to LCMV obviously would not help. Polymorphism diminishes the chance of extinction by (1) eliminating the possibility that viruses could adapt by mutation to mimic the species' self markers or could escape immune surveillance by other means, (2) restricting *H-2*-regulated low responsiveness or unresponsiveness to only few members of a species, and (3) causing heterozygosity, which in combination with duplication of certain *H-2* regions gives each individual maximal immune responsiveness and protection.

The performance of *MHC*-linked *Ir* genes in the virus models just described could relate to empirical associations found between *MHC* and susceptibility to disease (reviewed in McDevitt and Bodmer, 1974; Dausset and Svejgard, 1977).

We have summarized evidence that suggests (1) *MHC*-restricted T cells protect a host from intracellular parasites; the T-cell function is determined by the restriction specificity expressed by T cells. (2) The *MHC*-coded restricting self-H influences directly or indirectly the capacity of T cells to respond. Consequently, susceptibility to and maintenance of disease can be viewed as resulting from the balance between immunoprotective and immunodestructive effects of T cells, which in turn is influenced by the *MHC* and restriction-specificity-dependent capacity of T cells to respond.

From this point of view, susceptibility or resistance to disease falls into the following categories (Zinkernagel, 1978). High responsiveness results in relatively *increased* resistance to infectious *cytopathogenic virus* but *decreased* resistance to *poorly cytopathogenic* viruses, which tends to tip the balance of immune protection toward autoaggression since T-cell-mediated tissue damage is favored by the wider spread of virus. In contrast, low responsiveness results in relatively *great susceptibility to acute cytopathogenic virus* infection, and therefore has been eliminated by selection, but possibly *decreased susceptibility to virus-induced autoaggressive diseases*. For some time, chronic virus infections have been suspected as the cause of so-called autoimmune diseases. In fact, most of the associations between *MHC* and disease relate to autoaggressive (or autoimmune) disease, not to acute infections.

Increased susceptibility to acute virus infections would influence survival of the species dramatically, since acute infections can occur well
before an individual is reproductively mature. Natural selection would
tend to eliminate these types of low responders. In contrast, the more
chronic autoimmune types of diseases tend to become life-limiting
much later, after an individual reproduces; therefore, natural selection
need not discard susceptibility of this type, and *MHC*-associated
diseases are manifest.

ACKNOWLEDGMENTS

I thank Phyllis Minick for her great editorial collaboration in pre-
paring the manuscript and Annette Parson for her secretarial
assistance. Experimental work performed in this laboratory was
partially supported by USPHSG A1-07007, A1-13779, and A1-00273.
This publication was submitted in October 1978 and is Publication No.
1634 of the Immunopathology Department of Scripps Clinic and
Research Foundation.

6.   REFERENCES

Ada, G. L., Jackson, D. C., Blanden, R. V., Tha Hla, R., and Bowern, N. W., 1976,
    Changes in the surface of virus-infected cells recognized by cytotoxic T cells. I.
    Minimal requirements for lysis of ectromelia-infected P-815 cells, *Scand. J.
    Immunol.* **5**:23.
Alter, B. J., Schendel, D. H., Bach, M. L., Bach, F. H., Klein, J., and Stimpfling, J.
    H., 1973, Cell-mediated lympholysis: Importance of serologically defined *H-2*
    regions, *J. Exp. Med.* **137**:1303.
Bach, F. J., Bach, M. L., and Sondel, P. M., 1976, Differential function of major histo-
    compatibility complex antigens in T lymphocyte activation, *Nature (London)*
    259:273.
Benacerraf, B., and Germain, R., 1978, The immune response genes of the major histo-
    compatibility complex, *Immunol. Rev.* **38**:71.
Benacerraf, B., and Katz, D. H., 1975, The histocompatibility-linked immune response
    genes, *Adv. Cancer Res.* **21**:121.
Benacerraf, B., and McDevitt, H. O., 1972, Histocompatibility-linked immune response
    genes, *Science* **175**:273.
Bergholtz, B. O., and Thorsby, E., 1977, Macrophage-dependent response of immune
    human T lymphoytes to PPD *in vitro:* Influence of HLA-D histocompatibility,
    Scand. J. Immunol. **6**:779.
Bevan, M. J., 1975, Interaction antigens detected by cytotoxic T cells with the major
    histocompatibility complex as modifier, *Nature (London)* **256**:419.

Bevan, M. J., 1977, In radiation chimeras host H-2 antigen determine the immune responsiveness of donor cytotoxic cells, *Nature (London)* **269**:417.

Billings, P., Burakoff, S. J., Dorf, M. E., and Benacerraf, B., 1978, Genetic control of cytolytic T lymphocyte responses. II. The role of the host genotype in parental → F_1 radiation chimeras in the control of the specificity of cytolytic T lymphocyte responses to TNP-modified syngeneic cells. *J. Exp. Med.* **148**:353.

Binz, H., and Wigzell, H., 1977, Antigen-binding, idiotypic T-lymphocyte receptors, in: *Contemporary Topics in Immunobiology*, Vol. 7 (O. Stutman, ed.), Plenum Press, New York.

Blanden, R. V., 1974, T cell response to viral and bacterial infection, *Transplant. Rev.* **19**:5.

Blanden, R. V., and Langman, R. E., 1972, Cell-mediated immunity to bacterial infection in the mouse: Thymus derived cells as effectors of acquired resistance to *Listeria monocytogenes*, *Scand. J. Immunol.* **1**:379.

Blanden, R. V., Doherty, P. C., Dunlop, M. B. C., Gardner, I. D., Zinkernagel, R. M., and David, C. S., 1975, Genes required for T cell mediated cytotoxicity against virus infected target cells are in the *K* or *D* regions of the *H-2* gene complex, *Nature (London)* **254**:269.

Blanden, R. V., Hapel, A. J., and Jackson, D. C., 1976a, Mode of action of Ir genes and the nature of T cell receptors for antigen, *Immunochemistry* **13**:179.

Blanden, R. V., Hapel, A. J., Doherty, P. C., and Zinkernagel, R. M., 1976b, Lymphocyte–macrophage interactions and macrophage activation in the expression of antimicrobial immunity *in vivo*, in: *Immunobiology of the Macrophage* (D. S. Nelson, ed.), p. 367, Academic Press, New York.

Blanden, R. V., McKenzie, I., Kees, U., Melvold, R. W., and Kohn, H. I., 1977, Cytotoxic T cell response to ectomelia virus-infected cells. Different H-2 requirements for triggering precursor T-cell induction or lysis by effector T cells defined by the BALB/c H-2^{db} mutant, *J. Exp. Med.* **146**:869.

Blank, K. J., Freedman, H. A., and Lilly, F., 1976, T-lymphocyte response to friend virus-induced tumour cell lines in mice of strains congenic at *H-2*, *Nature (London)* **260**:250.

Bloom, B. R., and Rager-Zisman, B., 1975, Cell-mediated immunity in viral infections, in: *Viral Immunology and Immunopathology* (A. L. Notkins, ed.), p. 113, Academic Press, New York.

Bodmer, W. F., 1972, Evolutionary significance of the *HL-A* system, *Nature (London)* **237**:139.

Bodmer, W. F., 1973, A new genetic model of allelism at histocompatibility and other complex loci: Polymorphism for control of gene expression, *Transplant. Proc.* **5**:1471.

Bourgignon, L. Y. W., Hyman, R., Trowbridge, J., and Singer, S. J., 1978, Participation of histocompatibility antigens in capping of molecularly independent cell surface components by their specific antibodies, *Proc. Natl. Acad. Sci. USA* **75**:2406.

Braciale, T. J., 1977, Immunologic recognition of influenza virus-infected cells. II. Expression of influenza A matrix protein on the infected cell surface and its role in recognition by cross-reactive cytotoxic T cells, *J. Exp. Med.* **146**:673.

Bryere, E. J., and Williams, L. B., 1964, Antigens associated with a tumor virus: Rejection of isogenic skin grafts from leukemic mice, *Science* **146**:1055.

Bubbers, J. E., Steeves, R. A., and Lilly, F., 1977, Selective incorporation of antigenic determinants into Friend virus particles, *Nature (London)* **266**:458.

Bubbers, J. E., Chen, S., and Lilly, F., 1978, Nonrandom inclusion of *H-2K* and *H-2D* antigens in Friend virus particles from mice of various strains, *J. Exp. Med.* **147**:340.

Buchmeier, M., and Oldstone, M. B. A., 1978, personal communication.

Burnet, F. M., 1973, Multiple polymorphism in relation to histocompatibility antigens, *Nature (London)* **245**:359.

Callahan, G. J., Allison, J. P., 1978, H-2 antigens on a murine lymphoma are associated with additional proteins, *Nature (London)* **271**:165.

Cantor, H., and Boyse, E., 1977, Regulation of the immune response by T cell subclasses, in: *Contemporary Topics in Immunobiology*, Vol. 7 (O. Stutman, ed.), Plenum Press, New York.

Cartwright, B., and Brown, J., 1972, Serologic relationships between different strains of vesicular stomatitis virus, *J. Gen. Virol.* **16**:391.

Cerottini, J. C., and Brunner, K. T., 1974, Cell-mediated cytotoxicity, allograft rejection and tumor immunity, *Adv. Immunol.* **19**:67.

Cheers, C., and McKenzie, I. F. C., 1978, Resistance and susceptibility of mice to bacterial infection: Genetics of listeriosis, *Infect. Immun.* **19**:755.

Cohn, M., and Epstein, R., 1978, T cell inhibition of humoral responsiveness: II. Theory on the role of restrictive recognition in immune regulation, *Cell. Immunol.* **39**:125.

Cole, G. A., and Nathanson, N., 1975, Lymphocytic choriomeningitis: Pathogenesis, *Prog. Med. Virol.* **18**:94.

Dausset, J. F., and Svejgard, A., ed., 1977, *HLA and Disease*, Munksgaard, Copenhagen.

de Landazuri, M. O., and Herberman, R. B., 1972, Specificity of cellular immune reactivity to virus-induced tumors, *Nature (London) New Biol.* **238**:18.

Dickmeiss, E., Soeberg, B., and Svejgard, A., 1977, Human cell-mediated cytotoxicity against modified target cells restricted by HLA, *Nature (London)* **270**:526.

Doherty, P. C., and Bennink, J. R. 1979, Vaccinia-specific cytotoxic T cell responses in the context of *H-2* antigens not encountered in thymus may reflect aberrant recognition of a virus–H-2 complex, *J. Exp. Med.* **149**:150.

Doherty, P. C., and Zinkernagel, R. M., 1974, T cell-mediated immunopathology in viral infections, *Transplant. Rev.* **19**:89.

Doherty, P. C., and Zinkernagel, R. M., 1975, A biological role for the major histocompatibility antigens, *Lancet* **1**:1406.

Doherty, P. C., and Zinkernagel, R. M., 1976, Specific immune lysis of paramyxovirus infected cells by *H-2* compatible thymus-derived lymphocytes, *Immunology* **31**:27.

Doherty, P. C., Blanden, R. V., and Zinkernagel, R. M., 1976a, Specificity of virus-immune effector T cells for *H-2K* or *H-2D* compatible interactions: Implications for H-antigen diversity, *Transplant. Rev.* **29**:89.

Doherty, P. C., Gotze, D., Trinchieri, G., and Zinkernagel, R. M., 1976b, Models for recognition of virally modified cells by immune thymus derived lymphocytes, *Immunogenetics* **3**:517.

Doherty, P. C., Effros, R. B., and Bennink, J., 1977, Heterogeneity of cytotoxic response of thymus-derived lymphocytes after immunization with influenza viruses, *Proc. Natl. Acad. Sci. USA* **74**:1209.

Doherty, P. C., Biddison, W. E., Bennink, J. R., and Knowles, B. B., 1978, Cytotoxic T cell responses in mice infected with influenza and vaccinia viruses vary in magnitude with *H-2* type, *J. Exp. Med.* **148**:534.

Dorf, M. E., and Benacerraf, B., 1975, Complementation of *H-2* linked *Ir* genes in the mouse, *Proc. Natl. Acad. Sci.* **72**:3671.

Ennis, F. A., Martin, W. J., and Verbonitz, M. W., 1977, Hemagglutinin-specific cytotoxic T cell response during influenza infection, *J. Exp. Med.* **146**:893.

Erb, P., and Feldman, M., 1975, The role of macrophages in the generation of T helper cells. II. The genetic control of the macrophage-T-cell interaction for helper cell induction with soluble antigens, *J. Exp. Med.* **142**:460.

Ertl, H. C. J., and Koszinowski, U. H., 1976, Modification of H-2 antigenic sites by enzymatic treatment influences virus-specific target cell lysis, *J. Immunol.* **117**:2112.

Fenner, F. J., 1968, *The Biology of Animal Viruses*, Vol. III, Academic Press, New York.

Gardner, I., Bowern, N. A., and Blanden, R. V., 1974a, Cell-mediated cytotoxicity against ectromelia virus-infected target cells. I. Specificity and kinetics, *Eur. J. Immunol.* **4**:63.

Gardner, I., Bowern, N. A., and Blanden, R. V., 1974b, Cell-mediated cytotoxicity against ectromelia virus-infected target cells. II. Identification of effector cells and analysis of mechanism, *Eur. J. Immunol.* **4**:68.

Garrido, F., Schirrmacher, V., and Festenstein, H., 1976a, *H-2*-like specificities of foreign haplotypes appearing on a mouse sarcoma after vaccinia virus infection, *Nature (London)* **259**:228.

Garrido, F., Festenstein, H., and Schirrmacher, V., 1976b, Further evidence for derepression of *H-2* and *Ia*-like specificities of foreign haplotypes in mouse tumour cell lines, *Nature (London)* **261**:705.

Garrido, F., Schmidt, W., and Festenstein, H., 1977, Immunogenetic studies on meth-A-vaccinia tumour cells *in vivo* and *in vitro*, *J. Immunogenet.* **4**:115.

Gershon, R., 1974, T cell control of antibody production, in: *Contemporary Topics in Immunobiology*, Vol. 3, p. 1, Plenum Press, New York.

Gething, M. J., Koszinowski, U., and Waterfield, M., 1978, Fusion of Sendai virus with target cell membranes is required for T cell cytotoxicity, *Nature (London)* **274**:689.

Gomard, E., Duprez, V., Henin, Y., and Levy, J. P., 1976, H-2 product as determinant in immune cytolysis of syngeneic tumour cells by anti-MSV T lymphocytes, *Nature (London)* **260**:707.

Gomard, E., Duprez, V., Reme, T., Colombani, M. J., and Levy, J. P., 1977, Exclusive involvement of $H-2D^b$ or $H-2K^d$ product in the interaction between T-killer lymphocytes and syngeneic $H-2^b$ or $H-2^d$ viral lymphomas, *J. Exp. Med.* **146**:909.

Goulmy, E., Termijtelen, A., Bradley, B. A., and Van Rood, J. J., 1976, Y-antigen killing by T cells of women is restricted by HLA, *Nature (London)* **266**:544.

Hale, A. H., Owen, N. W., Baltimore, D., and Eisen, H. N., 1978, Vesicular stomatitis virus glycoprotein is necessary for *H-2*-restricted lysis of infected cells by cytotoxic T lymphocytes, *Proc. Natl. Acad. Sci. USA* **75**:970.

Hapel, A., Bablanian, R., and Cole, G. A., 1978, Inductive requirements for the generation of virus-specific T lymphocytes. I. Nature of the host cell–virus interaction that triggers secondary pox virus-specific cytotoxic T lymphocyte induction, *J. Immunol.* **121**:736.

Hecht, T. T., and Summers, D. F., 1972, Effect of vesicular stomatitis virus infection on the histocompatibility antigen of L cells, *J. Virol.* **10**:578.

Hecht, T. T., and Summers, D. F., 1976, Interactions of vesicular stomatitis virus with murine cell surface antigens, *J. Virol.* **19**:833.

Henning, R., Schrader, J. W., and Edelman, G. M., 1976, Antiviral antibodies inhibit the lysis of tumour cells by anti-*H-2* sera, *Nature (London)* **263**:689.

Herberman, R. B., Nunn, M. E., Lavrin, D. H., and Asofsky, R., 1973, Effect of antibody to antigen on cell-mediated immunity induced in syngeneic mice by murine sarcoma virus, *J. Natl. Cancer Inst.* **51**:1509.

Herberman, R. B., Nunn, M. E., Holden, H. T., Staal, S., and Djen, J. Y., 1977, Augmentation of natural cytotoxic reactivity of mouse lymphoid cells against syngeneic and allogeneic target cells, *Int. J. Cancer* **19**:555.

Holden, A. T., and Herberman, R. B., 1977, Cytotoxicity against tumor associated antigens not H-2 restricted, *Nature (London)* **268**:250.

Hotchin, J., 1971, Persistent and slow virus infection, *Monogr. Virol.*, **3**:1.

Invernizzi, G., and Parmiani, G., 1975, Tumour-associated transplantation antigens of chemically induced sarcomata cross reacting with allogeneic histocompatibility antigens, *Nature (London)* **254**:713.

Jackson, D. C., Ada, G. L., and Tha Hla, R., 1976, Cytotoxic T cells recognize very early minor changes in ectromelia virus-infected target cells, *Aust. J. Exp. Biol. Med. Sci.* **54**:349.

Janeway, C. A., Jr., Wigzell, H., and Binz, H., 1976, Two different V_H gene products make up the T-cell receptors, *Scand. J. Immunol.* **5**:993.

Jenner, E., 1798, An inquiry into the causes and effects of the variolae vaccinae, a disease discovered in some of the western counties of England, particularly Gloucestershire and known by the name of the Cow Pox, in: *Milestones in Microbiology* (T. H. Brock, ed.), p. 121, American Society of Microbiology.

Jerne, N. K., 1971, The somatic generation of immune recognition, *Eur. J. Immunol.* **1**:1.

Katz, D. H., 1977, *Lymphocyte Differentiation, Recognition and Regulation*, Academic Press, New York.

Katz, D. H., and Benacerraf, B., 1975, The function and interrelationship of T cell receptors: *Ir* genes and other histocompatibility gene products, *Transplant. Rev.* **22**:1975.

Katz, D. H., Hamaoka, T., Dorf, M. E., and Benacerraf, B., 1973a, Cell interaction between histocompatible T and B lymphocytes. II. Failure of physiologic cooperative interactions between T and B lymphocytes from allogeneic donor strains in humoral response to hapten protein conjugates, *J. Exp. Med.* **137**:1405.

Katz, D. H., Hamaoka, T., Dorf, M. E., Maurer, P. H., and Benacerraf, B., 1973b, Cell interactions between histoincompatible T and B lymphocytes. IV. Involvement of the immune response (*Ir*) gene in the control of lymphocyte interactions in responses controlled by the gene, *J. Exp. Med.* **138**:734.

Kees, U., and Blanden, R. V., 1976, A single genetic element in *H-2K* affects mouse T-cell antiviral function in pox virus infection, *J. Exp. Med.* **143**:450.

Kindred, B., and Shreffler, D. C., 1972, *H-2* dependence of cooperation between T and B cells *in vivo*, *J. Immunol.* **109**:940.

Klein, J., 1975, *Biology of the Mouse Histocompatibility-2 Complex*, Springer, New York.

Klein, P., 1975, Anomalous reactions of mouse alloantisera with culture tumor cells. I. Demonstration of widespread occurrence using reference typing sera, *J. Immunol.* **115**:1254.

Knipe, D. M., Baltimore, D., and Lodish, H. F., 1977, Maturation of viral proteins in cells infected with temperature-sensitive mutants of vesicular stomatitis virus, *J. Virol.* **21**:1149.

Koszinowski, U., and Ertl, H., 1975, Lysis mediated by T cells and restricted by *H-2* antigen of target cells infected with vaccinia virus, *Nature (London)* **255**:552.

Koszinowski, U., and Ertl, H., 1976, Role of early viral surface antigens in cellular immune response to vaccinia virus, *Eur. J. Immunol.* **6**:679.

Koszinowski, U., Wekerle, H., and Thomssen, R., 1976, Recognition of alteration induced by early vaccinia surface antigens and dependence of virus-specific lysis on *H-2* antigen concentration on target cells, *Cold Spring Harbor Symp. Quant. Biol.* **41**:529.

Koszinowski, U., Gething, M. J., and Waterfield, M., 1977, T-cell cytotoxicity in the absence of viral protein synthesis in target cells, *Nature (London)* **267**:160.

Lafay, F., 1974, Envelope proteins of vesicular stomatitis virus: Effect of temperature-sensitive mutants of vesicular stomatitis virus, *J. Virol.* **21**:1149.

Lane, F. C., and Unanue, E. R., 1972, Requirement of thymus (T) lymphocyte for resistance to listeriosis, *J. Exp. Med.* **135**:1104.

Langman, R. E., 1978, The role of the major histocompatibility complex in immunity: A new concept in the functioning of a cell-mediated immune system, *Rev. Physiol. Biochem. Pharmacol.* **81**:1.

Lavrin, D. H., Herberman, R. B., Nunn, M., and Soares, N., 1973, *In vitro* cytotoxicity studies of murine sarcoma virus-induced immunity in mice, *J. Natl. Cancer Inst.* **51**:1497.

Lawrence, H. S., 1959, Homograft sensitivity: An expression of the immunologic origins and consequences of individuality, *Physiol. Rev.* **39**:811.

Leclerc, J. C., Gomard, E., and Levy, J. P., 1972, Cell mediated reaction against tumors induced by oncornaviruses. I. Kinetics and specificity of the immune response in murine sarcoma virus (MSV) induced tumors and transplanted lymphomas, *Int. J. Cancer* **10**:589.

Leclerc, J. C., Gomard, E., Plata, F., and Levy, J. P., 1973. Cell-mediated immune reaction against tumors induced by oncornaviruses. II. Nature of the effector cells in tumor-cell cytolysis, *Int. J. Cancer* **11**:426.

Lehmann-Grube, F., 1972, Lymphocytic choriomeningitis virus monographs, *Virology* **10**:1.

Levine, B. B., Ojeda, A., and Benacerraf, B., 1963, Studies on artificial antigens. III. The genetic control of the immune response to hapten poly-L-lysine conjugates in guinea pigs, *J. Exp. Med.* **118**:953.

Lilly, F., Boyse, E. A., and Old, L. J., 1964, Genetic basis of susceptibility to viral leukemogenesis, *Lancet* **2**:1207.

Lindenmann, J., Deuel, E., Fanconi, S., and Haller, O., 1978, Inborn resistance of mice to myxoviruses: Macrophages express phenotype *in vitro*, *J. Exp. Med.* **147**:531.

Mackaness, G. B., 1964, The immunological basis of acquired cellular resistance, *J. Exp. Med.* **120**:105.

Mackaness, G. B., 1969, The influence of immunologically committed lymphoid cells on macrophage activity *in vivo*, *J. Exp. Med.* **129**:973.

Marshak, A., Doherty, P. C., and Wilson, D. B., 1977, The control of specificity of cytotoxic lymphocytes by the major histocompatibility complex (*Ag-B*) in rats and identification of a new alloantigen system showing no *Ag-B* restriction, *J. Exp. Med.* **146**:1773.

Martin, W. J., 1975, Immune surveillance directed against derepressed cellular and viral alloantigens, *Cell. Immunol.* **15**:1.

Matossian-Rogers, A., Garrido, F., and Festenstein, H., 1977, Emergence of foreign *H-2*-like cytotoxicity and transplantation targets on vaccinia and Moloney virus-infected meth. A tumour cells, *Scand. J. Immunol.* **6**:541.

McDevitt, H. O., and Bodmer, W. F., 1974, *HL-A*, immune response genes and disease, *Lancet* **1**:1269.

McDevitt, H. O., and Chinitz, A., 1969, Genetic control of antibody response: Relationship between immune response and histocompatibility (*H-2*) type, *Science* **163**:1207.

McDevitt, H. O., and Sela, M., 1965, Genetic control of the antibody response. I. Demonstration of determinant-specific differences in response to synthetic polypeptide antigens in two strains of inbred mice, *J. Exp. Med.* **122**:517.

McDevitt, H. O., Deak, B. D., Shreffler, D. C., Klein, J., Stimpfling, J. H., and Snell, G. D., 1972, Genetic control of the immune response. Mapping of the *Ir-l* locus, *J. Exp. Med.* **135**:1259.

McMichael, A. J., Ting, A., Zweerink, H. J., and Askonas, B. A., 1977, *HLA* restriction of cell mediated lysis of influenza virus-infected human cells, *Nature (London)* **270**:524.

Miller, J. F. A. P., Vadas, M. A., Whitlaw, A., and Gamble, J., 1975, *H-2* gene complex restricts transfer of delayed-type hypersensitivity in mice, *Proc. Natl. Acad. Sci. USA* **72**:5095.

Miller, J. F. A. P., Vadas, M. A., Whitlaw, A., and Gamble, J., 1976, Role of the major histocompatibility complex gene products in delayed-type hypersensitivity, *Proc. Natl. Acad. Sci. USA* **73**:2486.

Mims, C. A., and Blanden, R. V., 1972, Antiviral action of immune lymphocytes in mice infected with lymphocytic choriomeningitis virus, *Infect. Immun.* **6**:695.

Mitchison, N. A., 1954, Passive transfer of transplantation immunity, *Proc. R. Soc. London Ser. B* **142**:72.

Munro, A. J., and Bright, S., 1976, Products of the major histocompatibility complex and their relationship to the immune response, *Nature (London)* **264**:145.

Nabholz, M., Vives, J., Young, H. M., Meo, T., Miggiano, V., Rijnbeek, A., and Shreffler, D. C., 1974, Cell-mediated cell lysis *in vitro:* Genetic control of killer cell production and target specificities in the mouse, *Eur. J. Immunol.* **4**:378.

Notkins, A. L., 1975, Interferon as a mediator of cellular immunity in viral infections, in: *Viral Immunology and Immunopathology* (A. L. Notkins, ed.), p. 149, Academic Press, New York.

Paul, W. E., and Benacerraf, B., 1977, Functional specificity of thymus-dependent lymphocytes, *Science* **195**:1293.

Perlman, S. M., and Huang, A. S., 1974, Virus-specific RNA specified by the group I and IV temperature-sensitive mutants of vesicular stomatitis, *Intervirology* **2**:312.

Perlmann, R., Perlmann, H., and Wigzell, H., 1972, Lymphocyte mediated cytotoxicity *in vitro:* Introduction and inhibition by humoral antibody and nature of effector cells, *Transplant. Rev.* **13**:91.

Pfizenmaier, K., Starzinski-Powitz, A., Rollinghoff, M., Falke, D., and Wagner, H., 1977, T-cell-mediated cytotoxicity against herpes simplex virus-infected target cells, *Nature (London)* **265**:630.

Pfizenmaier, K., Trinchieri, G., Solter, D., and Knowles, B. B., 1978, Mapping of *H-2* genes associated with T cell-mediated cytotoxic responses to SV40-tumor associated specific antigens, *Nature (London)* **274**:691.

Plata, F., Gomard, E., Leclerc, J. C., and Levy, J. P., 1974, Comparative *in vitro* studies on effector cell diversity in the cellular immune response to murine sarcoma virus (MSV)-induced tumors in mice, *J. Immunol.* **112**:1477.

Plata, F., Cerottini, J. C., and Brunner, K. T., 1975, Primary and secondary *in vitro* generation of cytolytic T lymphocytes in the murine sarcoma virus system, *Eur. J. Immunol.* **5**:227.

Plata, F., Jongeneel, V., Cerottini, J. C., and Brunner, K. T., 1976, Antigenic specificity to the cytolytic T lymphocyte (CTL) response to murine sarcoma virus-induced tumors. I. Preferential reactivity of *in vitro* generated secondary CTL with syngeneic tumor cells, *Eur. J. Immunol.* **6**:823.

Pringle, C. R., 1970, Genetic characteristics of conditional lethal mutants of vesicular stomatitis virus induced by 5-fluorouracil, 5-azacytidine, and ethyl methane sulfonate, *J. Virol.* **5**:559.

Rager-Zisman, B., and Bloom, B. R., 1974, Immunological destruction of herpes simplex virus I infected cells, *Nature (London)* **251**:542.

Rajewsky, K., and Eichmann, K., 1977, Antigen receptors of T helper cells, in: *Contemporary Topics in the Immunobiology of T Cells*, Vol. 7 (O. Stutman, ed.), p. 69, Plenum Press, New York.

Ramseier, H., Aguet, M., and Lindenmann, J., 1977, Similarity of idiotypic determinants of T- and B-lymphocyte receptors for alloantigens, *Immunol. Rev.* **34**:50.

Röllinghoff, M., Starzinski-Powitz, A., Pfizenmaier, K., and Wagner, H., 1977, Cyclophosphamide-sensitive T lymphocytes suppress the *in vivo* generation of antigen-specific cytotoxic T lymphocytes, *J. Exp. Med.* **145**:455.

Rosenthal, A. S., and Shevach, E. M., 1973, Function of macrophages in antigen recognition by guinea pig T lymphocytes. I. Requirement for histocompatible macrophages and lymphocytes, *J. Exp. Med.* **138**:1194.

Rosenthal, A. S., Barcinski, M. A., and Blake, J. T., 1977, Determinant selection: A macrophage dependent immune response gene function, *Nature (London)* **267**:156.

Rothenberg, B. E., 1976, *The Self-Recognition Concept: An Active Function For the MHC Based On Protein-Carbohydrate Complementarity*, Billings and Rothenberg, Del Mar, Calif.

Schrader, J. W., and Edelman, G. M., 1977, Joint recognition by cytotoxic T cells of inactivated Sendai virus and products of the major histocompatibility complex, *J. Exp. Med.* **145**:523.

Schrader, J. W., Cunningham, B. A., and Edelman, G. M., 1975, Functional interactions of viral and histocompatibility antigens at tumor cell surfaces, *Proc. Natl. Acad. Sci. USA* **72**:5066.

Schrader, J. W., Henning, R., Milner, R. J., and Edelman, G. M., 1976, The recognition of *H-2* and viral antigens by cytotoxic T cells, *Cold Spring Harbor Symp. Quant. Biol.* **41**:547.

Schwartz, R. H., 1978, A clonal deletion model for *Ir* gene control of the immune response, *Scand. J. Immunol.* **7**:3.

Schwartz, R. N., and Paul, W. E., 1976, T-lymphocyte enriched murine peritoneal exudate cells. II. Genetic control of antigen induced T-lymphocyte proliferation, *J. Exp. Med.* **143**:529.

Shearer, G. M., 1974, Cell-mediated cytotoxicity to trinitrophenyl-modified syngeneic lymphocytes, *Eur. J. Immunol.* **4**:257.

Shearer, G. M., and Schmitt-Verhulst, A. M., 1977, Major histocompatibility complex restricted cell-mediated immunity, *Adv. Immunol.* **25**:55.

Shearer, G. M., Rehn, G. R., and Garbarino, C. A., 1975, Cell-mediated lympholysis of trinitrophenyl-modified autologous lymphocytes: Effector cell specificity to modified cell surface components controlled by the *H-2K* and *H-2D* regions of the murine major histocompatibility complex, *J. Exp. Med.* **141**:1348.

Shearer, G. M., Rehn, T. J., and Schmitt-Verhulst, A.-M, 1976, Role of the murine major histocompatibility complex in the specificity of *in vitro* T-cell mediated lympholysis against chemically-modified autologous lymphocytes, *Transplant. Rev.* **29**:222.

Shevach, E. M., and Rosenthal, A. S., 1973, Function of macrophages in antigen recognition by guniea pig T lymphocytes. II. Role of the macrophage in the regulation of genetic control of the immune response, *J. Exp. Med.* **138**:1213.

Shreffler, D. C., and David, C. S., 1975, The *H-2* major histocompatibility complex and the *I* immune response region: Genetic variation, function and organization, *Adv. Immunol.* **20**:125.

Simpson, E., and Gordon, R. D., 1977, Responsiveness to H-Y antigen: *Ir* gene complementation and target cell specificity, *Transplant. Rev.* **35**:51.

Sjögren, H. O., and Ringertz, N., 1961, Histopathology and transplantability of polyoma-induced tumors in strain A/Sn and three coisogeneic resistant substrains, *J. Natl. Cancer Inst.* **28**:859.

Snell, G. D., 1968, The *H-2* locus of the mouse: Observations and speculations concerning its comparative genetics and its polymorphism, *Folia. Biol.* **14**:335.

Stutman, O., Shen, F. W., and Boyse, E. A., 1977, *Ly* phenotype of T cells cytotoxic for syngeneic mouse mammary tumors: Evidence for T cell interactions, *Proc. Natl. Acad. Sci. USA* **74**:5669.

Sugamura, K., Shimizu, K., Zarling, D. A., and Bach, F. H., 1977, Role of Sendai virus fusion-glycoprotein in target cell susceptibility to cytotoxic T cells, *Nature (London)* **270**:251.

Sugamura, K., Shimizu, K., and Bach, F. H., 1978, Involvement of fusion activity of ultraviolet light-inactivated Sendai virus in formation of target antigens recognized by cytotoxic T cells, *J. Exp. Med.* **148**:276.

Svet-Moldavsky, G. A., and Hamburg, V. P., 1964, Quantative relationships in viral oncolysis and the possibility of artificial heterogenization of tumors, *Nature (London)* **202**:303.

Thomas, L., 1959, *Cellular and Humoral Aspects of the Hypersensitive States* (H. S. Lawrence, ed.), p. 529, Hoeber, New York.

Todaro, G. J., 1975, Type C virogenes: Genetic transfer and interspecies transfer, in: *Tumor Virus Infections and Immunity* (R. L. Crow, H. Friedman, and J. E. Prier, eds.), p. 35, University Park Press, Baltimore.

Toivanen, P., Toivanen, A., and Vainio, O., 1974*a*, Complete restoration of bursa-dependent immune system after transplantation of semiallogeneic stem cells into immunodeficient chicks, *J. Exp. Med.* **139**:1344.

Toivanen, P., Toivanen, A., and Sorvari, T., 1974*b*, Incomplete restoration of the bursa-dependent immune system after transplantation of allogeneic stem cells into immunodeficient chicks, *Proc. Natl. Acad. Sci. USA* **71**:957.

Trinchieri, G., Aden, D. P., and Knowles, B. B., 1976, Cell-mediated cytotoxicity to SV-40-specific tumor-associated antigens, *Nature (London)* **261**:312.

von Boehmer, H., 1977, *The Cytotoxic Immune Response Against Male Cells: Control by Two Genes in the Murine Major Histocompatibility Complex*, Basel Institute of Immunology, Basel.

von Boehmer, H., Haas, W., and Jerne, N. K., 1978, Major histocompatibility complex-linked immunoresponsiveness is acquired by lymphocytes of low-responder mice differentiating in thymus of high-responder mice, *Proc. Natl. Acad. Sci. USA* **75**:2439.

Wainberg, M. A., Markson, Y., Weiss, D. W., and Donjanski, F., 1974, Cellular immunity against Rouse sarcoma of chickens: Preferential reactivity against autochthonous target cells as determined by lymphocyte adherence and cytotoxicity tests *in vitro*, *Proc. Natl. Acad. Sci. USA* **71**:3565.

Ward, K., Cantor, H., and Boyse, E. A., 1977, Clonally restricted interactions among T and B cell subclasses, in: *The Immune System: Genetics and regulation*, Vol. 6 (E. Sercarz, L. A. Herzenberg, and C. F. Fox, eds.), p. 397, ICN-UCLA Symposium Molecular and Cellular Biology, Los Angeles, Calif.

Welsh, R. M., 1978, Cytotoxic cells induced during lymphocytic choriomeningitis virus infection of mice. I. Characterization of natural killer cell induction, *J. Exp. Med.* **147**.

Welsh, R. M., and Zinkernagel, R. M., 1977, Heterospecific cytotoxic cell activity induced during the first three days of acute lymphocytic choriomeningitis virus infection in mice, *Nature (London)* **268**:646.

Wiktor, T. J., Doherty, P. C., and Koprowski, H., 1977, *In vitro* evidence of cell-mediated immunity after exposure of mice to both live and inactivated rabies virus, *Proc. Natl. Acad. Sci. USA* **74**:334.

Wong, C. Y., Woodruff, J. J., and Woodruff, J. F., 1977, Generation of cytotoxic T lymphocytes during Coxsackie virus B-3 infection. I. Characteristics of effector cells and demonstration of cytotoxicity against viral infected myofibers, *J. Immunol.* **118**:1165.

Zarling, D. A., Keshet, I., Watson, A., and Bach, F., 1978, Association of mouse major histocompatibility and Rauscher murine leukemia virus envelope glycoprotein antigens on leukemia cells and their recognition by syngeneic virus-immune cytotoxic lymphocytes, *Scand. J. Immunol.* **2**:497.

Zavada, J., 1972, VSV pseudotype particles with the coat of avian myeloblastosis virus, *New Biol.* **240**:122.

Zinkernagel, R. M., 1977, Role of the *H-2* gene complex in cell-mediated immunity to infectious disease, *Transplant. Proc.* **9**:835.

Zinkernagel, R. M., 1978, Thymus and lymphohemopoietic cells: Their role in T cell maturation, in selection of T cell's *H-2* restriction specificity and in *H-2* linked *Ir* gene control, *Immunol. Rev.* **42**:224.

Zinkernagel, R. M., and Althage, A., 1977, Anti-viral protection by virus-immune cytotoxic T cells: Infected target cells are lysed before infectious virus progeny is assembled, *J. Exp. Med.* **145**:644.

Zinkernagel, R. M., and Doherty, P. C., 1974, Activity of sensitized thymus derived lymphocytes in lymphocytic choriomeningitis reflects immunological surveillance against altered self components, *Nature (London)* **251**:547.

Zinkernagel, R. M., and Doherty, P. C., 1975, *H-2* compatibility requirement for T cell mediated lysis of targets infected with lymphocytic choriomeningitis virus: Different cytotoxic T cell specificities are associated with structures coded in H-2K or H-2D, *J. Exp. Med.* **141:**1427.

Zinkernagel, R. M., and Doherty, P. C., 1977, Major transplantation antigens virus and specificity of surveillance T cells: The "altered self" hypothesis, *Contemp. Top. Immunobiol.* **7:**179.

Zinkernagel, R. M., Adler, B., and Althage, A., 1977a, The question of derepression of *H-2* specificities in virus-infected cells: Failure to detect specific alloreactive T cells after systemic virus infection or alloantigens detectable by alloreactive T cells on virus infected target cells, *Immunogenetics* **5:**367.

Zinkernagel, R. M., Althage, A., and Jensen, F. C., 1977b, Cell-mediated immune response to lymphocytic choriomeningitis and vaccinia virus in rats, *J. Immunol.* **119:**1242.

Zinkernagel, R. M., Althage, A., Adler, B., Blanden, R. V., Davidson, W. F., Kees, U., Dunlop, M. B. C., and Shreffler, D. C., 1977c, *H-2* restriction of cell-mediated immunity to an intracellular bacterium: Effector T cells are specific for *Listeria* antigen in association with *H-2I* region coded self-markers, *J. Exp. Med.* **145:**1353.

Zinkernagel, R. M., Adler, B., and Holland, J., 1977d, Cell-mediated immunity to vesicular stomatitis virus infections in mice, *Exp. Cell Biol.* **46:**53.

Zinkernagel, R. M., Callahan, G. N., Klein, J., and Dennert, G., 1978a, Cytotoxic T cells learn specificity for self-*H-2* during differentiation in the thymus, *Nature (London)* **271:**251.

Zinkernagel, R. M., Callahan, G. N., Althage, A., Cooper, S., Klein, P. A., and Klein, J., 1978b, On the thymus in the differentiation of *H-2* self-recognition by T cells: Evidence for dual recognition, *J. Exp. Med.* **147:**882.

Zinkernagel, R. M., Callahan, G. N., Althage, A., Cooper, J., Streilein, J. W., and Klein, J., 1978c, The lymphoreticular system in triggering virus-plus-self specific cytotoxic T cells: Evidence for T help, *J. Exp. Med.* **147:**897.

Zinkernagel, R. M., Althage, A., Cooper, S., Kreeb, G., Klein, P. A., Sefton, B., Flaherty, L., Stimpfling, J., Shreffler, D., and Klein, J., 1978d, *Ir* genes in *H-2* regulate generation of antiviral cytotoxic T cells: Mapping to *K* or *D* and dominance of unresponsiveness, *J. Exp. Med.* **148:**592.

Zinkernagel, R. M., Althage, A., Cooper, S., Callahan, G. N., and Klein, J., 1978e, In irradiation chimeras, *K* or *D* regions of the chimeric host, not of the donor lymphocytes determine immune responsiveness of antiviral cytotoxic T cells, *J. Exp. Med.* **148:**80.

Zinkernagel, R. M., Althage, A., and Holland, J., 1978f, Target antigens for *H-2* restricted vesicular stomatitis virus-specific cytotoxic T cells, *J. Immunol.* **121:**744.

Zweerink, H. J., Askonas, B. A., Millican, D., Courtneidge, S. A., and Skehel, J. J., 1977, Cytotoxic T cells to type A influenza virus; viral hemagglutinin induces A-strain specificity while infected cells confer cross-reactive cytotoxicity, *Eur. J. Immunol.* **7:**630.

CHAPTER 5

Interferons

E. De Maeyer and J. De Maeyer-Guignard

Institut Curie
Université de Paris-Sud
Campus d'Orsay, Bât. 110
91405—Orsay, France

1. INTRODUCTION

Over 20 years have elapsed since interferon was first described (Isaacs and Lindenmann, 1957*a,b*) and defined as a broad-spectrum antiviral substance (Isaacs, 1963). This definition was too restricted, and interferons now appear as a group of proteins displaying numerous biological activities. This does not mean that the antiviral activity has received less attention, as attested by the recent successful clinical applications (Desmyter *et al.*, 1976; Greenberg *et al.*, 1976; Merigan *et al.*, 1978). Lately, the pace of research on fundamental aspects of interferon has been accelerating considerably, and books have been edited on the subject. It is therefore not possible to consider all aspects of interferon in the same detail in a review like this, and we have restricted ourselves principally to aspects of interferon as they relate to virology. Emphasis has been placed on some of the newer developments, such as If-mRNA, mechanisms of antiviral action, purification, and interaction with the immune system. Many excellent reviews have been written on several particular aspects of interferon research, and the reader will be referred to these for an in-depth analysis.

The molecular characterization of interferon has quite recently made considerable progress, and it has become apparent that, for a given animal species, there exist several forms of interferon as distinguished by their antigenicity, size, degree of glycosylation, and pH stability. One major distinction is between two different classes of interferon molecules having quite distinct modes of induction. The first class comprises "classical" or virus-induced interferon, as originally discovered by Isaacs and Lindenmann (1957a,b), and the second class comprises mitogen- and antigen-induced lymphokines with antiviral activity, sometimes referred to as "immune interferons" (Falcoff, 1972). We have accepted the proposition of Youngner and Salvin (1973) to name the first group type I and the second group type II interferons, but we are aware that this distinction may eventually turn out to have been too dogmatic and simplistic. Nevertheless, for the time being it provides a useful framework for discussing interferon. To avoid confusion, type II interferon has been discussed separately, in Section 7. All other sections deal exclusively with type I interferon.

2. INTERFERON SYNTHESIS

Type I interferon production has been observed in all classes of vertebrates: birds,in which it was originally discovered, mammals, amphibiae, reptiles, and fish. Human, murine, rabbit, and chick cells have been used for the major part of studies on interferon induction, and we will not always refer to the species origin when discussing interferon induction.

2.1. Interferon Synthesis *in Vitro*

2.1.1. Induction

Most experiments to elucidate the basic mechanism of interferon induction and subsequent production have been performed in tissue culture, and therefore of necessity deal with averages obtained from a cell population in which the number of interferon-producing cells is usually an unknown. A few systems for studying interferon production by single cells have been reported (Fleischmann and Simon, 1974; Kronenberg, 1977), but such techniques have not been systematically used for the study of interferon production.

Cells of many different tissular origins are capable of producing interferon, and it is quite exceptional to find cells that cannot be induced to make interferon. This is the case for Vero cells, a continuous line of African green monkey cells (Desmyter *et al.*, 1968), and for a line of undifferentiated teratocarcinoma cells (Burke *et al.*, 1978). Under "normal" conditions, most cells do not make interferon: at least they do not release it in detectable quantities, nor can interferon be extracted from them. In view of the high sensitivity of most interferon assays, this means that, if cells do contain interferon which escapes detection, it must be in very small amounts indeed. Spontaneous interferon production has been described in macrophages, in cultures of normal bone marrow cells, in lymphoblastoid lines derived from Burkitt's lymphomas, and in leukemic and normal peripheral leukocyte cultures (Northrop and Deinhardt, 1967; Smith and Wagner, 1967; Swart and Young, 1969; Zajac *et al.*, 1969., Haase *et al.*, 1970; De Maeyer *et al.*, 1971a; Talas *et al.*, 1972; Adams *et al.*, 1975). Thus cells that are derived from hemopoietic stem cells often produce small amounts of interferon when put in tissue culture; this interferon has not always been characterized as either type I or type II, and one can only speculate as to the meaning of this "spontaneous" release of interferon. Other cells—including diploid cell lines—usually do not have spontaneous interferon production, although there are exceptions to this rule; we have, for example, consistently found low levels (between 1 and 10 units/ml) in a line of mouse L cells and also in cultures of the high-producer mouse C243 cell line first described by Oie *et al.* (1972). The mechanism of this spontaneous production is not known, nor is it known whether it is due to a few cells making much interferon or to many cells each of which makes very little.

If normally then there is either no or, occasionally, a very low interferon production, this situation very rapidly changes when cells are treated with an appropriate inducer. Not much is known of what happens between the first contact of the cell with an interferon inducer and the time of transcription of the interferon gene(s); there is as yet no compelling reason to suppose that, except for the first stages dealing with adsorption, penetration, and virus replication, different induction mechanisms are involved with different viral inducers, and we will discuss the general scheme of induction as it appears from studies in several systems. Interferon formation is inhibited by pretreatment of cells with actinomycin D (Heller, 1963; Wagner, 1963, 1964), and it was very soon concluded from studies with metabolic inhibitors that transcription of an interferon-specific mRNA is involved (Wagner and Huang, 1965). Actual measurement of mRNA extracted from induced cells has shown that interferon-mRNA activity increases for several hours after induction and that it reflects the increased levels of interferon released by the induced cells. Interferon mRNA leaves the nucleus after synthesis, as shown in studies with enucleated cells; enucleation of cells before induction prevents interferon formation, but when cells are enucleated after interferon formation has started, the cytoplasts continue to synthesize interferon (Burke and Veomett, 1977). Falcoff *et al.* (1976), in a study of poly(I·C)-induced interferon formation in human FS4 cells, arrived at the conclusion that most, if not all, interferon is synthesized on membrane-bound polysomes, discharged into the lumina of the rough endoplasmic reticulum, and then further processed during passage through various intracellular membrane compartments before being excreted by the cell. Active transport is involved in the latter stage (Tan *et al.*, 1972).

These findings are confirmed by studies on the intracellular location of human fibroblast interferon mRNA which have shown that most of the activity is membrane associated (Abreu and Bancroft, 1978).

Soon after reaching maximal levels, interferon synthesis decreases rapidly and then stops, in spite of the continued presence of inducer. Renewed induction results in lower interferon levels, and it can take up to several days before this state of "refractoriness" has disappeared (Cantell and Paucker, 1963a,b; Burke and Buchan, 1965; Billiau, 1970). The rapid decrease of interferon synthesis theoretically could be due to feedback by the interferon molecules themselves. There is, however, a great deal of experimental evidence, admittedly indirect, against feedback as the mechanism that stops interferon production, and this phenomenon will be more fully discussed in Section 2.1.3.

2.1.2. Inducers

2.1.2a. Viruses

The first known interferon inducers were viruses, since interferon was discovered by Isaacs and Lindenmann (1957a) during a study of viral interference. The original work was done with a strain of influenza virus, and it has since been shown that practically all viruses are capable of interferon induction when tested under appropriate conditions. These conditions can vary widely, depending on the virus–cell combination used, and it would be impossible to make a general statement concerning the optimal conditions for interferon induction by viruses. For example, live Newcastle disease virus (NDV) is a good interferon inducer in mouse or human cells, but it induces little or no interferon in chick cells unless it is first inactivated by heat at 56°C or by UV irradiation (Ho and Breinig, 1965; Gandhi and Burke, 1970; Sheaff *et al.*, 1972; Youngner *et al.*, 1966). Attenuated strains of some viruses can be better interferon inducers than virulent or wild strains, as is the case, for example, for measles virus in human cells (De Maeyer and Enders, 1965; Mirchamsy and Rapp, 1969; Volckaert-Vervliet and Billiau, 1977), for some influenza virus strains in human leucocyte suspensions (Polezhaev *et al.*, 1974), and for Sindbis virus in mouse cell cultures (Inglot *et al.*, 1973). Again, no general rule can be deduced (for example, the ability of NDV strains to induce interferon in chick cells is independent of their virulence in the animal) in that some virulent strains are more potent inducers than some avirulent ones (Lomniczi, 1970*a,b*, 1973). Often, interferon production can be directly correlated with virus replication rather than with virulence or attenuation (Lockart, 1963; McLaren and Potter, 1973), and it could conceivably be a reflection of the amount of viral RNA made during infection (Burke, 1971). As a rule, most RNA viruses, either single or double stranded, are efficient interferon inducers, and for many *in vitro* studies either myxoviruses or arboviruses have been used. The major exception is the oncornaviruses, and there are very few reports on *in vitro* interferon induction by oncornaviruses. Rous sarcoma virus is capable of inducing interferon in chick embryo cells (Bader, 1962). We are not aware of any similar report concerning the murine oncornaviruses, and, in fact, there are a number of reports indicating the failure of murine oncornaviruses to induce interferon formation in tissue culture (Peries *et al.*, 1964, 1965; Duc-Nguyen *et al.*, 1966).

2.1.2b. Nucleic Acids, Including Viral

The hypothesis that RNA is the stimulus to make interferon was first proposed by Isaacs (1961) but was then tacitly abandoned because of lack of convincing experimental evidence; it was also proposed by Isaacs that the RNA had to be "foreign" to the cell in order to induce. The interest in RNA as interferon inducer was rekindled when Lampson *et al.* (1967), Field *et al.* (1967), and Tytell *et al.* (1967) demonstrated that double-stranded RNAs from a wide variety of sources are potent interferon inducers, *in vitro* as well as *in vivo* (Nemes *et al.*, 1969*a,b*). Of the synthetic polyribonucleotides examined, the homopolymer pair, poly(I·C), is the most active. For double-stranded polyribonucleotides to be good interferon inducers, a stable secondary structure and a high molecular weight are prime requisites (Colby and Chamberlin, 1969; Tytell *et al.*, 1970). DNA–RNA hybrids do not induce (Colby *et al.*, 1971). A great number of studies have been performed comparing various structurally changed synthetic polyribonucleotides for their interferon–inducing capacity; for more details, the reader is referred to the very thorough review by Torrence and De Clercq (1977).

For an RNA to be an efficient interferon inducer, double strandedness is required, but the RNA does not necessarily have to be foreign to the cell, since cellular dsRNA can induce interferon in cells of the same origin that were used to extract the RNA (De Maeyer *et al.*, 1971*b*; Kimball and Duesberg, 1971; Stern and Friedman, 1971). Since many double-stranded RNAs are excellent interferon inducers, it is tempting to ascribe interferon induction by viruses to the formation of dsRNA during some stage of the replicative cycle. Although there is suggestive evidence that this is indeed the case, the overall situation is far from clear, and no general rule can be formulated. Double-stranded RNA viruses, regardless of their bacterial, fungal, plant, insect, or animal origin, as a rule are good interferon inducers when tested in murine or human cells, either as free double-stranded virion RNA or as intact virus particle, as has been shown with reovirus type 3 (Tytell *et al.*, 1967), with cytoplasmic polyhedrosis virus and with rice dwarf virus (Nemes *et al.*, 1969*b*), and with various *Penicillium* mycophages (Lampson *et al.*, 1967; Kleinschmidt *et al.*, 1968; Buck *et al.*, 1971). The double-stranded virion RNA of input virus appears to be sufficient to trigger interferon synthesis, as shown by Long and Burke (1971), who found reovirus type 3 capable of inducing interferon in chick cells without any concomitant production of infectious virus or even virus-specific RNA synthesis. Lai and Joklik (1973) similarly showed interferon induction by reovirus type 3, but comparison of the RNA synthesis and interferon induction of nine *ts* mutants with the wild-type virus at permissive and nonpermissive temperatures revealed no correlation between interferon synthesis and the amount of double-stranded RNA synthesized. The authors therefore conclude that reovirus can induce interferon synthesis while exercising none of the functions necessary for viral multiplication.

The hypothesis that single-stranded RNA viruses owe their interferon-inducing capacity to their replicative intermediates has received a great deal of attention. Falcoff and Falcoff (1970) showed that interferon induction in mouse L cells can be obtained by the replicative intermediate as well as the replicative form of mengovirus, and the amount of interferon induced is proportional to the amount of RNA added. However, formation of replicative intermediate does not always seem to be required to obtain interferon induction, as shown, for example, in studies with temperature-sensitive mutants of Sindbis or Semliki Forest viruses (Lockart *et al.*, 1968; Lomniczi and Burke, 1970). Interpretation of these studies is complicated by the fact that most of such mutants show a certain degree of leakiness, and, indeed, a minimum of RNA synthesis would seem to be required to obtain interferon induction in any case (Atkins *et al.*, 1974). This is furthermore borne out by studies with Newcastle disease virus. UV-inactivated NDV, not giving rise to infectious progeny, is still capable of interferon induction; this was taken as evidence that input single-stranded virion RNA can function as inducer (Gandhi and Burke, 1970; Gandhi *et al.*, 1970). However, it was then shown that even UV-inactivated virus, which has lost its infectivity, is still capable of inducing RNA synthesis, and that limited amounts of base-paired RNA associated with a transcriptive intermediate are involved in this RNA synthesis. With large doses of UV irradiation, RNA-synthesizing capacity and interferon-inducing capacity are lost in parallel (Clavell and Bratt, 1971). In addition, it should be emphasized that single-stranded polynucleotides can act as interferon inducers, but usually much less efficiently so than dsRNAs (Baron *et al.*, 1969; Pitha and Pitha, 1974; Thang *et al.*, 1977a; De Clercq *et al.*, 1978).

DNA viruses are, as a rule, much less efficient interferon inducers than are RNA viruses, although under suitable conditions they are capable of inducing. In general, virus replication would seem to be required; for example, *ts* mutants of adenovirus do not induce interferon in chick cells at nonpermissive temperatures (Ustacelebi and Williams, 1972). It has been suggested that, even in the case of DNA viruses, the formation of dsRNA is the signal for interferon synthesis, and Colby and Duesberg (1969) demonstrated the existence of a dsRNA intermediate for the replication of vaccinia virus in chick cells. Whether this dsRNA really is the trigger for interferon production in vaccinia-infected cells, and whether this is also true for other DNA viruses, is an unsettled problem (Bakay and Burke, 1972).

It is currently not possible to present unifying hypothesis accounting for a common interferon-inducing molecule or structure introduced into the cell or made during the replication of the various viruses that have been shown to induce interferon. On the other hand, since isolated dsRNA has been shown to be a very efficient interferon inducer, there is very little reason to doubt its contribution to interferon induction when it is introduced into the cell either as virion RNA or as a result of viral replication.

2.1.2c. Others

Several nonviral inducers have been described, and the reader is referred to Grossberg (1977) for an extensive analysis of all nonviral inducers.

2.1.3. Control Mechanisms: Regulation of Interferon Production

The fundamental questions pertaining to the mechanisms of onset and arrest of interferon synthesis remain unanswered, and even the best experiments in this domain have come up with only hypothetical explanations. This is not surprising, since the problem of control and regulation of interferon production reflects just one particular aspect of the complex problem of control and regulation of inducible proteins in vertebrate cells in general.

2.1.3a. Priming

In many systems, interferon treatment of cells affects their capacity to subsequently produce interferon. Pretreatment with low doses of interferon before induction in general enhances subsequent interferon production, a phenomenon called priming (Isaacs and Burke, 1958; Lockart, 1963; Stewart et al., 1971). Since priming is also obtained when poly(I·C) is subsequently used as inducer, and in systems in which the inducing virus does not replicate, it does not appear to act by merely preventing the inducing virus from replicating and destroying the protein-synthesizing apparatus of the cell. Paradoxically, about tenfold more If-mRNA activity was extracted from unprimed than from primed mouse L929 cells by Lebleu et al. (1978), but Saito et al. (1976) found more interferon mRNA activity in primed vs. nonprimed cells. No other attempts to study priming at the molecular level have been published. Priming may be the result of one or several of the biochemical changes brought about in cells by interferon (see Section 3), and, in a study using mouse–human hybrid cells, a correlation was observed between sensitivity of hybrid cells to the antiviral action of interferon and their ability to become primed (Frankfort *et al.*, 1978).

2.1.3b. Hyporeactivity

Cells that have produced interferon usually make considerably less on a second stimulation, a phenomenon of hyporesponsiveness that has also been observed in the animal. Thus the continued presence of an inducer does not lead to continued formation of interferon. There is some evidence that interferon itself can exert a negative feedback effect on its own synthesis (Youngner and Hallum, 1969; Cantell and Paucker, 1963*a,b*; Vilček and Rada, 1962; Paucker and Boxaca, 1967). Since these experiments have been performed with relatively crude interferon preparations, there is some discussion as to whether interferon itself is capable of provoking a state of hyporesponsiveness to a second induction; for example, Margolis *et al.* (1972) and Breinig *et al.* (1975) favor the idea that it is not interferon itself, but another substance, the synthesis of which is also triggered by interferon inducers, whereas Barmak and Vilček (1973) do not exclude the possibility that it is interferon itself. Recent experiments in the authors' laboratory, using electrophoretically pure mouse interferon, have shown that preincubation of C-243 cells for 24 hr with amounts of interferon ranging from 16 to 160,000 units does not inhibit subsequent poly(I·C)-induced interferon synthesis by these cells. In fact, even at the highest dose of interferon used for preincubation, priming rather than blocking is observed. The fact that interferon does not inhibit its own synthesis indicates that negative feedback is not the mechanism responsible for the cessation of interferon synthesis after induction.

2.1.3c. Superinduction

The regulation of poly(I·C)-induced interferon production has been studied to a great extent, especially by Vilček and his co-workers. When applied at suitable interval and dosages after onset of induction, various inhibitors of protein and of RNA synthesis, as well as a combination of these, can increase interferon production induced by poly(I·C) (Youngner *et al.*, 1965; Vilček *et al.*, 1969; Tan *et al.*, 1970, 1971*a*). Based on a certain analogy with enzyme superinduction in rat liver cells (Garren *et al.*, 1964), the phenomenon has been called "superinduction." Superinduction of interferon synthesis is essentially due to the inhibition of the shutoff mechanism of interferon production. Vilček has proposed that a rapidly turning over repressor system is induced coordinately with interferon; this repressor system would cause irreversible inactivation of interferon mRNA and hence be responsible for the shutoff of interferon production as well as for the phenomenon of hyporesponsiveness to repeated interferon induction (Kohase and Vilček, 1977; Vilček and Ng, 1971). The existence of a repressor of interferon synthesis induced at the same time as interferon itself has also been postulated by Borden and Murphy (1971), based on the observation that interferon preparations derived from mice soon after induction were less efficient inhibitors of interferon synthesis than were preparations obtained late after induction, implying that the inhibitor appeared later than did interferon. Treatment of interferon-producing cells with inhibitors of RNA or protein synthesis could then possibly block or decrease the synthesis of such a repressor, with the result that interferon synthesis would go on. In line with this hypothesis is the observation by Tan and Berthold (1977) that some inhibitors of protein synthesis—e.g., cycloheximide—when put on human cells provoke a low level of interferon synthesis; this is interpreted to suggest that the synthesis of the proposed repressor substance is inhibited and therefore interferon synthesis is triggered.

Another possibility—not necessarily exclusive of the foregoing— would be that, by inhibiting the synthesis of certain mRNAs of rapid turnover, more of the protein-synthesizing apparatus of the cell would become accessible to interferon mRNA. In accord with this explanation is the observation that treatment of chick embryo cells with actinomycin D increases their capacity to translate heterologous mouse interferon mRNA (De Maeyer et al., 1975a).

One intriguing aspect of the superinduction phenomenon is the fact that it is usually significantly pronounced only when poly(I·C) is employed as inducer, whereas in the case of viral induction it either is not operative at all or hardly enhances the interferon yields. This raises the additional question of how much—or how little—one can generalize about the control mechanism of interferon synthesis from studies in superinduced cells. This problem has been discussed to some extent by Vilček et al. (1976). Based on differential effects of UV irradiation on poly(I·C) and NDV-induced interferon synthesis in rabbit cells, Mozes and Vilček (1974, 1975) propose that whereas poly(I·C)-induced interferon production is under negative control of the translational repressor, this repressor is either completely absent or plays a much less important role in virus-induced interferon synthesis. A combination of cytogenetic and biochemical studies will be required to obtain satisfactory answers to this difficult problem (Cassingena *et al.*, 1971; Tan *et al.*, 1977). A correlation between human chromosome 16 and superinducibility has been suggested by Creagan *et al.* (1975), and human interferon loci have been assigned to chromosomes 2 and 5 (Tan *et al.*, 1974*a*). Using this approach, it has been possible to isolate high-interferon-producing lines of human cells (Tan *et al.*, 1977), and such cell lines will be instrumental in the study of the fundamental mechanisms of interferon production. The existence of separate structural genes for human fibroblast interferon on chromosomes 2, 5, and 9 has now been unequivocally established (Slate and Ruddle, 1979; Meager *et al.*, 1979). It is not known whether the gene products are identical or different.

2.1.4. Interferon mRNA

Interferons are cellular proteins, and their induction is characterized by *de novo* synthesis of mRNA, as first described by Wagner and Huang (1965) from work with metabolic inhibitors. Interferon mRNA can now be assayed directly, by using cells that have been induced as a source of interferon mRNA. Three different techniques have been developed for translating interferon mRNA. The first one takes advantage of the relative species specificity of interferon and involves translation of the RNA by whole heterologous cells (De Maeyer-Guignard *et al.*, 1972). In order to obtain optimal results, the recipient cells have to be pretreated with actinomycin D, and DEAE-dextran has to be present during incubation of the cells with the RNA. Both mouse and human interferon mRNAs have been translated under these conditions (De Maeyer-Guignard *et al.*, 1972; Reynolds and Pitha, 1974; Orlova *et al.*, 1974; Kronenberg and Friedmann, 1975; Greene *et al.*, 1978). Mouse and human interferon mRNA have also been translated in cell-free systems: mouse interferon mRNA in a wheat germ and a rabbit reticulocyte system (Thang *et al.*, 1975; Lebleu *et al.*, 1978) and human interferon mRNA in a cell-free system prepared from either wheat germ, rabbit reticulocytes, or mouse ascites cells (Reynolds *et al.*, 1975; Pestka *et al.*, 1975; Raj and Pitha, 1977). A third translational system that has been used successfully is the *Xenopus laevis* oocyte, both for mouse and for human interferon mRNA (Raj and Pitha 1977; Cavalieri *et al.*, 1977*a*; Sehgal *et al.*,

1977; Lebleu *et al.*, 1978). Within rather narrow limits, the different translational systems can be made quantitative, and thus information relevant to rate of synthesis and rate of disappearance of interferon mRNA from induced cells can be obtained. So far, it has not been possible to obtain interferon mRNA from uninduced cells using any of the translational systems mentioned above, thus confirming earlier results with metabolic inhibitors indicating that induction of interferon involves derepression of gene function and *de novo* synthesis of interferon mRNA. Shortly after contact of the cells with an inducer [poly(I·C) or NDV has been used in most studies], interferon mRNA can be extracted. The amount of interferon mRNA activity that is thus obtained increases with time and is by and large a reflection of the rate of interferon synthesis in the RNA donor cells; at the time time of shutoff of interferon synthesis, mRNA activity can no longer be recovered from the cells (Fig. 1) (De Maeyer-Guignard *et al.*, 1972; De Maeyer *et al.*, 1975*a*; Reynolds and Pitha, 1974; Cavalieri *et al.*, 1977*a*; Greene *et al.*, 1978). Studies with metabolic inhibitors have suggested that a posttranscriptional event is involved in the shutoff of interferon synthesis (Tan *et al.*, 1970; Vilček *et al.*, 1969; Sehgal *et al.*, 1975).

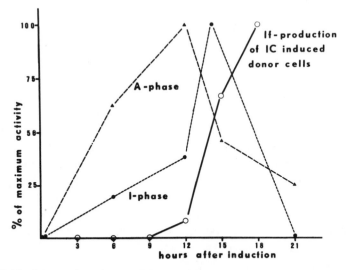

Fig. 1.   Yield of mouse interferon mRNA activity as a function of time after induction of mRNA donor cells. Messenger activity is expressed as percentage of maximal mouse interferon yields obtained from translation in heterologous cells (chick). For comparison, the kinetics of interferon production in the mRNA donor cells is also represented. A phase, mainly cytoplasmic RNA; I phase, mainly membrane-bound RNA. From De Maeyer *et al.* (1975*a*).

Sehgal and Tamm (1976) have shown that interferon shutoff in human diploid cells induced with poly(I·C) can be prevented by giving an RNA inhibitor such as actinomycin D or 5,6-dichloro-β-D-ribofuranosylbenzimidazole to the cells after induction. Under these conditions, interferon synthesis does not stop at the usual time, but goes on, suggesting that the interferon mRNA is a stable species with relatively long half-life. It is therefore possible that the rapid decline in interferon mRNA activity extracted from interferon-producing cells is the result of a specific inactivation event, such as suggested by the studies of Vilček and Ng (1971), postulating the existence of a specific repressor of interferon-mRNA function. The isolation and characterization of such a repressor would be relevant to the control of protein synthesis in eukaryotic systems in general. In any case, the fact that more interferon is produced when cells are superinduced with poly(I·C) in the presence of cycloheximide compared to ordinary induction with poly(I·C) only does not yet have a clear explanation. Determination of the level of interferon mRNA at various times after induction in induced and superinduced cells will be useful to explain the phenomenon in terms of posttranscriptional control. Reynolds and Pitha (1974) and Raj and Pitha (1977) found very little difference in the level of interferon mRNA in superinduced cells as compared to induction in the absence of cycloheximide. Cavalieri *et al.* (1977*b*), on the contrary, found much greater amounts of mRNA activity in superinduced than induced cells (Fig. 2), and similar findings have been reported by Sehgal *et al.* (1978). It should be realized, however, that all these studies suffer from the drawback that quantitation of interferon mRNA—regardless of the translational system used—is still quite unreliable in that linearity is not always obtained and to some extent is influenced by the purity of the RNA preparations used. Purification of interferon mRNA has been based mainly on retention by oligo(dT)-cellulose or poly(U)-Sepharose columns, followed by velocity sedimentation. Mouse and human interferon mRNA have been found to have $s_{20,w}$ sedimentation values between 9 and 12 S (Reynolds and Pitha, 1974; De Maeyer *et al.*, 1975*a*; Lebleu *et al.*, 1978; Sehgal *et al.*, 1978). The fact that interferon mRNA can be assayed should permit its isolation and total purification. The purified mRNA provides a handle with which the interferon gene can be isolated and manipulated, a great advantage for fundamental studies. It is also conceivable that the interferon genes may eventually be inserted into bacteria. These could then be utilized to produce human interferon in the amounts necessary for therapeutic uses.

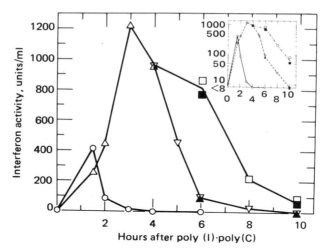

Fig. 2. Effect of superinduction on interferon mRNA. Translatable interferon mRNA in cells induced with poly(I·C), poly(I·C) and cycloheximide, and poly(I·C), cycloheximide, and actinomycin D as a function of time. Cultures were induced at time 0 with poly (I·C) (5 μg/ml) alone (O) or with poly(I·C) in the presence of cycloheximide (50 μg/ml) ($\triangle,\triangledown,\blacktriangle,\square,\blacksquare$). In addition, some of these cultures were treated with actinomycin D (1 μg/ml) for 4–5 hr ($\square,\blacksquare$). The inducing medium with cycloheximide (and actinomycin D, if applicable) was removed at 5 hr; the cells were thoroughly washed and further incubated in the absence of inducer in inhibitor-free medium. The data were obtained for three experiments performed at different times. The following sets of symbols represent data from experiments performed concurrently: (O,$\triangle$), ($\triangledown,\square$), and ($\blacktriangle,\blacksquare$). At the times indicated, the medium was removed, the cell monolayers were washed, and the cells were harvested. Poly(A)-containing mRNA was prepared from each cell pellet and injected into oocytes. Experimental values represent interferon yields obtained with 25 ng of mRNA injected per oocyte. (Inset) Logarithmic plot of the same data. From Cavalieri *et al.* (1977*b*).

2.2. In the Animal

2.2.1. Cells That Produce Interferon

Interferon can be isolated from various tissues in the organism during acute viral infections, and the production of interferon is one of the very first lines of antiviral defense. Any doubts that may have remained as to the importance of the interferon system as an antiviral mechanism have been removed by the studies of Gresser and collaborators, who showed that by treating mice with a potent anti-interferon serum some rather benign virus infections can be transformed into fulminant and sometimes lethal disease (Gresser *et al.*, 1976*b,c*;

Virelizier and Gresser, 1978), confirming and extending an earlier observation by Fauconnier (1970) (Fig. 3).

Probably all cells in the body are capable of interferon synthesis (Sutton and Tyrrell, 1961; Ho and Ke, 1970); for example, interferon can be isolated from mouse brains during infection with arboviruses (Vilček and Stanček, 1963). However, the attention of most investigators has been focused on cells derived from the hemopoietic system. Human peripheral blood leukocytes stimulated by Sendai or measles virus (Gresser, 1961), mouse peritoneal leukocytes infected with vaccinia virus (Glasgow and Habel, 1963), and rabbit spleen or peritoneal exudate cells stimulated with NDV (Kono and Ho, 1965; Smith and Wagner, 1967) were all shown to produce interferon. Practically pure suspensions of human peripheral blood lymphocytes are excellent interferon producers when stimulated by NDV (Wheelock, 1966).

Cells that are derived from the hemopoietic system, such as lymphocytes and macrophages, appear to make a significant contribution to the total interferon synthesis of the body in the case of those infections that at one stage or another are characterized by viremia or when virus is administered directly into the bloodstream. Under these conditions, interferon is released into the bloodstream (Baron and Buckler, 1963), and this method has been extensively used to study

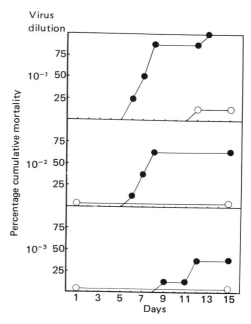

Fig. 3. Effect of anti-interferon globulin on infection of mice with herpes simplex virus type I. Only one mouse died of 19 mice treated with normal serum globulin and injected subcutaneously with a 10^{-1} dilution of HSV, and none died when injected with either 10^{-2} or 10^{-3} dilution of virus. In contrast, the mortality in mice treated with anti-interferon globulin was very pronounced at all three virus dilutions. ●, Mice treated with anti-interferon globulin; ○, mice treated with normal sheep globulin. From Gresser *et al.* (1976*b*).

interferon production *in vivo*. The potential contribution of circulating interferon to the antiviral defense is important, since this interferon can reach all organs of the body and thus increases their resistance to the spread of the viral infection (Baron *et al.*, 1966). The cells that are responsible for the production of circulating interferon are not always the same but vary depending on the virus involved.

The lymphocyte is the cell source of *in vivo* circulating interferon in the mouse after intravenous NDV challenge (De Maeyer *et al.*, 1967, 1969; De Maeyer-Guignard *et al.*, 1969; De Maeyer-Guignard and De Maeyer, 1971; Jullien *et al.*, 1974). Production of circulating interferon after *in vivo* NDV challenge is markedly depressed in mice following total-body X-irradiation, even after only 125 R. The depressed interferon response is due to radiation-induced depression of hematopoietic function, since it can be corrected by either syngeneic or xenogeneic bone marrow transplants to lethally irradiated recipients. In xenogeneic radiation chimeras, the circulating interferon induced by NDV is of donor origin, and hence from some line of hemopoietic cells. Since both lymphocytes and granulocytes are radiosensitive, anti-lymphocyte serum can be used to identify the actual cells producing interferon; this points to the lymphocyte as the main source of NDV-induced circulating interferon (De Maeyer-Guignard and De Maeyer, 1971). T cells have been implicated in synthesis of NDV-induced circu-lating interferon in mice by Pantelouris and Pringle (1976), who found a decreased production in nude mice of early-appearing circulating interferon but not of later (10 hr) production. T cells have also been implicated as main producers *in vitro* in spleen cells from C3H mice induced with influenza virus (Tsukui, 1977). Studies with other viruses indicate that the lymphocyte is not the only cell type in the mouse that responds to viremia with the production of circulating interferon. For example, whereas induction of interferon by NDV, a paramyxovirus, is a very radiosensitive process, induction by encephalomyocarditis virus (EMC), vaccinia virus, or poly(I·C) is relatively insensitive to radiation or antilymphocyte serum. In fact, EMC virus-induced interferon remains of recipient type in xenogeneic chimeras up to 3 months after lethal irradiation and xenogeneic chimeras up to 3 months after lethal irradiation and xenogeneic bone marrow transplantation, indicating that a mjaor part of the interferon observed after EMC challenge originates from a cell population not derived from the hemopoietic system at all. In contrast, interferon induced by poly(I·C) becomes donor type within 3 months after xenogeneic bone marrow grafting, indicating that it is made by cells from the hemopoietic system. When xenogeneic chimeras are subjected to reirradiation 1 month after the initial bone marrow transplant, interferon production by donor cells in response to poly(I·C) is not affected, thus implicating a hemopoietic cell more radioresistant than a lymphocyte, i.e., the macrophage, as the cell source of this type of interferon (Jullien *et al.*, 1974). Stebbing *et al.* (1978) report further evidence in support of the notion that macrophages are the principal cells producing serum interferon after administration of poly(I·C) to mice, since silica treatment or treatment with aurothiomalate reduces the production of serum interferon by 85–90%.

The determination of interferon-producing cells *in vivo* is obviously a complex undertaking; the fact that a given cell type has been implicated in interferon production for a given virus reflects, of course, the clearance of the virus and does not exclude the possibility that other cells in the body can be induced by this virus when given the opportunity.

2.2.2. Factors Influencing Interferon Production

Several physiological parameters have been shown to affect interferon synthesis *in vivo*.

2.2.2a. Age

In many instances, the interferon production of embryos and very young animals is lower than that of adult individuals (Baron and Isaacs, 1961; Heineberg *et al.*, 1964). When challenged with NDV, mice less than 1 month old and mice older than 8 months produce less circulating interferon than 2- to 6-month-old animals (De Maeyer and De Maeyer-Guignard, 1968). Since the bulk of this interferon comes from lymphocytes and macrophages, the decrease of production with age would seem to be a reflection of the diminishing functions of the immune system with age in general. When interferon production is the result of virus replication, sometimes an inverse correlation is found, with more virus and more interferon being produced by fetal or neonatal tissues, as is the case for Sindbis virus in mice (Vilček, 1963) and for Chikungunya virus in fetal lambs (Overall and Glasgow, 1970).

2.2.2b. Hormones

Little or nothing is known about possible interactions between the endocrine system and the interferon system except that several steroid hormones are capable of decreasing interferon production, in the animal and in tissue culture (Kilbourne *et al.*, 1961; De Maeyer and De Maeyer-Guignard, 1963; Mendelson and Glasgow, 1966; Rytel and Kilbourne, 1966).

2.2.2c. Animal Genotype

Circulating interferon levels of mice after intravenous administration of some viruses are under genetic control. A detailed study comparing NDV-induced interferon production of different inbred mouse strains using Mendelian analysis, has shown that one autosomal locus, *If-1*, is responsible for the difference in interferon production. Mice having the low-producer allele, *l*, have circulating interferon levels about tenfold lower than mice belonging to strains with the high-producer allele, *h* (De Maeyer and De Maeyer-Guignard, 1969). Similarly, circulating interferon induced by mMTV (mouse mammary tumor virus) is quantitatively controlled by the *If-2* locus, which segregates independently from *If-1* (De Maeyer *et al.*, 1974). Sendai- and influenza-virus-induced circulating interferon levels also can differ tenfold or more when different inbred strains of mice are compared. However, with Sendai virus the situation is more complex than with NDV and mMTV, and at least two genes, different from the foregoing, are involved for this virus. In all instances, the difference is a real difference in production and not due to secondary effects such as different inactivation or different clearance rates for interferon in high and low producers (De Maeyer and De Maeyer-Guignard, 1970). How these different *If* loci affect interferon production is not known. Low-responder animals can be converted into high responders by X-irradiation followed by restoration with bone marrow of high responders; this indicates that *If-1* acts on or through cells derived from the hemopoietic system (De Maeyer *et al.*, 1975*b*). *In vitro* the *If-1* locus is expressed in macrophage cultures, and this system should allow for an easier approach to the study of its mode of action. Regardless of how interferon levels are affected, mouse strains congenic at the alleles of the *If-1* locus (De Maeyer *et al.*, 1975*c*) have proved to be a useful tool for the study of the effect of interferon *in vivo* (see Section 5).

2.2.3. Hyporeactivity

Mice infected with cytomegalovirus and lymphocytic choriomeningitis virus develop a state of hyporesponsiveness to the induction of interferon (Osborn and Medearis, 1967; Holtermann and Havell, 1970). The same is true for mice with Friend leukemia or AKR lymphomas; the degree of hyporesponsiveness to viral and nonviral inducers of these leukemic animals is proportional to the extent of their leukemia (De Maeyer-Guignard, 1972). This phenomenon has been studied in some detail by Stringfellow (1975, 1976) and by Stringfellow et al. (1977), who find that mice infected with one of several viruses (EMC, Semliki Forest, influenza A2, herpesvirus hominis type 2, or murine cytomegalovirus) have in their serum a factor capable of mediating hyporeactivity to interferon induction in tissue culture. Although the factor resembles mouse interferon in that it is species specific, acid stable, and of about the same molecular weight, it is devoid of antiviral activity. Comparable findings have been reported by Borden et al. (1975) and by Tarr et al. (1978). Hyporeactivity to interferon production as a result of leukemia or viral infection could be related to the earlier observed hyporeactivity to repeated induction of interferon, first described by Ho and Kono (1965) and Ho et al. (1965), and Youngner and Stinebring (1965), using rabbits and mice, respectively. In any case, it appears that, as a result of various pathological conditions, the organism produces substances that inhibit the synthesis of interferon. Whether these are the factors that are involved in the normal control and regulation of interferon synthesis in the cell remains to be seen.

3. MECHANISMS OF THE ANTIVIRAL ACTIVITY

3.1. Establishment of the Antiviral State

Interferons inhibit viral replication indirectly by bringing about changes in the interferon-treated cells. Before they develop significant resistance, cells have to be exposed for a certain time to interferon; the period necessary varies with the dose of interferon used and has been reported to be from 1 to 6 hr (Dianzani and Baron, 1975; Dianzani et al., 1977). Some active metabolic process is required, since cells that have been treated with interferon in the cold become resistant only after they have been brought back to 37°C, and pretreatment with actinomycin D prevents the establishment of resistance, as does treatment with inhibitors of protein synthesis such as cycloheximide and parafluorophenylalanine (Taylor, 1964; Friedman and Sonnabend, 1964, 1965; Dianzani et al., 1969). Additional confirmation that an active process is required comes from studies using enucleated cells, which show that the establishment but not the maintenance of the antiviral state requires the presence of the nucleus (Radke et al., 1974;

Young *et al.*, 1975). The antiviral state is not permanently established but decays after a few days if interferon is removed from the cells. There exists as yet no definite proof for a specific interferon receptor at the cell surface, but several observations are in favor of such a receptor, and of its importance in the induction of the antiviral state (Chany, 1976). Studies by Pitha *et al.* (1976*a*) have provided evidence that for interferon to be active it has first to be secreted by the interferon-producing cells, so that it can interact with the external part of the cellular membrane (Vengris *et al.*, 1975; Pitha *et al.*, 1976*a*). Interferon covalently bound to Sepharose beads is active, suggesting that it need only bind to the cell surface and not enter the cell (Ankel *et al.*, 1973; Chany *et al.*, 1974; Knight, 1974). Such experiments are unfortunately not foolproof, and a slow, undetectable leakage of interferon molecules from the beads cannot be excluded, especially since the specific activity of electrophoretically pure interferon indicates that a few molecules per cell are sufficient to induce the antiviral state. Interferon binding involves both cellular gangliosides and glycoproteins, and treatment of cells with exogenous gangliosides blocks interferon action; possibly the interferon receptor is a ganglioside on the outside of the cell membrane (Besançon and Ankel, 1974 *a,b*; Besançon *et al.*, 1976; Vengris *et al.*, 1976; Friedman and Kohn, 1976; Pitha *et al.*, 1976*a*). Pretreatment of cells with glycoprotein hormones can inhibit interferon action, and this has been attributed to competition for ganglioside-binding sites (Besançon and Ankel, 1976; Friedman and Kohn, 1976; Kohn *et al.*, 1976). In mouse–human hybrid cells, the presence of a gene(s) located on the distal part of the long arm of human chromosome 21 is necessary for the antiviral action of human interferon, and cells trisomic for chromosome 21 have been found to be 3–7 times more sensitive to protection by interferon than the normal diploid cells (Tan *et al.*, 1973, 1974*a,b*; Tan, 1975; Chany *et al.*, 1975; Tan and Greene, 1976). Furthermore, some correlation between the number of chromosome 21 copies and the amount of interferon bound to the cell was observed (Wiranoswska-Stewart and Stewart, 1977). Chany *et al.* (1975) and Revel *et al.* (1976) have suggested that a gene on chromosome 21 codes for an interferon receptor site, and Revel *et al.* (1976) have shown that antibodies to a cell-surface component coded by human chromosome 21 inhibit the action of interferon. Thus, although the physical existence of a specific interferon receptor site at the cell membrane has not been demonstrated, many different approaches, cytogenetical, biochemical, and immunological, point to the existence of such a receptor, and, at the least, demonstrate the importance of a first step in which interferon interacts with some structure at the cell surface. The species specificity of interferon appears to be determined at an early stage of interaction with the cell, maybe at the receptor level, as suggested by both cytogenetic and biochemical studies (Stewart *et al.*, 1972; Berman and Vilček, 1974). In monkey–mouse hybrid cells, human interferon under certain conditions can inhibit virus replication, but the antiviral state induced in these hybrids can be of mouse origin (Chany *et al.*, 1973). Samuel and Farris (1977) have isolated from interferon-treated cells a ribosome-associated inhibitor of viral mRNA translation that can inhibit the translation of viral mRNA in a heterologous cell-free system, and the interferon-induced phosphorylation of a specific mouse protein of molecular weight 67,000 is triggered by human interferon in mouse–human hybrid cells (Revel, 1977; Blalock and Baron, 1977*b*; Slate *et al.*, 1978).

3.2. Nature of the Antiviral State

All viruses, DNA or RNA, single or double stranded, enveloped or not, with or without virion-associated polymerase, and replicating in the nucleus or in the cytoplasm, are sensitive to interferon. There are differences in degree of sensitivity between different viruses, and these can be quite pronounced as there are differences between variants or mutants of the same virus, but none has been found completely resistant. It has been impossible to select interferon-resistant mutants, in spite of the fact that theoretically this would be a technically very easy task. Many people have tried to isolate such mutants, and some have published their failure to do so (Metz and Douglas, 1977; Takemoto and Baron, 1966). On the other hand, interferon-sensitive mutants, i.e., more sensitive than the wild-type virus, can be isolated (Simon *et al.*, 1976). The fact that all viruses, in spite of their widely divergent mechanisms of replication, are sensitive to the antiviral action of interferon suggests that the effect of interferon on viral replication is pleiotropic. Moreover, the various other biological activities of interferon, such as the effects on different manifestations of cell-mediated and humoral immunity, or on the cell surface, or on cell growth, all have to be considered when looking at the mechanism of action of interferon. Such nonantiviral activities could be conveniently ignored as long as they had not been observed with pure interferon, but this is now no longer possible since it has been demonstrated recently that they are due to the same molecules that induce the antiviral state. Therefore, it would not be very logical to adopt the hypothesis of one mechanism for the antiviral state and another for all nonantiviral effects. The different stages of viral infection that theoretically could be affected by interferon are adsorption and penetration, uncoating, transcription, translation, assembly, and release. In general, there is no effect on adsorption and penetration, but there is some suggestive evidence now that uncoating may sometimes be affected. The most significant changes in interferon-treated cells, however, occur at the level of translation of virus RNA, with some effect also on transcription. For oncornaviruses there is also evidence for an effect on assembly and release.

3.2.1. Transcription vs. Translation

Transcription of viral mRNA in interferon-treated cells has been examined in cells infected with viruses that have virion-associated polymerases such as vaccinia, vesicular stomatis virus (VSV), and reovirus, and also with SV40, which depends for its transcription on a cellular polymerase. Marcus *et al.* (1971) reported inhibition of transcription of VSV in interferon-treated cells, but Repik *et al.* (1974) have suggested that it was not the primary transcription that was affected but rather secondary transcription, dependent on translation of input VSV mRNA. These studies were performed in intact cells, and the use of protein synthesis inhibitors such as cycloheximide, necessary to isolate primary transcription from subsequent replicative events, may have introduced complicating factors, such as aberrations, in the regulation of virus transcription. Therefore, Marcus and Sekellick (1978) studied the effect of interferon treatment on the transcription of a temperature-sensitive VSV mutant, *tsG41* (IV), in Vero cells, at the nonpermissive temperature in order to exclude the possibility of secondary transcription (at the nonpermissive temperature, the *ts* mutant is defective in all synthetic activities subsequent to primary transcription). Treatment of the cells with interferon reduces the initial rate of transcription about fourfold, irrespective of the presence or absence of cycloheximide. The mRNA transcripts in interferon-treated cells are equal in size to those made in control cells, and eventually as much RNA accumulates as in control cells, indicating that only the rate of transcription is affected. Although this is certainly evidence for an effect on transcription, the effect would not appear sufficiently pronounced to explain the high sensitivity of VSV to the antiviral state. This is borne out by the work of Baxt *et al.* (1977), who arrive at the conclusion that the primary effect of interferon in human cells is on translation of VSV mRNA and that there is little or no effect on transcription. Recently, an interesting *in vitro* system was developed, coupling transcription and translation of VSV (Ball and White, 1978); this system was then used to study the effect of interferon. In extracts of interferon-treated cells, viral transcription is not affected, but the rate of translation is reduced by up to 70%, the extent of inhibition being dependent on the interferon dose; however, translation of host-cell mRNA is equally inhibited.

Studies with SV40 virus in monkey cells have provided evidence for an effect of interferon on transcription. Oxman and Levin (1971) found a marked inhibition of early RNA synthesis under conditions where the formation of late RNA was blocked by preventing viral DNA synthesis through treatment of cells with cytosine arabinoside, and additional evidence was provided in a follow-up study (Metz *et al.*, 1976). Furthermore, the accumulation of virus-specific RNA in isolated nuclei from SV40-infected cells was inhibited by pretreatment of the cells with interferon (Metz *et al.*, 1977). However, the possibility that the reduced accumulation of viral RNA was due to enhanced degradation by a specific ribonuclease could not be excluded. These results were confirmed by Yakobson *et al.* (1977a,b), who found that pretreatment with interferon reduces the amount of early RNA transciption. Postinfection interferon treatment, however, inhibits *de novo* synthesis of all SV40 viral proteins without any detectable inhibition of viral RNA synthesis; this is probably the major effect of interferon on SV40 replication. Comparable results have been reported using a double-stranded RNA virus. Wiebe and Joklik (1975) examined the expression of a variety of reovirus-specified functions in interferon-treated cells and found absorption, penetration, and uncoating to be unaffected. An interferon dose-dependent effect on transcription of all ten species of reovirus mRNA was observed, with inhibition of transcription ranging from 15% to 60%, depending on how much interferon had been used to treat the cells. However, the translation of early mRNA was inhibited much more severely, ranging from 36% to 72%, for the lowest dose of interferon used. Some species of early reovirus mRNA were found to be more inhibited than others (Wiebe and Joklik, 1975), thus suggesting the interesting possibility that different mRNAs display differential sensitivities to interferon.

Thus it appears that under certain conditions early viral mRNA synthesis can be affected by interferon; the relative contribution of this effect to the antiviral action of interferon remains to be established and is probably rather slight; there is presently no indication as to its possible molecular mechanism. Possibly, some step in the uncoating process is impeded in interferon-treated cells, and this interferes with the

conversion of incoming virions to functional transcription templates
(Yamamoto *et al.*, 1975). It is indeed conceivable that changes of the
cell surface, described in interferon-treated cells (Knight and Korant
1977), can affect virus penetration and uncoating. Studies with the
electron microscope might be helpful in elucidating this question.
Nevertheless, translation appears to be the major target of interferon
for the establishment of the antiviral state, as is already evident from
the results discussed in the foregoing and from the additional evidence
that will be presented now.

3.2.2. Effects on Translation

Over the past few years, considerable evidence, coming from many
directions, has pointed to translation of mRNA into viral proteins as
one of the major sites of interferon action.

3.2.2a. Studies in Intact Cells

In addition to the results obtained with VSV, SV40, and reovirus,
discussed in the previous section, the replication of vaccinia virus has
been used as a model by several groups. Interferon treatment does not
inhibit transcription of vaccinia mRNA but inhibits subsequent translation of this mRNA into vaccinia polypeptides. As a result of this, vaccinia DNA fails to replicate, and no viral progeny are formed (Joklik
and Merigan, 1966; Metz and Esteban, 1972). The polysomes of
interferon-treated vaccinia-infected cells are found to be disaggregated,
and this has been ascribed to an inhibition of the initiation of virus
polypeptide synthesis; inhibition of polypeptide chain elongation also
occurs (Metz *et al.*, 1975). A block in translation of early viral mRNAs
has also been described for mengovirus in L cells (Levy and Carter,
1968) and for Semliki Forest virus in chick embryo fibroblasts
(Friedman, 1968).

3.2.2b. Studies in Cell-Free Systems

Studies in cell-free systems have confirmed and extended the
notion that translation is affected in interferon-treated cells and have
revealed the existence of differences between interferon-treated and
control cells, such as degradation of RNA by an interferon-activated
nuclease and impairment of mRNA methylation.

The translational inhibitory activity of crude cell sap from interferon-treated cells has been described for many different cell systems and various viral and nonviral mRNAs (Kerr, 1971; Friedman *et al.*, 1972*a,b*; Falcoff *et al.*, 1972, 1973; Gupta *et al.*, 1973). Kinetic studies of the translation of mengo RNA and rabbit hemoglobin mRNA in extracts from interferon-treated L cells show that both initiation and elongation are affected. Messenger RNA still binds to ribosomes, but initiator met-tRNA^{fMet} is inhibited, and the block in initiation appears to be secondary to the block in elongation (Content *et al.*, 1975). The elongation block can be overcome by addition of certain minor tRNA species (Gupta *et al.*, 1974; Zilberstein *et al.*, 1976*a*; Mayr *et al.*, 1977), and fMet-tRNA has been reported to restore the initiation block. Apparently, the presence of the abnormal formyl group on the initiator fMet-tRNA somehow allows bypass of the interferon-induced initiation block (Kerr *et al.*, 1974*a*). The *in vivo* relevance of some of these results, especially of the tRNA effects, has not yet been established.

The 5′ termini of many eukaryotic mRNAs are capped and methylated, and it has been reported that methylated, capped reovirus mRNAs are more efficiently translated *in vitro* than unmethylated RNAs (Both *et al.*, 1975). Impairment of methylation may be another expression of the antiviral state, since reovirus mRNA methylation is decreased in extracts from interferon-treated cells as well as in intact cells (Sen *et al.*, 1977). A virus specificity of the interferon-induced change in mRNA cap methylation seems unlikely, since Kroath *et al.* (1978) have found that vaccinia mRNA was less methylated in interferon-treated chick cells, but so were other nonviral poly(A)-containing RNAs. Methylation of ribosomal and transfer RNA was not affected in these cells.

Addition of double-stranded RNA (synthetic or viral) to extracts of interferon-treated cells significantly enhances the translational inhibition of these extracts (Kerr *et al.*, 1974*b*). This observation undoubtedly has physiological significance in that double-stranded RNA is frequently present in cells as a result of infection with many viruses. Extracts from interferon-treated cells plus dsRNA are therefore probably a better *in vitro* reflection of the situation as it occurs in the interferon-treated, virus-infected cells. The study of cell-free extracts from interferon-treated cells in the presence of dsRNA has revealed some interesting mechanisms that may be active during the antiviral state as it exists in intact cells.

Activation of a dsRNA-Dependent Protein Kinase System: One of the characteristic changes induced by interferon is the dsRNA-stimulated phosphorylation of several ribosome-associated proteins, among which are a protein of molecular weight 67,000 (Fig. 4) and the 35,000 molecular weight initiation factor eIF-2 subunit. The modification of eIF-2 could possibly be related to the inhibition of protein synthesis initiation and the loss of 40 S Met-tRNA$_F$ complexes found in interferon-treated cell extracts (Roberts *et al.*, 1976*b*; Zilberstein *et al.*, 1976*b*, 1978; Lebleu *et al.*, 1976; Samuel *et al.*, 1977). The exact role that the other phosphorylated proteins play in the inhibition of virus replication is presently unclear, but the fact that interferon modulates protein kinase activity is certainly relevant to explain the wide diversity of its biological effects.

Activation of an Endonuclease: Addition of dsRNA and ATP to cell-free extracts from interferon-treated cells activates an endonuclease that degrades reovirus mRNA. dsDNA or RNA–DNA hybrids do not substitute for dsRNA in activating the endonuclease (Brown *et al.*, 1976; Sen *et al.*, 1976; Ratner *et al.*, 1977; Shaila *et al.*, 1977). It is not known at the present time how selective exactly the endonuclease is, and cellular mRNAs may also be degraded (Kerr *et al.*, 1976). Clemens and Williams (1978) have evidence indicating that the nuclease is activated by the low molecular weight oligonucleotide described below.

Synthesis of a Low Molecular Weight Inhibitor of Translation: Extracts of interferon-treated mouse L cells, on addition of dsRNA, synthesize from ATP a low molecular weight oligonucleotide, pppA2'-p5'A2'p5'A, which is highly active in inhibiting protein synthesis

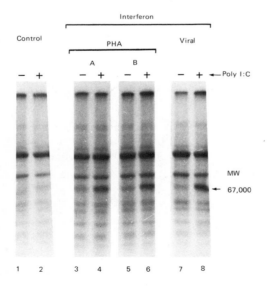

Fig. 4. Autoradiograph of electrophoresis of phosphorylated proteins from control extracts and from extracts derived from cells treated with either type II interferon (PHA induced) or type I interferon (NDV induced). Tracks 1 and 2, untreated cell extracts. PHA interferon-treated cell extracts: (A) haired control mouse interferon; (B) nude mouse interferon; Tracks 7 and 8, NDV L-cell interferon-treated cell extracts. Doses of interferon were 80 IU/ml, with (+) or without (−) polyinosinic acid–polycytidylic acid. From Wietzerbin *et al.* (1978).

(Roberts *et al.*, 1976*a*,*b*; Kerr *et al.*, 1977; Hovanessian *et al.*, 1977; Kerr and Brown, 1978). The activity does not appear to be species specific, cell-type specific, or mRNA specific, at least not between rabbit and mouse. Possibly, this oligonucleotide is the activator of the endonuclease appearing in extracts from interferon-treated cells as discussed above, since this endonuclease requires dsRNA and ATP for its activation. Reticulocyte lysate and L-cell extracts derived from cells that have not been treated with interferon also respond to the addition of 2′5′ppp(A)3, suggesting that the precursor of the putative endonuclease is already present in these cells without interferon treatment (Hovanessian and Kerr, 1978). Furthermore, and in contrast to mouse L cells, rabbit reticulocyte lysates synthesize the inhibitor on addition of dsRNA and ATP without previous treatment of the cells with interferon; this is an indication that the role of the inhibitor appearing in interferon-treated cells on addition of dsRNA is not limited to the interferon system and strongly suggests that interferon induces the antiviral state by activating one of the natural control mechanism of protein synthesis of eukaryotic cells. In favor of this possibility is the observation by Baglioni *et al.* (1978) that nuclease activity of HeLa cell extracts, on activation by 2′5′ppp(A)3, degrades both cellular and viral (VSV) mRNAs. The apparent lack of toxicity of interferon at doses that inhibit virus replication is attributed by these workers to the fact that the enzyme responsible for the synthesis of 2′5′ppp(A)3 and which is activated in interferon-treated cells binds only to the replicative complexes of RNA and thus restricts the presence of 2′5′ppp(A)3 at the sites of viral RNA replication. When the oligonucleotide inhibitor is added to intact cells in hypertonic medium to stimulate its uptake, protein synthesis is inhibited, thus showing conclusively that its activity is not limited to cell-free systems (Williams and Kerr, 1978).

Based on these multiple effects by which interferon affects protein synthesis, Revel *et al.* (1978) have recently proposed the "multiphase antiviral state hypothesis" as summarized in Fig. 5.

3.2.3. Oncornaviruses—A Special Case?

Both replication and cellular transformation caused by MLV and MSV are inhibited by interferon (Gresser *et al.*, 1967*a*,*b*,*c*; Peries *et al.*, 1968; Sarma *et al.*, 1969). Interferon does not affect transcription of the viral genome once it is integrated, and it affects translation of viral mRNA only marginally, at least for those virus-specific antigens that can be measured (Friedman *et al.*, 1975, 1976; Pitha *et al.*, 1976*b*, 1977;

Shapiro *et al.*, 1977). In contrast to the effect of interferon observed in other virus–cell systems, the inhibition of MLV replication apparently then would not be due to inhibition of viral protein synthesis but rather to an effect on later steps in the virus growth cycle; effects both on virus assembly and on release of virus particles from infected cells have been described (Billiau *et al.*, 1974, 1975, 1976; Chang *et al.*, 1977a). Furthermore, many of the released virus particles are defective (Chang *et al.*, 1977b). It has been proposed that this effect on virus maturation reflects interferon-induced changes in the properties of the plasma membrane (Friedman, 1977). On the other hand, in theory, all the observed effects on maturation and release could still be due to an inhibition of the translation of one or several viral proteins as yet not characterized, and therefore escaping detection, but necessary for assembly or release (Billiau *et al.*, 1978).

4. MOLECULAR CHARACTERIZATION OF INTERFERONS

4.1. General Considerations

Early after its discovery, interferon was characterized as a protein since its antiviral activity was destroyed by trypsin (Lindenmann *et al.*, 1957), and yet the first preparations of interferon purified to homogeneity as shown by SDS-polyacrylamide gel electrophoresis have been obtained only recently. They were derived from human fibroblast interferon induced with poly(I·C) (Fig. 6) (Knight, 1976a), from mouse C243 cell interferon induced with NDV (Fig. 7) (De Maeyer-Guignard *et al.*, 1978), and from human leukocytes induced with NDV (Rubinstein *et al.*, 1979). The main obstacle to the total purification of interferon is its high specific activity, and, even in preparations with considerable biological activity, the amount of interferon protein is very low. A specific activity of 2.4×10^9 has been found for mouse interferon (De Maeyer-Guignard *et al.*, 1978), which means for a molecular weight of 22,000 that 1 unit of interferon corresponds to 0.4 pg. Interferon purification to homogeneity is now feasible, largely through the development of techniques of mass production of interferon of high specific activity, combining priming and superinduction of selected cells. To obtain 1 mg, one would presently need about 25 liters of a crude preparation titering 10^5 units/ml, and one would have needed 250,000 liters of preparations available 20 years ago! Interferon preparations are difficult to handle. Progress was made when it was found that the antiviral activity is greatly stabilized by anionic

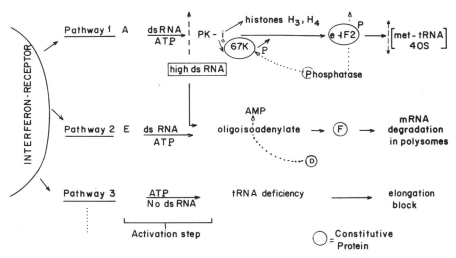

Fig. 5. "Multiphase antiviral state" hypothesis of Revel *et al.* The multiple effects by which interferon affects protein synthesis could each have its function in the cells. The tRNA-sensitive inhibition, seen in the absence of dsRNA, may play its role mainly in the noninfected cell, where dsRNA is very low or absent. After infection, in the case of many viruses, dsRNA is formed and accumulates. The protein kinase pathway is activated at low dsRNA concentrations, but at higher levels it is switched off and the isoadenylate-nuclease system may act. This "multiphase antiviral state" could ensure that the interferon-induced control of gene expression is appropriate to .the state of the cell. It is striking that the three pathways of translation control share a common requirement for ATP and are regulated by antagonists. What is not understood is how these regulations discriminate between host and viral functions. Work has to be continued, in intact cells and in cell-free systems, to determine how the pathways already found or additional effects of interferon control viral replication and cell proliferation. From Revel *et al.* (1978).

detergents; this also presents the advantage of dissociating interferon from contaminants to which it sometimes sticks (Stewart *et al.*, 1974*a,b*). The analysis of interferon by polyacrylamide gel electrophoresis in the presence of SDS (SDS-PAGE) has become an important tool, and, although usually there is not enough interferon protein to be stained, one can measure the antiviral activity by eluting it from the gel (Stewart, 1974; Stewart and Desmyter, 1975).

Another significant complication for the characterization of interferon at the molecular level has been its heterogeneity, due to three factors: the species specificity, the presence of several interferon genes within a given species—for example, human leukocyte and fibroblast interferons are coded for by two distinct genes (Cavalieri *et al.*, 1977*a*)—and posttranslational modifications of interferon molecules (glycosylation).

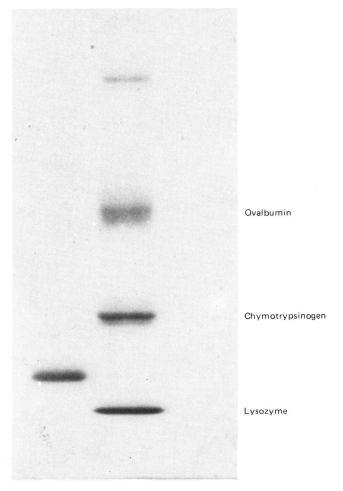

Fig. 6. Electrophoretic analysis of human diploid fibroblast interferon by SDS-PAGE. Molecular weight markers are ovalbumin, chymotrypsinogen, and lysozyme. Approximately 0.5 μg of protein was analyzed. From Knight (1976a).

Only recent results obtained with human and mouse interferon will be considered in this section.

4.2. Human Interferon

The characterization of human interferon has focused on three different systems that have been developed for mass production:

1. Human leukocyte interferon, usually induced by Sendai virus in buffy coat cells (Cantell *et al.*, 1974; Cantell and Hirvonen, 1977).
2. Human diploid fibroblasts induced with poly(I·C) (Havell and Vilček, 1972; Billiau *et al.*, 1973).
3. Human lymphoblastoid cells, usually induced with a myxo- or paramyxovirus (Strander *et al.*, 1975; Zoon and Buckler, 1977).

The use of antisera prepared in rabbits immunized with either leukocyte or fibroblast interferon has revealed the exitence of two anti-genically distinct types of human interferon (Berg *et al.*, 1975; Havell *et al.*, 1975; Paucker *et al.*, 1975). Furthermore, translational studies in *Xenopus* oocytes show that each of these two types is coded for by a different mRNA, thus suggesting the existence of two distinct structural genes (Cavalieri *et al.*, 1977a). Human Le interferon represents the major form produced by leukocytes and lymphoblastoid cells, and F

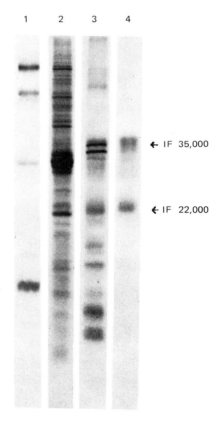

Fig. 7. SDS-PAGE in a 15% gel of mouse C243 cell interferon preparations of different degrees of purity. Input per channel was 20 μl in each case. Channel 1, molecular weight markers, from top to bottom: bovine serum albumin, ovalbumin, chymotrypsinogen, and cytochrome *c*. Channel 2, after purification on poly(U)-agarose; input was 1×10^7 U. Channel 3, after purification on antibody–agarose; input was 1.3×10^7 U. Channel 4, after combination of the two methods; input was 1.2×10^7 U. From De Maeyer-Guignard *et al.* (1978).

interferon is the major form synthesized by fibroblasts. The relative proportion of the two types varies with the cell system and inducer used. For example, NDV-induced interferon in lymphoblastoid Namalva cells consists of 85% Le and 15% F type (Havell *et al.*, 1978*a*); FS4 fibroblasts, on the other hand, produce only F type when induced with poly(I·C), and 20% type Le and 80% F type if the inducer is NDV or VSV (Havell *et al.*, 1978*b*). In addition to antigenicity, F and Le interferon differ by other biological and physicochemical properties, as will be discussed in the following sections.

4.2.1. Fibroblast Interferon (F Type)

Only F-type interferon derived from poly(I·C)-induced FS4 cells has been completely purified (Knight, 1976*a*). Using classical methods of protein purification, Knight was able to purify human fibroblast interferon in three stages, with a final yield of 8%. Analysis on SDS-PAGE reveals one band migrating at 20,000 molecular weight, stainable with Coomassie brilliant blue. Antiviral activity can be eluted from the same zone, and the specific activity of the thus obtained product is 2 $\times$ 10^8 units. The band stains with periodic acid–Schiff reagent, indicating that it is a glycoprotein. The purified product also has cell multiplication inhibitory activity (Knight, 1976*b*), and recently it has been iodinated (Knight, 1978). The amino acid composition of this interferon is presently being determined.

Results from several laboratories have shown that the antiviral activity of F interferon migrates on SDS-PAGE to a zone corresponding to 19,000–20,000 molecular weight (Vilček et al., 1977; Berthold *et al.*, 1978). The peak fraction of antiviral activity from preparative SDS-PAGE can be concentrated by lyophilization and labeled *in vitro* with [^{125}I]iodine, with sodium [^{3}H]borohydride, and with [^{3}H]dansyl chloride. All three types of labeled interferon comigrate with the purified interferon preparation as a single protein component with a molecular weight of 19,000. Antiviral activity is retained after tritium labeling but not after iodination (Berthold *et al.*, 1978).

When crude F-type interferon is analyzed by electrofocusing, a broad peak of activity is recovered ranging from pH 6.8 to 7.8, indicating a certain degree of heterogeneity of glycosylation (Havell *et al.*, 1977*a*). Some of this heterogeneity disappears if the interferon is made by cells that have been treated with inhibitors of glycosylation, such as 2-desoxy-D-glucose or D-glucosamine. The interferon thus obtained, when analyzed by SDS-PAGE, shows two peaks of activity, one migrating with an apparent molecular weight of 16,000, and a second one migrating with an apparent molecular weight of 20,000; the latter is normally found for interferon produced in the absence of inhibitors of glycosylation (Havell *et al.*, 1977*b*). These results suggest that the sugar moiety of F-type interferon is responsible for about 20% of its apparent molecular weight as determined by SDS-PAGE and, furthermore, that the antiviral activity does not require the presence of the sugar moiety, a conclusion also arrived at by Bose *et al.* (1976). The presence of sialic acid in human F-type interferon was recently demonstrated indirectly by Fung and Ng (1978), who found that neuraminidase can be used as ligand to purify F-type interferon by affinity chromatography. Obviously, only the chemical analysis of pure F-type interferon will reveal the relative importance of sialic acid residues in the composition of the sugar moiety. The glycoprotein nature of F-type interferon has made it possible to use for its purification several ligands with affinity for sugars, such as, for example, concanavalin A (Davey *et al.*, 1974, 1976*a*; Berthold *et al.*, 1978) and horseshoe crab and lotus lectins (Jankowski *et al.*, 1975). The affinity for Con A would also seem to be the result of hydrophobic bonding (Davey *et al.*, 1974, 1976*a*). In general, affinity chromatography methods based on hydrophobic bonding result in significant purification of F-type interferon. Such ligands are BSA (Huang *et al.*, 1974; Jankowski *et al.*, 1975), ω-carboxypentylagarose (CH-sepharose 4B) (Davey *et al.*, 1975; Jankowski *et al.*, 1975), ω-aminohexylagarose (AH-sepharose 4B) (Jankowski *et al.*, 1975), as well as the hydrophobic amino acids and dipeptides (Sulkowski *et al.*, 1976). F-type interferon attached to any of these ligands can be desorbed by ethylene glycol. F-type interferon made by FS4 cells that have been induced with NDV seems to be more hydrophobic than when the same cells are induced by poly(I·C), as shown by its affinity for AH-Sepharose 4B (Jankowski *et al.*, 1975). Indeed, under these conditions, NDV-induced interferon can only be desorbed by ethylene glycol, whereas poly(I·C)-induced interferon can be desorbed by an aqueous solution of high molarity (1 M NaCl). It is impossible to evaluate at present the various degrees of purification obtained with these various ligands, since relatively small quantities of interferon have been used to describe these methods, and the authors were therefore not able to analyze electrophoretically the purified preparations at concentrations that would allow for staining of the interferon band and for assessing the number of other contaminating polypeptides.

Another ligand that can be used for the purification of F-type interferon is Cibacron blue F3GA (De Maeyer-Guignard and De Maeyer, 1976; Jankowski et al., 1976; Cesario et al., 1976). De Maeyer-Guignard and De Maeyer could desorb the interferon from this ligand by increasing the molarity, whereas Jankowski et al. had to use ethylene glycol, indicating that they were dealing with a hydrophobic bond. The reason for this different behavior is not clear, since in both cases the interferon was obtained from poly(I·C)-induced cells.

F interferon can be purified also by adsorption to controlled-pore glass (Edy et al., 1976) and by zinc chelate affinity chromatography (Edy et al., 1977).

Anti-F-type-interferon globulin would certainly be the most specific ligand for purification by affinity chromatography. Although monospecific antiserum is not yet available, this will be only a matter of time, either through immunization with pure interferon or by the use of hybridomas to produce such antibodies. Antibodies made in animals immunized with leukocyte interferon have also been used as ligands for purification of F interferon by affinity chromatography on immuno-sorbent columns (Anfinsen et al., 1974; Berg et al., 1975, 1977). The efficacy of those columns is striking in view of the small amounts (± 1%) of F interferon reported to be present in the preparations of Le interferon that were used as antigen (Havell et al., 1975; Paucker et al., 1975; Vilček et al., 1977). Either the relative importance of F component in Le interferon has been underestimated or, in spite of the many adsorption steps, the immunoglobulins used as ligands are retain-ing contaminants to which both F and Le interferon are sticking; another possibility would be that Le and F share some common anti-genic determinant(s).

4.2.2.   Leukocyte Interferon (Le type)

Leukocyte interferon is currently used in large-scale clinical trials, and we will therefore consider its purification in some detail. Most clinical studies are presently carried out with semipurified preparations derived from buffy coats induced with Sendai virus (Cantell et al., 1974). Partial purification is obtained as follows: crude interferon derived from buffy coats is precipitated in the presence of KSCN at pH 3.5 (Fantes, 1974), and is dissolved in acid ethanol. Impurities are selec-tively precipitated from the ethanolic solution around neutrality, concentrated further, and fractionated into two preparations, P-IF B and P-IF A, by KSCN precipitation at pH 4.7 and 3.0, respectively (Cantell and Hirvonen, 1977). The most concentrated P-IF A and P-IF B preparations obtained by this method contain $1-3 \times 10^7$ reference interferon units ml (in terms of the Medical Research Council standard for leukocyte interferon, 69/19). Their specific activities are 3×10^5 to 1×10^6 units. The P-IF B preparations are somewhat purer than the P-IF A preparations. The main contaminant of P-IF A is albumin. Slight modifications of this method (Cantell and Hirvonen, 1978) now permit the large-scale preparation of P-IF A containing over 10^8 units/ml with a specific activity around 2×10^6 (recovery over 50%). Despite their high protein content ($\pm$ 50 mg/ml), these P-IF A preparations present the advantage of not forming precipitates during storage at 4°C or after freezing and thawing.

Le-type interferon is much more stable than F-type interferon; it is more resistant to changes in temperature and pH (pH 2–10), and conserves its activity in the presence of a wide variety of denaturing agents such as urea, guanidine, thiocyanate, ethanol, and SDS (Cantell *et al.*, 1974; Mogensen and Cantell, 1974). Le-type interferon, on the other hand, is quite sensitive to inactivation by β-mercaptoethanol (Mogensen and Cantell, 1974; Stewart *et al.*, 1975). Evidently, results concerning physicochemical properties of human leukocyte interferon must await complete purification of the molecules to be accepted without reservation.

Contrary to the situation observed with human F interferon, affinity chromatography on hydrophobic ligands in general cannot be applied in the case of human leukocyte interferon (Jankowski *et al.*, 1975, 1976; Chen *et al.*, 1976). The most promising ligand is the anti-human Le antibody. Important degrees of purification on immunosorbant columns have been reported by Anfinsen *et al.* (1974) and Berg *et al.* (1975, 1977). Recovery of the antiviral activity is about 100%. The main problem is to clean the antiserum from the antibodies directed against the numerous contaminating proteins present in the crude preparations. To this end, Berg *et al.* (1977) adsorbed it by 13 passages on a column of crude leukocyte interferon covalently bound to Sepharose. They thus obtained immunoglobulins, which, when in their turn were covalently linked proved very efficient in the purification of the three types of human interferon, namely, leukocyte, fibroblast, and Namalva interferon. All preparations can be purified in this system to $2-20 \times 10^7$ units/mg of protein with full recovery.

Analysis by SDS-PAGE of crude and semipurified Le interferon preparations gives two rather broad peaks with antiviral activity, corresponding to molecular weights 21,000 (± 20%) and 15,000 (± 80%) Stewart and Desmyter, 1975; Desmyter and Stewart, 1976; Stewart *et al.*, 1976; Törma and Paucker, 1976; Vilček *et al.*, 1977; Chadha *et al.*, 1978). Both forms can be renaturated after boiling in the presence of urea and SDS, but only the minor peak of antiviral activity (21,000) remains active under reducing conditions (1% β-mercaptoethanol) (Stewart and Desmyter, 1975). In general, human Le interferon displays more cross-species antiviral activity than F interferon (Gresser *et al.*, 1974*b*). The degree of cross-species antiviral activity is distinct for the two components obtained after SDS-PAGE. The 21,000 molecular weight component is as active in rabbit kidney cells as in human diploid cells, while the 15,000 component is twentyfold less active in rabbit kidney cells than in human cells (Stewart and Desmyter, 1975). Each of the two molecular weight components has about the same antiviral activity on cat cells; however, after treatment with SDS under reducing conditions, interferon migrating in the faster band retains full activity on cat cells, although it becomes totally inactive on human cells (Desmyter and Stewart, 1976).

Human Le interferon presents a rather broad profile on isoelectric focusing (pH 5.7–7) (Mogensen *et al.*, 1974; Bose *et al.*, 1976; Havell *et al.*, 1977*a*; Lin *et al.*, 1978). Distinct degrees of cross-species antiviral activity have been described for distinct charge components (Lin *et al.*, 1978).

Opinions are still divided on whether human Le interferon is a glycoprotein or not. According to Jankowski *et al.* (1975) and Davey *et al.*, (1976*a*), leukocyte interferons induced with NDV or poly(I·C) do not bind either to concanavalin A or to other lectins, which suggests an absence of carbohydrate moieties recognizable by the lectins, or, if present, they are masked. This is in contrast to an observation by Besançon and Bourgeade (1974), who reported that NDV-induced human Le interferon did bind to Con A sepharose and that the reaction did not take place in the presence of β-methyl-D-mannoside. According to Mogensen *et al.* (1974), isoelectric profiles of Sendai-induced human Le interferon do not significantly differ before and after treatment with neuraminidase, an enzyme known to cleave sialic acid chains. By contrast, Bose *et al.* (1976) reported that on treatment with a mixture of glycosidases, including neuraminidase, the heterogeneous character of semipurified Le interferon, as revealed by isoelectric focusing, is significantly reduced. Concomitantly, the molecular weight of interferon as determined by gel filtration is reduced by about 4000 (26,000 → 22,000), but antiviral activity is fully preserved. The controversy for and against the presence of carbohydrates on leukocyte interferon still goes on. Observing that the molecular weight of human Le interferon, as determined by molecular sieving, can be diminished by 5000 (26,000 → 21,000) when the preparation is subjected to denaturation by guanidine hydrochloride under reducing conditions and reactivated by dialysis, and that the product gives a single component with antiviral activity (18,000) on SDS-PAGE, Chadha *et al.* (1978) ascribe their results to a proteolytic cleavage of interferon molecules. Noticing that treatment of Le interferon with sodium periodate results in conversion of the preparation to a single band of antiviral activity in SDS-PAGE, and to charge homogeneity (pH 5) on isoelectric focusing, Stewart *et al.* (1977*a*) concluded that carbohydrates are responsible for size and charge heterogeneity.

4.2.3. Lymphoblastoid Interferon

Lymphoblastoid cell lines, especially Namalva cells, can be grown to high densities in suspension culture and produce fairly high interferon titers when stimulated with paramyxoviruses (Strander *et al.*, 1975; Zoon and Buckler, 1977). As stated before, Namalva interferon is antigenically mostly of Le type but contains also a component of F type amounting to about 13% (Havell *et al.*, 1978*a*).

When analyzed by SDS-PAGE and by isoelectric focusing, crude Namalva interferon qualitatively resembles crude leukocyte interferon (Havell *et al.*, 1978*a*). The Le and F subspecies can be separated by antibody affinity chromatography and tested for their heterospecific activities on bovine cells (Havell *et al.*, 1978*a*).

An important degree of purification (35,000 ×) of Namalva interferon has been achieved by a three-step procedure, using anti-leukocyte interferon affinity chromatography, sulfopropyl Sephadex ion exchange chromatography, isoelectric focusing, and SDS-PAGE (Bridgen *et al.*, 1977). Two components of antiviral activity are found, corresponding to molecular weights of 22,000 and 18,000. Treatment with glycosidases results in all the activity being associated with the lower molecular weight species. The specific activity corresponds to 1.1 × 10^7 units in the lower molecular weight fraction. Total recovery is 11–33%, based on the original crude material.

4.3. Mouse Interferon

Mouse interferon derived from C243 cells induced with NDV has recently been purified to homogeneity with 100% recovery (De Maeyer-

Guignard *et al.*, 1978). Two polypeptide bands are obtained on SDS-PAGE, one migrating at 35,000 daltons and representing 80% of the antiviral activity of the starting material, the other migrating at 22,000 daltons and representing the rest of the antiviral activity (Fig. 7). The slower-migrating component stains almost as intensely with Schiff's reagent as with Coomassie blue; the faster-migrating component hardly stains with Schiff's reagent at all. Treatment of the purified interferon preparation with β-mercaptoethanol after boiling does not affect migration of either band, excluding the possibility that the 35,000 molecular weight component is a dimer of the 22,000 molecular weight component. The specific activity is 2.4×10^9 NIH reference units.

Other SDS-PAGE studies carried out with crude or highly purified mouse interferon derived from L, C243, or Ehrlich ascites tumor cells induced with NDV also have shown two distinct molecular weight forms with antiviral activity (Stewart, 1974; Yamamoto and Kawade, 1976; Stewart *et al.*, 1977*b*; Iwakura *et al.*, 1978; Kawakita *et al.*, 1978). Treatment of interferon under reducing conditions does not affect the biological activity of the high molecular weight component but results in a 90% or more reduction of the antiviral activity in the low molecular weight component (Stewart, 1974; De Maeyer-Guignard *et al.*, 1978).

Knight (1975) reports the purification of mouse L cell interferon induced with M-M virus and, within the 20,000–32,000 molecular weight range, finds ten or eleven distinct bands with antiviral activity, all staining with Coomassie blue, six of them with Schiff. The specific activity of this purified preparation is 2.5×10^8 NIH reference units. Further work is needed to determine whether the type of virus used as inducer of interferon can affect the extent of glycosylation of interferon molecules, hence the heterogeneity, or whether the preparation obtained by Knight was less purified than that obtained by De Maeyer-Guignard *et al.* (1978). When partially purified L-cell interferon is briefly exposed to acidic periodate buffer, the larger molecular weight component is apparently converted to the smaller form, since the activity at 38,000 is completely eliminated, while the activity at 22,000 increases significantly. On further oxidative cleavage, antiviral activity becomes detectable, migrating at 15,000 (Stewart *et al.*, 1978). This suggests that the slower-migrating interferons are glycosylated forms of a common low molecular weight protein (Stewart *et al.*, 1978). Relevant to this observation is the previously reported finding that mouse interferon mRNA, when translated by chick cells, codes for the synthesis of interferon of multiple molecular weights, among which is a 13,000 molecular weight component as measured by gel filtration (De Maeyer *et al.*, 1975*a*). Moreover, when L-cell interferon produced in the presence of inhibitors of glycosylation (either D-glucosamine or 2-deoxy-D-glucose) is analyzed by SDS-PAGE, less than 10% of the antiviral activity migrates in either the 38,000 or the 22,000 molecular weight region, while about 90% of the antiviral activity is found as a narrow band at 15,000 molecular weight (Stewart *et al.*, 1978). Those results suggest that the 35,000–38,000 and 22,000 molecular weight components have the same polypeptide component (15,000 or less) and are coded for by a single gene. The alternative would be that several interferon genes code for different products of the same size, which would then be substituted with different amounts of carbohydrates.

It will be important to determine whether the numerous biological effects attributed to interferon preparations are obtained with the pure material; such studies are presently being carried out. A good correlation between antiviral and cell multiplication inhibitory activities has been reported with the pure preparation (De Maeyer-Guignard *et al.*, 1978).

Furthermore, electrophoretically pure mouse interferon has been examined for a number of biologic effects previously ascribed to crude or partially purified interferon preparations. The effects obtained with pure interferon include (1) inhibition of the growth of a transplantable tumor in the mouse; (2) inhibition of cell multiplication of mouse tumor cells *in vitro;* enhancement of the expression of histocompatibility antigens on mouse tumor cells *in vitro;* (3) inhibition of antibody formation *in vitro;* (4) inhibition of sensitization to sheep erythrocytes and the expression of delayed type hypersensitivity in mice; (5) enhancement of NK cell activity *in vivo* and *in vitro;* (6) enhancement of cell sensitivity to the toxicity of poly(I)·poly(C) and enhanced production ("priming") of interferon production *in vitro*. These results establish that the same molecules responsible for the antiviral action of interferon are also responsible for these varied biologic effects (Gresser *et al.*, 1979).

Several affinity chromatography procedures have been described for purification of mouse interferon. Ligands such as bovine serum albumin and hydrocarbons terminated with a polar head make use of hydrophobic bonding properties of mouse interferon molecules (Davey *et al.*, 1976*b,c*). An extensive degree of purification is achieved, with 100% recovery, if one uses as ligands Cibacron blue F3GA (De Maeyer-Guignard and De Maeyer, 1976), synthetic polynucleotides, especially poly(U) or poly(I) (De Maeyer-Guignard *et al.*, 1977), and natural polynucleotides such as tRNAs of various origins (Thang *et al.*, 1977*b*).

Evidently, the most specific ligand for purification of mouse interferon by affinity chromatography is anti-interferon antibody. Monospecificity has not yet been reached despite extensive purification of the potent antiserum raised in sheep by Gresser *et al.* (1976*a*). The use of antibody columns for purification of interferon by affinity chromatography was first described by Sipe *et al.* (1973) for mouse interferon. The method has since been used extensively not only for purification of mouse interferon (Ogburn *et al.*, 1973; Hajnicka *et al.*, 1976; De Maeyer-Guignard *et al.*, 1978) but also for human interferon, as mentioned above.

4.4. Concluding Remarks

The totally purified interferon preparations obtained so far make it possible to determine whether the various biological properties attributed to interferon preparations are due to interferon itself. The availability of radioactive interferon will facilitate the study of the interaction of interferon with cell membranes and probably lead to the characterization of cellular receptors for interferon. Since there is now enough pure material available, amino acid analysis and sequencing is being done. The observation that the heterogeneity of some interferons can be drastically reduced by appropriate treatment is encouraging for the characterization of the moiety responsible for the antiviral activity. From a physiological point of view, however, it would be too simplistic to consider this heterogeneity as a superfluous embellishment by carbohydrates. In the organism, this heterogeneity may well have a physiological function in that different degrees of glycosylation and different affinities for other molecules may determine clearance rates and uptake by the various specialized cells of the body. This problem has by and large been neglected, and only some evidence for different tissue specificities of human leukocyte and fibroblast interferon has been reported (Einhorn and Strander, 1977).

5. INTERACTION WITH THE IMMUNE SYSTEM

5.1. Introduction

None of the published work concerning the effects of interferon on the immune system was carried out with pure material, since pure mouse interferon was not available at that time. Most investigators, however, have been careful to use interferon preparations of different cellular origins and of varying degrees of purity, all of which have comparable effects on antibody formation. In addition, mock interferon preparations are devoid of effect, as are interferon preparations derived from different species. Furthermore, anti-interferon serum abolishes the effect, but it should be realized that the serum used is far from being monospecific for mouse interferon. In spite of these restrictions, when all evidence available is combined and analyzed, there is little doubt left that the antiviral activity is closely correlated with the effects on antibody formation and that the same molecules possess both these effects. However, only experiments with electrophoretically pure interferon are able to give an unequivocal answer to this question. Using pure mouse interferon, the authors of the present chapter, in collaboration with I. Gresser and M. Tovey, of Villejuif, France, have been able to reproduce a number of effects of interferon on the immune system described in this section (Gresser *et al.*, 1979).

In addition to its function as a direct inhibitor of viral replication, it is clear from what will follow that type I interferon contributes in several ways to the outcome of the complex interplay between immune cells and antigens and target cells. In this respect, type I interferon is in a rather unique situation, since it is made not only by the specialized cells of the immune system such as lymphocytes and macrophages, but by any nucleated cell of the body that is virally infected; hence, interferon production is a way by which these cells can influence immune reactions.

5.2. Antibody Formation

5.2.1. *In Vivo*

Braun and Levy (1972) reported that small amounts of interferon given intraperitoneally to mice at the time of immunization with sheep erythrocytes (SRBC) slightly stimulate the number of antibody-forming cells measured 48 hr later. On the other hand, higher doses of interferon significantly inhibit the number of antibody-forming cells. These experiments had been prompted by the known immunostimulating effects of certain double-stranded RNAs that are also interferon inducers. The same reasoning was behind the experiments of Chester *et al.* (1973), who tried to mimic the stimulation of antibody formation induced by poly(I·C) by administering interferon to mice. The interferon was given 48 hr before the antigen, at a dose of about 1×10^5 units per mouse, and antibody production was measured by the number of spleen cells making antibody to SRBC 6 days after immunization. Under those conditions, no stimulation but rather a significant inhibition of the number of antibody-forming cells was obtained (Fig. 8). In mice infected with murine hepatitis virus (MHV3), interferon production can be followed and correlated with effects on SRBC-induced antibody formation. Infecting the mice before administration of antigen leads to immunodepression, whereas simultaneous infection and inoculation of SRBC leads to immunostimulation, and the presence of circulating interferon correlates well with these phenomena (Virelizier *et al.*, 1976).

5.2.2. *In Vitro*

Mouse interferon of different origins inhibits anti-SRBC antibody-forming cells in a Mishell and Dutton (1967) system. The application of

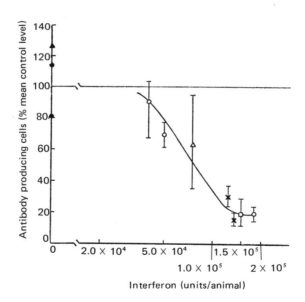

Fig. 8.   Relationship of interferon dose and number of antibody-producing spleen cells. Various doses of interferon, of different cellular origins, were administered 2 days before administration of antigen (sheep erythrocytes). Antibody-producing capability was measured by the number of spleen cells producing antibody to sheep erythrocytes 6 days after antigen administration. Antibody-producing cells were assayed by the plaque technique. From Chester *et al.* (1973).

a mosaic cell culture system as developed by Gisler and Dukor (1972) suggests that the effect of interferon is due to an action on B cells (mesenteric lymph node cells of *nu/nu* mice) and not on T cells (derived from cortisone-treated *nu/+* mice) or macrophages. In low-responder composite cultures, low doses of interferon stimulate the number of antibody-forming cells. In all cultures, *late* addition of interferon (day 4 of culture) results in stimulation of the number of antibody-forming cells if the latter are counted on day 4, but not on day 5. These studies show that the effects of interferon are complex and are influenced by the time of addition to the system and the dose used (Gisler *et al.*, 1974). Similarly, Johnson *et al.* (1974) and Johnson and Baron (1976) found that mouse L-cell interferon and also some rather pure preparations of mouse ascites tumor-cell interferon inhibit primary antibody formation in a Mishell-Dutton system. Interferon has to be present at an early stage (day O), and the inhibitory effect is obtained regardless of whether a T-cell-dependent antigen (SRBC) or a thymus-independent antigen (*Escherichia coli* 0127 LPS) is used. These same authors also show that interferon is capable of blocking the antibody response of cells that have been primed *in vivo*, suggesting that interferon can block the response of memory lymphocytes. Additional evidence that interferon acts at an early stage in the development of the *in vitro* antibody response to SRBC has been obtained by Booth *et al.* (1976a). This timing experiment consisted of adding 800 units of mouse interferon to different cultures at 12-hr intervals, following SRBC addition. After a total of 4 days, all cultures were assayed for anti-SRBC antibody-forming cells. The greatest inhibition of plaque-forming cells occurs when interferon is added at the beginning of the culture period. Interferon seems to inhibit the *in vitro* antibody response by affecting clonal initiation or activation and has little effect on dividing B cells in a developing clone (Booth *et al.*, 1976b).

5.3. Cell-Mediated Immunity

Experiments on interferon and cell-mediated immunity (CMI) were prompted by the possibility that circulating interferon contributes to the decreased intensity of cell-mediated immune reactions which is sometimes observed during and immediately after viral infections. This was first reported by von Pirquet (1908), who described a decreased skin reactivity to tuberculin in patients with measles, and has been repeatedly observed since and confirmed for many other virus infections (Notkins *et al.*, 1970).

5.3.1. Allograft Rejection

Different viral and nonviral interferon inducers, as well as interferon preparations, can prolong allograft survival across the *H-2* barrier in the mouse. The most pronounced prolongation is obtained when interferon is administered right after grafting, and the effect can not be enhanced by giving interferon daily until the time of graft rejection (Mobraaten *et al.*, 1973; De Maeyer *et al.*, 1973, 1975*d*). Prolongation after interferon treatment of skin graft survival in the mouse has also been observed by Hirsch *et al.* (1974), and Imanishi *et al.* (1977) have observed this in a rabbit corneal allograft system.

5.3.2. Delayed Hypersensitivity

The delayed hypersensitivity system makes it possible to examine the afferent and efferent pathways separately, so that effects on sensitization on the one hand and on expression of the sensitized state on the other hand can be readily distinguished. Mice sensitized by either SRBC, NDV, or picryl chloride do not react on challenge with the same antigen if they have been treated with at least 10^5 units of interferon during the 24 hr preceding the challenge. When less than 10^5 units of interferon is given, some reaction occurs, but to a significantly lesser extent than in control animals. Interferon can be administered systemically and does not have to be injected into the organ that receives the challenge dose of antigen (ear or footpad) (De Maeyer *et al.*, 1975*e*; De Maeyer, 1976, 1977). Interferon also has an effect on the afferent arc, i.e., sensitization. Experiments using either SRBC or NDV as antigen have shown that interferon is capable of either completely inhibiting or decreasing sensitization. In order to obtain this effect, interferon has to be administered 24 hr before the antigen (De Maeyer-Guignard *et al.*, 1975). The timing of interferon administration is crucial, because when interferon is given at the same time as or after the antigen, there either is no effect or even enhancement of delayed hypersensitivity. These results show that exogenous interferon can affect the afferent and the efferent pathways of the delayed hypersensitivity reaction.

The use of *If-1* congenic mice has unequivocally demonstrated that endogenous interferon, produced as a result of viral infection, has the same effect. *If-1* congenic mice differ exclusively by their levels of NDV-induced circulating interferon (De Maeyer *et al.*, 1975*c*), cellular immune reactions, after inoculation of NDV, ought to be more depressed in the high than in the low producers, if interferon is involved. This is exactly what is observed when, for example, the effect on expression to SRBC delayed hypersensitivity is measured (Fig. 9) (De Maeyer *et al.*, 1975c).

5.4. Effects on Lymphocyte and Macrophage Activity as Monitored *in Vitro*

5.4.1. Lymphocytes

Interferon enhances the specific cytotoxicity of sensitized mouse lymphocytes against allogeneic tumor cells. The effect is rapid, occur-

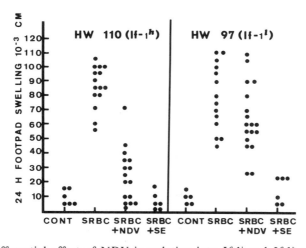

Fig. 9. Differential effect of NDV inoculation into *If-1^l* and *If-1^h* congenic mice on the expression of delayed hypersensitivity to sheep erythrocytes. The figure summarizes an experiment demonstrating that the effect of the inoculation of a virus on the expression of delayed hypersensitivity is directly related to the amount of interferon induced by the virus. Sensitized high- or low-interferon-producing congenic mice were divided each into three groups. Six hours before inoculation of SRBC into the left footpad, the first group was inoculated with NDV, the second with Sendai virus, and the third, serving as control, with allantoic fluid. The amount of NDV inoculated induced peak levels of about 55,000 units/ml of serum interferon in HW110 and 4500 units/ml in HW97 mice. The dose of Sendai virus used results in peak interferon levels of about 40,000 units/ml in both strains. Footpad swelling was measured 24 hr later in all groups. The results show unequivocally that the decreased responsiveness is influenced by the *If-1* locus, since in the *If-1^l* congenic strain NDV is without effect, as opposed to the *If-1^h* strain, in which it provokes a significant inhibition of DH reaction. On the other hand, the inoculation of Sendai virus decreases footpad swelling to the same extent in both strains, since interferon induction by Sendai virus is not influenced by the *If-1* locus and is identical in both strains. From De Maeyer *et al.* (1975e).

ring within several hours (Lindahl *et al.*, 1972). In addition, recently it has been shown that interferon or its inducers significantly increase the activity of natural killer (NK) lymphocyte activity in murine as well as in human cells (Gidlund *et al.*, 1978; Trinchieri *et al.*, 1978). Interferon can cause alterations in H-2 expression on DBA/2 mouse thymocytes without affecting cell proliferation, whereas the expression of θ antigen is not affected (Lindahl *et al.*, 1974).

Enhancement of the expression of H-2 antigens on mouse thymocytes also occurs after *in vivo* administration of interferon and after the endogenous induction of interferon by NDV (Lindahl *et al.*, 1976). Lonai and Steinman (1977) find that interferon treatment results in the enhanced expression of H-2 K and H-2 D on spleen cells, splenic T lymphocytes, and thymic lymphocytes, but does not affect the expression of Ia antigen on these cells. Brief interferon treatment of T lymphocytes from genetic high-responder animals also results in cellular-specific enhanced binding of synthetic polypeptide antigens.

5.4.2. Macrophages

Interferon can produce functional and morphological changes in mononuclear phagocytes. Huang *et al.* (1971) first reported enhanced uptake of colloidal carbon by mouse peritoneal macrophages treated with interferon *in vitro*. Previous to these direct experiments on the effect of interferon on phagocytosis, it had been reported by Gresser *et al.* (1970b) that, in RC14-tumor-bearing mice, tumor-cell phagocytosis by macrophages in ascitic fluid is enhanced by interferon treatment of the animals. Subsequent reports by Kishida *et al.* (1973) and Imanishi *et al.* (1975) have confirmed the fact that interferon treatment can activate murine peritoneal macrophages and human peripheral mono-cytes, as measured by increased uptake of Latex particles. Levy and Wheelock (1975) have extended this finding and have shown that interferon can stimulate the activity of macrophages derived from mice with Friend leukemia. Macrophages have depressed phagocytic and migratory functions in these leukemic animals, but interferon treatment restores normal function of these cells. Resting mouse macrophages are transformed to activated cells by interferon treatment, either *in vitro* or *in vivo*, and are rendered cytotoxic for syngeneic lymphoblastic leukemia cells (Schultz *et al.*, 1976, 1977, 1978).

Manejias *et al.* (1978) have shown in recombinant inbred strains that, after intravenous inoculation of NDV, the alleles of the *If-1* locus influence the degree of macrophage activation, as measured by the uptake of antibody-coated sheep erythrocytes, in that activation is more pronounced in $If-1^h$ than in $If-1^l$ animals. Most likely this occurs through the effect of $If-1$ on interferon production.

Taken together, these studies offer compelling evidence for an effect of interferon on mononuclear phagocytes and indicate that not only lymphocyte function but also monocyte activity can be influenced by interferon. However, it should be emphasized that in most of the studies concerning the effect of interferon on macrophage or lymphocyte activity the activity of these cells was measured under very special conditions, *in vitro*, and it is presently not possible to know to what extent these findings can be extrapolated to the normal activity of these cells *in vivo*.

5.5. Concluding Remarks

A few hundred units of interferon is sufficient to influence antibody synthesis *in vitro*, and, in the mouse, one inoculation of 10^5–10^6 interferon units can have significant effects on antibody formation, cell-mediated immunity, natural killer cells, and other lymphocyte and macrophage functions. Many of these effects are either stimulatory or inhibitory, depending on timing and dosage. This indicates that, at concentrations that are normally present as a result of infection with many viruses, interferon is capable of modulating various aspects of the immune response. Through interferon production, the organism not only directly limits virus replication but also influences the different lymphocyte and macrophage populations that are mobilized as a result of the infection. Several important questions are therefore raised. For example, it is conceivable that interaction of lymphocytes with virus-infected target cells is directly influenced by the amount of interferon produced by these cells or by cells in their neighborhood. In addition, the physiological contribution of the interferon induced by a given virus to the establishment of immunity to that virus merits our attention, and the possible interplay between various effects of type I and type II interferons on the immune system adds yet another degree of complexity to this fascinating problem (Fig. 10).

An excellent review of the effects of interferon on the immune system has been published by Epstein (1977*b*), and Gresser (1977*b*) has considered this in the more general context of the various nonantiviral effects of interferon.

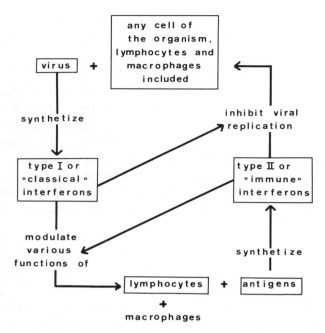

Fig. 10.   Schematic view of the interplay of the cells belonging to the immune system and the other cells of the organism through the production of type I and type II interferons.

6.   ANTITUMOR AND CELL MULTIPLICATION INHIBITORY EFFECTS

6.1.   Antitumor Effect

Atanasiu and Chany (1960) showed that pretreatment of hamsters with interferon preparations prior to inoculation of polyoma virus delays the appearance of tumors and decreases the number of tumor-bearing animals. Comparable observations were reported by Lampson *et al.* (1963) in chicks infected with RSV. Gresser and his co-workers have published a series of papers describing in great detail the various effects of interferon on the development of several murine leukemias. Continued administration of interferon to either Friend-virus-infected Swiss and DBA/2 mice or to Rauscher-virus-infected BALB/c mice inhibits or delays the evolution of various manifestations of the disease and prolongs the mean survival time (Gresser *et al.*, 1967a,b,c, 1968). Interferon also delays the onset and decreases the incidence of spontaneous lymphoid leukemia in AKR mice, even when treatment is started after onset of the leukemia (Gresser *et al.*, 1969a, 1976a). The evolution of another spontaneously appearing murine tumor of viral origin, the mouse mammary tumor, is similarly delayed by the repeated administration of interferon (Came and Moore, 1971). Gresser and co-workers have established that repeated daily administration of mouse interferon inhibits or delays the development of various types of allogeneic and syngeneic transplantable tumors of viral and nonviral origin (Gresser *et al.*, 1969*b*; Gresser and Bourali, 1969, 1970). The multiplication of transplantable Friend leukemia cells can similarly be inhibited by daily treatment of recipient mice with interferon (Rossi *et al.*, 1975). Furthermore, daily intravenous inoculation of interferon into mice results in the inhibition of the growth of the Lewis lung carcinoma and inhibits the development of pulmonary metastases. Interferon treatment can be delayed until 6 days after tumor inoculation and still be inhibitory for both primary tumor and metastases (Gresser and Bourali-Maury, 1972).

6.2. Cell Multiplication Inhibitory Effect

Paucker *et al.* (1962) first reported that mouse interferon preparations inhibited the multiplication of mouse L cells in suspension cultures. This observation has since been confirmed for many different systems, and it is now well established that interferon affects cell multiplication. Gresser *et al.* (1970*a*) reported that the cell multiplication inhibitory activity of different mouse interferon preparations on mouse leukemia L1210 cells is directly proportional to the antiviral activity; a subline of L1210 cells resistant to the anticellular effect of interferon also is resistant to the antiviral effect (Gresser *et al.*, 1974*a*). The *in vitro* inhibitory effect of interferon on cell multiplication is not limited to malignant cells, and mouse interferon affects multiplication of mouse embryo cell cultures, as well as *in vitro* blast formation of mouse lymphocytes (Lindahl-Magnusson *et al.*, 1972). There is no evidence that interferon is cytotoxic, but it delays the rate of cell multiplication (Tovey *et al.*, 1975) by causing an extension of different phases of the cell cycle (Balkwill and Taylor-Papadimitriou, 1978).

6.3. Mechanism of the Antitumor Effect

The antiviral effect obviously contributes to the inhibition by interferon of virus-induced leukemias and solid tumors, but additional mechanisms must be involved in the overall antitumor effect. The cell multiplication inhibitory effect on normal and tumor cells observed *in vitro* offers one possible mechanism, but there is no direct evidence that this mechanism is operative *in vivo*. On the other hand, interferon does act by enhancing in some way the capacity of the host to reject tumors, as shown by Gresser *et al.* (1972), who injected mice with leukemia L1210 cells derived from a line that is resistant *in vivo* to the antiviral and anticellular effect of interferon (Gresser *et al.*, 1974a,b). In spite of this, interferon treatment increases the survival of these mice, clearly suggesting an effect through the host rather than a direct effect on the cells. Such an effect could be mediated through the various actions of interferon on lymphocyte and monocyte function that have been discussed in Section 5. The action of interferon as an antitumor agent, and the clinical trials that are presently going on to this effect, have been discussed in detail by Gresser (1977a).

7. TYPE II INTERFERON

7.1. Introduction

Type II interferon still represents an operational concept since it has not yet been characterized molecularly. Thus it cannot be ascertained presently whether one is dealing with one or several substances, and whether mitogen- and antigen-induced type II interferons are identical. Some relationship between type II interferon and the immune system was evident as soon as it was discovered, since this interferon is made only by immune-stimulated lymphocytes and macrophages. Its relationship to other lymphokines is not clear, but it does seem to be different from MIF (Bartfeld and Vilček, 1975; Block *et al.*, 1978), and its production is not merely a result of blast formation, since there are data indicating that different cell types are involved in blast formation and type II interferon production (Epstein *et al.*, 1971a; Wallen *et al.*, 1973). Like type I interferon, it has a broad-spectrum antiviral activity which is relatively species specific and not limited to the type of cell that produced it (Epstein *et al.*, 1971a; Babiuk and Rouse, 1976). It is not neutralized by sera that neutralize type I interferon and *vice versa*. In addition to the antigenic difference, it differs from type I interferon by the destruction of its antiviral activity at pH 2. The lack of neutralization by anti-type-I interferon sera and the acid lability are the two most widely used criteria for distinguishing between type I and type II interferons (Falcoff, 1972; Valle *et al.*, 1975a; Wietzerbin *et al.*, 1977). The effects of type I and type II interferon on various functions of B and T cells and macrophages are gradually emerging from studies by several groups of investigators. Type II interferon is a lymphokine made by T cells on an immune-specific basis. It has immunosuppressive and enhancing properties as revealed by studies on antibody formation; its effect on CMI remains to be determined. Type I interferon, made by all nucleated cells as a result of viral infection or of the presence of dsRNA, has immunoenhancing and suppressive effects on antibody formation as well as on CMI. It is too early for a coherent picture to be drawn; the concept that type II interferon is a natural immunoregulator substance with adventitious antiviral effect, whereas type I interferon is a natural antiviral substance with adventious immunoregulatory effects, is probably too simple.

7.2. Production

7.2.1. *In Vitro*

Mitogen-stimulated interferon production in spleen cell suspensions was first reported by Wheelock (1965). It was subsequently shown by Epstein *et al.* (1971*b*) that lymphocytes, and not macrophages, are the source of mitogen-stimulated interferon and that a lymphocyte–macrophage collaboration is necessary for optimal production. No interferon is demonstrable in cultures containing 96–100% pure macrophages, with or without phytohemagglutinin, whereas in pure lymphocyte cultures low levels of interferon are induced. A fivefold increase in titer occurs when the lymphocytes are combined with macrophages. The first evidence that type II interferon is produced in lymphocyte cultures on an immune-specific basis came from Green *et al.* (1969), who found that, after addition of either PPD, diphtheria, or pertussis toxoid to human lymphocyte suspensions, interferon appears only in the supernatants of lymphocytes derived from individuals having been immunized with the corresponding antigens; thus the production of interferon reflects the immune status of the lymphocyte donor. This was subsequently confirmed by Epstein *et al.* (1972) and Rasmussen *et al.* (1974) and extended to viral antigens. Sensitized human lymphocytes produce interferon *in vitro* if challenged with viral antigens in the presence of macrophages. The antigens studied were vaccinia and herpesvirus hominis (herpes simplex), and the amount of interferon produced reflected the immune status of the donor. T. lymphocytes are the source of this interferon (Valle *et al.*, 1975*b*). As with mitogens, macrophages are an essential part of the culture system, but the memory for the interferon production resides in the T cells; when macrophages are omitted from the culture system, only type I interferon is made (Haahr *et al.*, 1976). A requirement for T cells also exists for mitogen-induced interferon production in the mouse, and θ-bearing spleen cells—but not thymocytes—are necessary, suggesting that type II interferon may be produce by mature T cells (Stobo *et al.*, 1974).

This conclusion is reinforced by the findings of Sonnenfeld *et al.* (1979) in that T cells appear to be the significant cell for production of type II interferon induced by tuberculin. Suppressor or cytotoxic (Ly-2,3+) T lymphocytes appear to be of particular importance, and cooperation of the T lymphocytes with another cell type, possibly B lymphocytes and/or macrophages, is required for production of murine type II interferon. The mechanism by which macrophages stimulate type II interferon, or lymphocyte mediator production in general, is not understood. Human macrophages derived from different sources are effective. T-lymphocyte interferon production in response to phyto-hemagglutinin (PHA), for example, is enhanced by macrophages derived from peripheral blood and by peritoneal macrophages obtained from ascitic fluid (Epstein, 1977a). This is in contrast to the finding that mouse peritoneal macrophages are not capable of restoring mitogen-induced interferon formation by nylon wool column purified lympho-cytes, whereas either spleen or bone marrow derived macrophages are equally capable of doing so (Neumann and Sorg, 1977). The contribu-tion of macrophages to interferon production in general has been dis-cussed in detail by Epstein (1976).

Cellular antigens also stimulate type II interferon formation, and Virelizier *et al.* (1977a) observed production of type II interferon in one-way-mixed lymphocyte cultures. The viral inhibitor previously observed by Gifford *et al.* (1971) in mixed lymphocyte cultures of mice was acid stable, so that it is not certain whether these authors were dealing with type I or type II interferon.

7.2.2. *In Vivo*

Mice previously infected with *Mycobacterium tuberculosis*, strain BCG, make large amounts of circulating type II interferon and MIF when inoculated intravenously with either old tuberculin or BCG. This induction is immune specific, since the production of NDV- or poly(I·C)-induced interferon is not enhanced in these animals (Stine-bring and Absher, 1970; Salvin *et al.*, 1973). The correlation between the release of MIF and type II interferon was confirmed in a sub-sequent study by the same group, and it was furthermore shown that tuberculin-induced type II interferon is produced by a heterogenous population of lymphocytes comprising both B and T cells. The authors arrived at the conclusion that type II interferon and MIF are closely related substances that are produced by the same or closely related cells (Salvin *et al.*, 1975; Sonnenfeld *et al.*, 1977a). The conclusion of this study is somewhat at variance with that reached in a study by Bartfeld and Vilček (1975) in which it was found that leukocyte cultures of rab-bits sensitized with Freund's complete adjuvant made interferon (pre-sumably of type II, but it was not characterized) when challenged with PPD, whereas peripheral lymphocyte cultures of the same rabbits, when challenged with PPD, made MIF. There was furthermore no correla-tion between interferon titer and MIF activity. Viral antigens have also been implicated as inducers of type II interferon *in vivo*. Rytel and Hooks (1977) showed that murine cytomegalovirus induces the forma-tion of type II interferon in lymphocytes of mice that had been infected 7 days earlier with the same virus: the authors suggest that immune interferon constitutes an important effector moiety by which cell-mediated immunity counteracts infection with viruses which spread directly from cell to cell. Lodmell and Notkins (1974) and also Fujiba-yashi *et al.* (1975) arrived at similar conclusions in a study of herpes simplex virus (HSV) infection in rabbits. An interesting and unexpected aspect of this study was the observation that HSV–anti-HSV antibody complexes were capable of stimulating type II interferon formation in immune rabbit lymphocytes; this suggests that the host can protect cells from destruction by neutralizing infectious virus while at the same time allowing virus–antibody complexes to stimulate immune lymphocytes to produce interferon for additional protection. This observation, however, awaits confirmation, since in human macrophage–lymphocyte cultures the presence of anti-HSV antibody reduced the formation of HSV-induced type II interferon (Haahr *et al.*, 1976).

It is thus quite evident from the aforementioned work that the production of type II interferon is a specialized function of T cells and that the stimulus for its production is the contact of "sensitized" or "immunized" T cells with antigen, not necessarily of viral origin. The relationship of this lymphokine to type I interferon, if any, is far from clear. Indeed, the best yields of this type of interferon have so far been obtained with nonviral antigens; whether all antigens are capable of inducing its production is not clear. Although antigenically and physically it appears to be different from type I interferon as mentioned before, it is possible that the antiviral moieties of type I and type II interferons are identical. This is suggested by the work of Epstein and Epstein (1976) showing that, as is the case for human type I interferon, the *AVG* locus of chromosome 21 is also necessary for the antiviral activity of human type II interferon.

In addition, like type I interferon, type II interferon enhances the specific phosphorylation of a 67,000 molecular weight protein *in vitro* in the presence of double-stranded RNA (Wietzerbin *et al.*, 1978) (Fig. 4). If these findings are confirmed and extended, it would appear that the biochemical changes brought about in interferon-treated cells are similar for type I and type II.

7.3. Interaction with the Immune System

Interferon produced by T cells on renewed contact with viral antigen can obviously be of benefit to the host. As such, the production of type II interferon is a useful component of cell-mediated immunity against viral infections, especially in the case of DNA viruses that are usually not very efficient inducers of type I interferon. In this respect, it may be relevant to mention the observation of Rasmussen *et al.* (1974) that subjects with HSV disease who failed to produce a detectable type II interferon response within 2–6 weeks after infection had more frequent recurrence of lesions than subjects producing greater quantities of interferon after disease. However, the induction of type II interferon on an immune-specific basis by nonviral antigens, as well as its induction by mitogens, suggests that its function is not merely—or maybe not even primarily—antiviral, but of a more general nature, and it seems likely that type II interferon plays a role in the modulation of the immune response. In BCG-sensitized mice, a correlation is found between the subsequent induction of type II interferon with old tuberculin and the suppression of antibody formation to sheep erythrocytes; the greatest reduction is obtained when type II interferon is induced 24 hr before the SRBC are administered. Furthermore, preparations containing type II interferon also suppress antibody formation against SRBC *in vitro*, and, in fact, are about 250 times more active in doing so than type I interferon if the antiviral titer is taken as the basis of comparison (Sonnenfeld *et al.*, 1977*b*). Similar results were obtained by Virelizier *et al.* (1977). These authors compared the immunosuppressive effects of type II and type I interferon and found type II interferon about 20 times more active than type I. Antibody formation *in vitro* is inhibited if type II interferon is added to the system before or at the same time as the antigen; if, however, the interferon is added to the system 48 hr after the antigen, a definite stimulation of the antibody response is obtained. Furthermore, the immunoenhancing effect of type II interferon on antibody responses is produced by an effect on T lymphocytes in contrast with the immunosuppressive effect which appears to be mediated through an effect on B lymphocytes (Sonnenfeld *et al.*, 1978). Thus type II interferon preparations contain one or several substances capable of either enhancing or depressing antibody formation; whether this or these factor(s) are identical with the antiviral factor(s) will have to await complete purification of this lymphokine. The latter will be a formidable undertaking if the specific activity comes anywhere near that of type I interferon, especially since the systems for production of type II interferon are several orders of magnitude less efficient than are the systems for the production of type I interferon, and furthermore the starting material contains much more protein.

8. SUMMARY AND CONCLUSIONS

Interferons are a group of vertebrate glycoproteins which, by definition, exert a broad antiviral activity in the species they derive from; they also have numerous other species-specific biological effects. Within a given animal species, interferon heterogeneity can be ascribed to the presence of several interferon genes and to different degrees of glycosylation of interferon molecules. Spontaneous interferon synthesis is exceptional. As a rule, interferon is induced by viruses in any nucleated cell of the organism (type I interferon) or by renewed contact of sensitized T cells with the antigen (type II interferon). The molecular characterization is quite advanced for type I but has hardly started for type II interferons, which are lymphokines.

In susceptible cells, interferon triggers a cascade of biochemical changes that are responsible for the antiviral activity and also for the multitude of other effects. This amplification explains the high specific activity of interferons and why they can be considered as some of the biologically most active proteins.

Interferons represent the first line of defense of the organism against virus infection. In addition to their direct antiviral effect, they have modulating effects on various specialized functions of the immune system, such as antibody formation, cell-mediated immunity, and several other activities of lymphocytes and macrophages. How these various effects integrate at the level of the organism is subject to further study (Fig. 10).

ACKNOWLEDGMENTS

The personal work of the authors was supported by the Centre National de la Recherche Scientifique, the Fondation pour la Recherche Médicale Française, and the Ligue Nationale Française contre le Cancer. We are grateful to Dr. T. C. Merigan for critically reading the sections on interaction with the immune system and on type II interferon, and to Dr. R. M. Friedman for critically reading the section on the mechanisms of the antiviral activity. Drs. I. Gresser, E. Knight, M. Revel, and J. Wietzerbin kindly provided the photographs for Figs. 3, 4, 5, and 6. We are also grateful to Dr. Jan Vilček, who kindly read the section of this chapter on interferon synthesis.

9.   REFERENCES

Abreu, S. L., and Bancroft, F. C., 1978, Intracellular location of human fibroblast interferon messenger RNA, *Biochem. Biophys. Res. Commun.* **82**:1300–1305.

Adams, A., Lidin, B., Strander, H., and Cantell, K., 1975, Spontaneous interferon production and Epstein–Barr virus antigen expression in human lymphoid cell lines, *J. Gen. Virol.* **28**:219–223.

Anfinsen, C. B., Bose, S., Corley, L., and Gurari-Rotman, D., 1974, Partial purification of human interferon by affinity chromatography, *Proc. Natl. Acad. Sci. USA* **71**:3139–3142.

Ankel, H., Chany, C., Galliot, B., Chevalier, M. J., and Robert, M., 1973, Antiviral effect of interferon covalently bound to sepharose, *Proc. Natl. Acad. Sci. USA* **70**:2360–2363.

Atanasiu, P., and Chany, C., 1960, Action d'un interféron provenant de cellules malignes sur l'infection expérimentale du hamster nouveau-né par le virus du polyome, *C. R. Acad. Sci.* **251**:1687–1689.

Atkins, G. J., Johnston, M. D., Westmacott, L. M., and Burke, D. C., 1974, Induction of interferon in chick cells by temperature-sensitive mutants of Sindbis virus, *J. Gen. Virol.* **25**:381–390.

Babiuk, L. A., and Rouse, B. T., 1976, Immune interferon production by lymphoid cells: Role in the inhibition of herpes viruses, *Infect. Immun.* **13**:1567–1578.

Bader, J. P., 1962, Production of interferon by chick embryo cells exposed to Rous sarcoma virus, *Virology* **16**:436–443.

Baglioni, C., Minks, M. A., and Maroney, P. A., 1978, Interferon action may be mediated by activation of a nuclease by pppA2′p5′A2′p5′A, *Nature (London)* **273**:684–687.

Bakay, M., and Burke, D. C., 1972, The production of interferon in chick cells infected with DNA viruses: A search for double-stranded RNA, *J. Gen. Virol.* **16**:399–403.

Balkwill, F., and Taylor-Papadimitriou, J., 1978, Interferon affects both G_1 and $S + G_2$ in cells stimulated from quiescence to growth, *Nature (London)* **274**:798–800.

Ball, L. A., and White, C. N., 1978, Effect of interferon pretreatment on coupled transcription and translation in cell-free extracts of primary chick embryo cells, *Virology* **84**:496–508.

Barmak, S. L., and Vilček, J., 1973, Altered cellular responses to interferon induction by poly I·poly C: Priming and hyporesponsiveness in cells treated with interferon preparations, *Arch. Gesamte Virusforsch.* **43**:272–283.

Baron, S., and Buckler, C. E., 1963, Circulating interferon in mice after intravenous injection of virus, *Science* **141**:1061–1063.

Baron, S., and Isaacs, A., 1961, Mechanism of recovery from viral infection in the chick embryo, *Nature (London)* **191**:97–98.

Baron, S., Buckler, C. E., Friedman, R. M., and McCloskey, R. V., 1966, Role of interferon during viremia. II. Protective action of circulating interferon, *J. Immunol.* **96**:17–24.

Baron, S., Bogomolova, N. N., Billiau, A., Levy, H. B., Buckler, C. E., Stern, R., and Naylor, R., 1969, Induction of interferon by preparations of synthetic single-stranded RNA, *Proc. Natl. Acad. Sci. USA* **64**:67–74.

Bartfeld, H., and Vilček, J., 1975, Immunologically specific production of interferon in cultures of rabbit blood lymphocytes: Association with *in vitro* tests for cell-mediated immunity, *Infect. Immun.* **12**:1112–1115.

Baxt, B., Sonnabend, J. A., and Bablanian, R., 1977, Effects of interferon on vesicular stomatitis virus transcription and translation, *J. Gen. Virol.* **35**:325–334.

Berg, K., Ogburn, C. A., Paucker, K., Mogensen, E. K., and Cantell, K., 1975, Affinity chromatography of human leukocyte and diploid cell interferons on sepharose-bound antibodies, *J. Immunol.* **114**:640–644.

Berg, K., Alacam, R., Hamilton, R. D., and Heron, I., 1977, Purification of human interferons by antibody affinity chromatography, *Tex. Rep. Biol. Med.* **35**: 187–192.

Berman, B., and Vilček, J., 1974, Cellular binding characteristics of human interferon, *Virology* **57**:378–386.

Berthold, W., Tan, C., and Tan, Y. H., 1978, Purification and *in vitro* labeling of interferon from a human fibroblastoid cell line, *J. Biol. Chem.* **253**:5206–5212.

Besançon, F., and Ankel, H., 1974a, Inhibition of interferon action by plant lectins, *Nature (London)* **250**:784–786.

Besançon, F., and Ankel, H., 1974b, Binding of interferon to gangliosides, *Nature (London)* **252**:478–480.

Besançon, F., and Ankel, H., 1976, Inhibition de l'action de l'interféron par les hormones glycoprotéiques, *C. R. Acad. Sci.* **283**:1807–1810.

Besançon, F., and Bourgeade, M. F., 1974, Affinity of murine and human interferon for concanavalin A, *J. Immunol.* **113**:1061–1063.

Besançon, F., Ankel, H., and Basu, S., 1976, Specificity and reversibility of interferon ganglioside interaction, *Nature (London)* **259**:576–578.

Billiau, A., 1970, The refractory state after induction of interferon with double-stranded RNA, *J. Gen. Virol.* **7**:225–232.

Billiau, A., Joniau, M., and De Somer, P., 1973, Mass production of human interferon in diploid cells stimulated by poly(I·C), *J. Gen. Virol.* **19**:1–8.

Billiau, A., Edy, V. G., Sobis, H., and De Somer, P., 1974, Influence of interferon on virus-particle synthesis in oncornavirus-carrier lines. II. Evidence for a direct effect on particle release, *Int. J. Cancer* **14**:335–340.

Billiau, A., Edy, V. G., De Clercq, E., Heremans, H., and De Somer, P., 1975, Influence of interferon on the synthesis of virus particles in oncornavirus carrier cell lines. III. Survey of effects on A-, B- and C-type oncornaviruses, *Int. J. Cancer* **15**:947–953.

Billiau, A., Heremans, H., Allen, P. T., De Maeyer-Guignard, J., and De Somer, P., 1976, Trapping of oncornavirus particles at the surface of interferon-treated cells, *Virology* **73**:537–542.

Billiau, A., Heremans, H., Allen, P. T., Baron, S., and De Somer, P., 1978, Interferon inhibits C-type virus at a post-transcriptional prerelease step, *Arch. Virol.* **57**:205–220.

Blalock, J. E., and Baron, S., 1977a, Interferon-induced transfer of viral resistance between animal cells, *Nature (London)* **269**:422–425.

Blalock, J. E., and Baron, S., 1977b, The transfer of interferon-induced viral resistance between animal cells, *Tex. Rep. Biol. Med.* **35**:307–315.

Block, L. H., Cantell, K., Bamberger, S., Ruhenstroth-Bauer, G., and Strander, H., 1978, Lack of correspondence between virus-induced human leukocyte interferon and concanavalin A-induced human migration inhibitory factor (MIF), *Arch. Virol.* **56**:341–343.

Booth, R. J., Rastrick, J. M., Bellamy, A. R., and Marbrook, J., 1976a, Modulating effects of interferon preparations on an antibody response *in vitro*, *Aust. J. Exp. Biol. Med. Sci.* **54**:11–25.

Booth, R. J., Booth, J. M., and Marbrook, J., 1976b, Immune conservation: A possible consequence of the mechanism of interferon-induced antibody suppression, *Eur. J. Immunol.* **6**:769–772.

Borden, E. C., and Murphy, F. A., 1971, The interferon refractory state: *In vivo* and *in vitro* studies of its mechanism, *J. Immunol.* **106**:134–142.

Borden, E. C., Prochownik, E. V., and Carter, W. A., 1975, The interferon refractory state. II. Biological characterization of a refractoriness-inducing protein, *J. Immunol.* **114**:752–756.

Bose, S., Gurari-Rotman, D., Ruegg, U. T., Corley, L., and Anfinsen, C. B., 1976, Apparent dispensability of the carbohydrate moiety of human interferon for antiviral activity, *J. Biol. Chem.* **251**:1659–1662.

Both, G. W., Furuichi, Y., Muthukrishnan, S., and Shakin, A. J., 1975, Ribosome binding to reovirus mRNA in protein synthesis requires 5' terminal 7-methylglyanosine, *Cell* **6**:185–195.

Braun, W., and Levy, H. B., 1972, Interferon preparations as modifiers of immune responses, *Proc. Soc. Exp. Biol. Med.* **141**:769–773.

Breinig, M. C., Armstrong, J. A., and Ho, M., 1975, Rapid onset of hyporesponsiveness to interferon induction on reexposure to polyribonucleotide, *J. Gen. Virol.* **26**:149–158.

Bridgen, P. J., Anfinsen, C. B., Corley, L., Bose, S., Zoon, K. C., Ruegg, U. T., and Buckler, C. E., 1977, Human lymphoblastoid interferon, large scale production and partial purification, *J. Biol. Chem.* **252**:6585–6587.

Brown, G. E., Lebleu, B., Kawakita, M., Shaila, S., Sen, G. C., and Lengyel, P., 1976, Increased endonuclease activity in an extract from mouse Ehrlich ascites tumor cells which had been treated with a partially purified interferon preparation dependence on double-stranded RNA, *Biochem. Biophys. Res. Commun.* **69:** 114–122.

Buck, K. W., Chain, E. B., and Himmelweit, F., 1971, Comparison of interferon induction in mice by purified penicillium chrysogenum virus and derived double-stranded RNA, *J. Gen. Virol.* **12:**131–139.

Burke, D. C., 1971, The production of interferon by animal viruses, *Proc. R. Soc. London Ser. B* **177:**17–22.

Burke, D. C., and Buchan, A., 1965, Interferon production in chick embryo cells. I. Production by ultraviolet inactivated virus, *Virology* **26:**28–35.

Burke, D. C., and Veomett, G., 1977, Enucleation and reconstruction of interferon-producing cells, *Proc. Natl. Acad. Sci USA* **74:**3391–3395.

Burke, D. C., Graham, C. F., and Lehman, J. M., 1978, Appearance of interferon inducibility and sensitivity during differentiation of murine teratocarcinoma cells *in vitro*, *Cell* **13:**243–248.

Came, P. E., and Moore, D. H., 1971, Inhibition of spontaneous mammary carcinoma of mice by treatment with interferon and poly(I·C), *Proc. Soc. Exp. Biol. Med.* **137:**304–305.

Cantell, K., and Hirvonen, S., 1977, Preparation of human leukocyte interferon for clinical use, *Tex. Rep. Biol. Med.* **35:**138–144.

Cantell, K., and Hirvonen, S., 1978, Large-scale production of human leukocyte interferon containing 10^8 units per ml, *J. Gen. Virol.* **39:**541–543.

Cantell, K., and Paucker, K., 1963a, Studies on viral interference in two lines of Hela cells, *Virology* **19:**81–87.

Cantell, K., and Paucker, K., 1963b, Quantitative studies on viral interference in suspended L cells. IV. Production and assay of interferon, *Virology* **21:**11–21.

Cantell, K., Hirvonen, S., Mogensen, K. E., and Pyhala, L., 1974, Human leucocyte interferon: Production, purification stability and animal experiments, *In Vitro* (Publication of the Tissue Culture Association) *Monog.* **3:**35–38.

Cassingena, R., Chany, C., Vignal, M., Suarez, H., Estrade, S., and Lazar, P., 1971, Use of monkey–mouse hybrid cells for the study of the cellular regulation of interferon production and action, *Proc. Natl. Acad. Sci. USA* **68:**580–584.

Cavalieri, R. L., Havell, E. A., Vilcek, J., and Pestka, S., 1977a, Synthesis of human interferon by *Xenopus laevis* oocytes: Two structural genes for interferons in human cells, *Proc. Natl. Acad. Sci. USA* **74:**3287–3291.

Cavalieri, R. L., Havell, E. A., Vilcek, J., and Pestka, S., 1977b, Induction and decay of human fibroblast interferon mRNA, *Proc. Natl. Acad. Sci. USA* **74:**4415–4419.

Cesario, T. C., Schryer, P., Mandel, A., and Tilles, J. G., 1976, Affinity of human fibroblasts interferon for blue dextran, *Proc. Soc. Exp. Biol. Med.* **153:**486–489.

Chadha, K. C., Sclair, M., Sulkowski, E., and Carter, W. A., 1978, Molecular size heterogeneity of human leukocyte interferon, *Biochemistry* **17:**196–200.

Chang, E. H., Mims, S. J., Triche, T. J., and Friedman, R. M., 1977a, Interferon inhibits mouse leukemia virus release: An electron microscope study, *J. Gen. Virol.* **34:**363–367.

Chang, E. H., Myers, M. W., Wong, P. K. Y., and Friedman, R. M., 1977b, The inhibitory effect of interferon on a temperature sensitive mutant of Moloney murine leukemia virus, *Virology* **77:**625–636.

Chany, C., 1976, Membrane-bound interferon specific cell receptor system: Role in the establishment and amplification of the antiviral state, *Biomedicine* **24:**148–157.

Chany, C., Gregoire, A., Vignal, M., Lemaitre-Moncuit, J., Brown, P., Besançon, F.,

Suarez, H., and Cassingena, R., 1973, Mechanism of interferon uptake in parental and somatic monkey–mouse hybrid cells, *Proc. Natl. Acad. Sci. USA* **70**:557–561.

Chany, C., Ankel, H., Galliot, B., Chevalier, M. J., and Gregoire, A., 1974, Mode of action and biological properties of insoluble interferon, *Proc. Soc. Exp. Biol. Med.* **147**:293–299.

Chany, C., Vignal, M., Couillin, P., Nguyen van Cong, Boué, J., and Boué, A., 1975, Chromosomal localization of human genes governing the interferon-induced antiviral state, *Proc. Natl. Acad. Sci. USA* **72**:3129–3133.

Chen, J. K., Jankowski, W. J., O'Malley, J. A., Sulkowski, E., and Carter, W. A., 1976, Nature of the molecular heterogeneity of human leukocyte interferon, *J. Virol.* **19**:425–434.

Chester, T. J., Paucker, K., and Merigan, T. C., 1973, Suppression of mouse antibody producing spleen cells by various interferon preparations, *Nature (London)* **246**:92–94.

Clavell, L. A., and Bratt, M. A., 1971, Relationship between the ribonucleic acid-synthesizing capacity of ultraviolet-irradiated Newcastle disease virus and its ability to induce interferon, *J. Virol.* **8**:500–508.

Clemens, M. J., and Williams, B. R. G., 1978, Inhibition of cell-free protein synthesis by pppA2′p5′p5′A: A novel oligonucleotide synthesized by interferon-treated L cell extracts, *Cell* **13**:565–572.

Colby, C., and Chamberlin, M. J., 1969, The specificity of interferon induction in chick embryo cells by helical RNA, *Proc. Natl. Acad. Sci. USA* **63**:160–167.

Colby, C., and Duesberg, P. H., 1969, Double-stranded RNA in vaccinia virus infected cells, *Nature (London)* **222**:940–944.

Colby, C., Stollar, B. D., and Simon, M. I., 1971, Interferon induction: DNA-RNA hybrid or double stranded RNA? *Nature (London) New Biol.* **229**:172–174.

Content, J., Lebleu, B., Nudel, U., Zilberstein, A., Berissi, H., and Revel, M., 1975, Blocks in elongation and initiation of protein synthesis induced by interferon treatment in mouse L cells, *Eur. J. Biochem.* **54**:1–10.

Creagan, R. P., Tan, Y. H., Ghen, S., and Ruddle, F. H., 1975, Somatic cell genetic analysis of the interferon system, *Fed. Proc.* **34**:2222–2226.

Davey, M. W., Huang, J. W., Sulkowski, E., and Carter, W. A., 1974, Hydrophobic interaction of human interferon with concanavalin A-agarose, *J. Biol. Chem.* **249**:6354–6355.

Davey, M. W., Huang, J. W., Sulkowski, E., and Carter, W. A., 1975, Hydrophobic binding sites on human interferon, *J. Biol. Chem.* **250**:348–349.

Davey, M. W., Sulkowski, E., and Carter, W. A., 1976a, Binding of human fibroblast interferon to concanavalin A-agarose. Involvement of carbohydrate recognition and hydrophobic interaction, *Biochemistry* **15**:704–713.

Davey, M. W., Sulkowski, E., and Carter, W. A., 1976b, Purification and characterization of mouse interferon with novel affinity sorbents, *J. Virol.* **17**:439–445.

Davey, M. W., Sulkowski, E., and Carter, W. A., 1976c, Hydrophobic interaction of human, mouse, and rabbit interferons with immobilized hydrocarbons, *J. Biol. Chem.* **251**:7620–7625.

De Clercq, E., Stollar, B. D., and Thang, M. N., 1978, Interferon inducing activity of polyinosinic acid, *J. Gen. Virol.* **40**:203–212.

De Maeyer, E., 1976, Interferon and delayed-type hypersensitivity to a viral antigen, *J. Infect. Dis.* **133**:A63–A65.

De Maeyer, E., and De Maeyer-Guignard, J., 1963, Two-sided effect of steroids on interferon in tissue culture, *Nature (London)* **197:**724–725.

De Maeyer, E., and De Maeyer-Guignard, J., 1968, Influence of animal genotype and age on the amount of circulating interferon induced by Newcastle disease virus, *J. Gen. Virol.* **2:**445–449.

De Maeyer, E., and De Maeyer-Guignard, J., 1969, Gene with quantitative effect on circulating interferon induced by Newcastle disease virus, *J. Virol.* **3:**506–512.

De Maeyer, E., and De Maeyer-Guignard, J., 1970, A gene with quantitative effect on circulating interferon induction. Further studies, *Ann. N.Y. Acad. Sci.* **173:** 228–238.

De Maeyer, E., and De Maeyer-Guignard, J., 1977, Effect of interferon on cell-mediated immunity, *Tex. Rep. Biol. Med.* **35:**370–374.

De Maeyer, E., and Enders, J. F., 1965, Growth characteristics, Interferon production and plaque formation with different lines of Edmoston measles virus, *Arch. Gesamte Virusforsch.* **16:**151–167.

De Maeyer, E., Jullien, P., and De Maeyer-Guignard, J., 1967, Interferon synthesis in X-irradiated animals. II. Restoration by bone-marrow transplantation of circulating interferon production in lethally-irradiated mice, *Int. J. Rad. Biol.* **13:**417–431.

De Maeyer, E., De Maeyer-Guignard, J., and Jullien, P., 1969, Interferon synthesis in X-irradiated animals, III. The high radiosensitivity of myxovirus-induced circulating interferon production, *Proc. Soc. Exp. Biol. Med.* **131:**36–41.

De Maeyer, E., De Maeyer-Guignard, J., and Jullien, P., 1970, Circulating interferon production in the mouse. Origin and nature of cells involved and influence of animal genotype, *J. Gen. Physiol.* **56:**43s–56s.

De Maeyer, E., Fauve, R. M., and De Maeyer-Guignard, J., 1971*a*, Production d'interféron au niveau du macrophage, *Ann. Inst. Pasteur* **120:**438–446.

De Maeyer, E., De Maeyer-Guignard, J., and Montagnier, L., 1971*b*, Double-stranded RNA from rat liver induces interferon in rat cells, *Nature (London) New Biol.* **229:**109–110.

De Maeyer, E., Mobraaten, L, and De Maeyer-Guignard, J., 1973, Prolongation par l'interféron de la survie des greffes de peau chez la souris, *C. R. Acad. Sci.* **277D:**2101–2103.

De Maeyer, E., De Maeyer-Guignard, J., Hall, W. T., and Bailey, D. W., 1974, A locus affecting circulating interferon levels induced by mouse mammary tumor virus, *J. Gen. Virol.* **23:**209–211.

De Maeyer, E., Montagnier, L., De Maeyer-Guignard, J., and Collandre, H., 1975*a*, Assay for interferon messenger RNA in heterologous cells, in: *Effects of Interferon on Cells, Viruses and the Immune System* (A. Geraldes, ed.), pp. 191–209, Academic Press, New York.

De Maeyer, E., Jullien, P., De Maeyer-Guignard, J., and Démant, P., 1975*b*, Effect of mouse genotype on interferon production. Distribution of *If-1* alleles among inbred strains and transfer of phenotype by grafting bone marrow cells, *Immunogenetics* **2:**151–160.

De Maeyer, E., De Maeyer-Guignard, J., and Bailey, D. W., 1975*c*, Effect of mouse genotype on interferon production: Lines congenic at the *If-1* locus, *Immunogenetics* **1:**438–445.

De Maeyer, E., Mobraaten, L. E., and De Maeyer-Guignard, J., 1975*d*, Prolongation of allograft survival in mice by interferon inducers and interferon preparations, in:

Effects of Interferon on Cells, Viruses and the Immune Systems (A. Geraldes, ed.),
pp. 367–379, Academic Press, New York.

De Maeyer, E., De Maeyer-Guignard, J., and Vandeputte, M., 1975e, Inhibition by
interferon of delayed-type hypersensitivity in the mouse, *Proc. Natl. Acad. Sci
USA* **72**:1753–1757.

De Maeyer-Guignard, J., 1972, Mouse leukemia: Depression of serum interferon
production, *Science* **177**:797–799.

De Maeyer-Guignard, J., and De Maeyer, E., 1971, Effect of antilymphocytic serum on
circulating interferon in mice as a function of the inducer, *Nature (London) New
Biol.* **229**:212–214.

De Maeyer-Guignard, J., and De Maeyer, E., 1976, Le chromophore du bleu dextran:
Un ligand puissant pour la purification de l'interféron par chromatographie
d'affinité, *C.R. Acad. Sci.* **283D**:709–711.

De Maeyer-Guignard, J., De Maeyer, E., and Jullien, P., 1969, Interferon synthesis in
X-irradiated animals. IV. Donor-type serum interferon in rat-to-mouse radiation
chimeras injected with Newcastle disease virus, *Proc. Natl. Acad. Sci. USA*
63:732–739.

De Maeyer-Guignard, J., De Maeyer, E., and Montagnier, L., 1972, Interferon
messenger RNA: Translation in heterologous cells, *Proc. Natl. Acad. Sci. USA*
69:1203–1207.

De Maeyer-Guignard, J., Cachard, A., and De Maeyer, E., 1975, Delayed-type
hypersensitivity to sheep red blood cells: Inhibition of sensitization by interferon,
Science **190**:574–576.

De Maeyer-Guignard, J., Thang, M. N., and De Maeyer, E., 1977, Binding of mouse
interferon to polynucleotides, *Proc. Natl. Acad. Sci. USA* **74**:3787–3790.

De Maeyer-Guignard, J., Tovey, M. G., Gresser, I., and De Maeyer, E., 1978, Purification of mouse interferon by sequential affinity chromatography on poly(U)- and
antibody–agarose columns, *Nature (London)* **271**:622–625.

Desmyter, J., and Stewart, W. E., II, 1976, Molecular modification of interferon:
Attainment of human interferon in a conformation active on cat cells but inactive
on human cells, *Virology* **70**:451–458.

Desmyter, J., Melnick, J. L., and Rawls, W. E., 1968, Defectiveness of interferon
production and of rubella virus interference in a line of african green monkey
kidney cells (Vero), *J. Virol.* **2**:955–961.

Desmyter, J., De Groote, J., Desmet, V. J., Billiau, A., Ray, M. B., Bradburne, A. F.,
Edy, V. G., De Somer, P., and Mortelmans, J., 1976, Administration of human
fibroblast interferon in chronic hepatitis-B infection, *Lancet* **2**:645–647.

Dianzani, F., and Baron, S., 1975, Unexpectedly rapid action of human interferon in
physiological conditions, *Nature (London)* **257**:682–684.

Dianzani, F., Buckler, C. E., and Baron, S., 1969, Effect of cycloheximide on the
antiviral action of interferon, *Proc. Soc. Exp. Biol. Med.* **130**:519–523.

Dianzani, F., Viano, I., Santiano, M., Zucca, M., and Baron, S., 1977, Effect of cell
density on development of the antiviral state in interferon-producing cells: A possible model of "*in vivo*" conditions, *Proc. Soc. Exp. Biol. Med.* **155**:445–448.

Duc-Nguyen, H., Rosenblum, E. N., and Zeigel, R. F., 1966, Persistent infection of a
rat kidney cell line with Rauscher murine leukemia virus, *J. Bacteriol.*
92:1133–1140.

Edy, V. G., Braude, I. A., De Clercq, E., Billiau, A., and De Somer, P., 1976, Purification of interferon by adsorption chromatography on controlled pore glass, *J. Gen. Virol.* **33**:517–521.

Edy, V. G., Billiau, A., and De Somer, P., 1977, Purification of human fibroblast interferon by zinc chelate affinity chromatography, *J. Biol. Chem.* **252**:5934–5935.

Einhorn, S., and Strander, H., 1977, Is interferon tissue specific? Effect of human leukocyte and fibroblast interferons on the growth of lymphoblastoid and osteosarcoma cell lines, *J. Gen. Virol.* **35**:573–577.

Epstein, L. B., 1976, The ability of macrophages to augment *in vitro* mitogen- and antigen-stimulated production of interferon and other mediators of cellular immunity by lymphocytes, in: *Immunobiology of the Macrophage*, Vol. 8, pp. 201–234, Academic Press, New York.

Epstein, L. B., 1977*a*, Mitogen and antigen induction of interferon *in vitro* and *in vivo*, *Tex. Rep. Biol. Med.* **35**:42–56.

Epstein, L. B., 1977*b*, The effects of interferons on the immune response *in vitro* and *in vivo*, in: *Interferons and Their Actions* (W. Stewart, II, ed.), pp. 92–132, CRC Press, Cleveland.

Epstein, L. B., and Epstein, C. J., 1976, Localization of the gene AVG for the antiviral expression of immune and classical interferon to the distal portion of the long arm of chromosome 21, *J. Infect. Dis.* **133**:A56–A62.

Epstein, L. B., Cline, M. J., and Merigan, T. C., 1971*a*, The interaction of human macrophages and lymphocytes in the phytohemagglutinin-stimulated production of interferon, *J. Clin. Invest.* **50**:744–753.

Epstein, L. B., Cline, M. J., and Merigan, T. C., 1971*b*, PPD-stimulated interferon: *In vitro* macrophage-lymphocyte interaction in the production of a mediator of cellular immunity, *Cell. Immunol.* **2**:602–613.

Epstein, L. B., Stevens, D. A., and Merigan, T. C., 1972, Selective increase in lymphocyte interferon response to vaccinia antigen after revaccination, *Proc. Natl. Acad. Sci. USA* **69**:2632–2636.

Falcoff, E., Falcoff, R., Lebleu, B., and Revel, M., 1972, Interferon treatment inhibits Mengo RNA and haemoglobin mRNA translation in cell-free extracts of L cells, *Nature (London) New Biol.* **240**:145–147.

Falcoff, E., Falcoff, R., Lebleu, B., and Revel, M., 1973, Correlation between the antiviral effect of interferon treatment and the inhibition of *in vitro* mRNA translation in noninfected L cells, *J. Virol.* **12**:421–430.

Falcoff, E., Havell, E. A., Lewis, J. A., Lande, M. A., Falcoff, R., Sabatini, D. D., and Vilcek, J., 1976, Intracellular location of newly synthesized interferon in human FS-4 cells, *Virology* **75**:384–393.

Falcoff, R., 1972, Some properties of virus and immune-induced human lymphocyte interferons, *J. Gen. Virol.* **16**:251–253.

Falcoff, R., and Falcoff, E., 1970, Induction de la synthèse d'interféron par des RNA bicaténaires. II. Etude de la forme intermédiaire de réplication du virus Mengo, *Biochim. Biophys. Acta* **199**:147–158.

Fantes, K. A., 1974, Human leucocyte interferon: Properties and purification, in: *The Production and Use of Interferon for the Treatment and Prevention of Human Virus Infections, In Vitro*, Monograph 3 (C. Waymouth, ed.), p. 48.

Fauconnier, B., 1970, Augmentation de la pathogénicité virale par l'emploi de sérum anti-interféron *in vivo*, *C. R. Acad. Sci.* **271**:1464–1466.

Field, A. K., Tytell, A. A., Lampson, G. P., and Hilleman, M. R., 1967, Inducers of interferon and host resistance. II. Multistranded synthetic polynucleotide complexes, *Proc. Natl. Acad. Sci. USA* **58**:1004–1010.

Fleischmann, W. R., and Simon, E. H., 1974, Mechanism of interferon induction by NDV: A monolayer and single cell study, *J. Gen. Virol.* **25**:337–349.

Frankfort, H. M., Havell, E. A., Croce, C. M., and Vilcek, J., 1978, The synthesis and actions of mouse and human interferons in mouse-human hybrid cells, *Virology* **89**:45–52.

Friedman, R. M., 1968, Inhibition of arbovirus protein synthesis by interferon, *J. Virol.* **2**:1081–1085.

Friedman, R. M., 1977, Antiviral activity of interferons, *Bacteriol. Rev.* **41**:543–567.

Friedman, R. M., and Kohn, L. D., 1976, Cholera toxin inhibits interferon action, *Biochem. Biophys. Res. Commun.* **70**:1078–1084.

Friedman, R. M., and Sonnabend, J. A., 1964, Inhibition of interferon action by *p*-fluoro-phenylalanine, *Nature (London)* **203**:366–367.

Friedman, R. M., and Sonnabend, J. A., 1965, Inhibition of interferon action by puromycin, *J. Immunol.* **95**:696–703.

Friedman, R. M., Esteban, R. M., Metz, D. H., Tovell, D. R., Kerr, I., and Williamson, R., 1972*a*, Translation of RNA by L cell extracts: Effect of interferon, *FEBS Lett.* **24**:273–277.

Friedman, R. M., Metz, D. H., Esteban, R. M., Tovell, D. R., Ball, L. A., and Kerr, I. M., 1972*b*, Mechanism of interferon action: Inhibition of viral messenger ribonucleic acid translation in L cells extracts, *J. Virol.* **10**:1184–1198.

Friedman, R. M., Chang, E. H., Ramseur, J. M., and Myers, M. W., 1975, Interferon-directed inhibition of chronic murine leukemia virus production in cell cultures: Lack of effect on intracellular viral markers, *J. Virol.* **16**:569–574.

Friedman, R. M., Costa, J. C., Ramseur, J. M., Myers, M. W., Jay, F. T., and Chang, E. H., 1976, Persistence of the viral genome in interferon-treated cells infected with oncogenic or nononcogenic viruses, *J. Infect. Dis.* **133**:A43–A50.

Fujibayashi, T., Hooks, J. J., and Notkins, A. L., 1975, Production of interferon by immune lymphocytes exposed to herpes simplex virus-antibody complexes, *J. Immunol.* **115**:1191–1193.

Fung, K. P., and Ng, M. H., 1978, Purification of human diploid fibroblast interferon by immobilized neuraminidase, *Arch. Virol.* **56**:1–6.

Gandhi, S. S., and Burke, D. C., 1970, Interferon production by myxoviruses in chick embryo cells, *J. Gen. Virol.* **6**:95–103.

Gandhi, S. S., Burke, D. C., and Scholtissek, C., 1970, Virus RNA synthesis by ultraviolet-irradiated Newcastle disease virus and interferon production, *J. Gen. Virol.* **9**:97–99.

Garren, L. D., Howell, R. R., Tomkins, G. M., and Crocco, R. M., 1964, A paradoxical effect of actinomycin D: The mechanism of regulation of enzyme synthesis by hydrocortisone, *Proc. Natl. Acad. Sci. USA* **52**:1121–1129.

Gidlund, M., Orn, A., Wigzell, H., Senik, A., and Gresser, I., 1978, Enhanced NK cell activity in mice injected with interferon and interferon inducers, *Nature (London)* **273**:759–761.

Gifford, G. E., Tibor, A., and Peavy, D. L., 1971, Interferon production in mixed lymphocyte cell cultures, *Infect. Immun.* **3**:164–166.

Gisler, R. H., and Dukor, P., 1972, A three cell mosaic culture: *In vitro* immune response by combination of pure B- and T-cells with peritoneal macrophage, *Cell. Immunol.* **4**:341–350.

Gisler, R. H., Lindahl, P., and Gresser, I., 1974, Effects of interferon on antibody synthesis *in vitro*, *J. Immunol.* **113**:438–444.

Glasgow, L. A., and Habel, K., 1963, Interferon production by mouse leucocytes *in vitro* and *in vivo*, *J. Exp. Med.* **117**:149–160.

Green, J. A., Cooperband, S. R., and Kibrick, S., 1969, Immune specific induction of interferon production in cultures of human blood lymphocytes, *Science* **164**: 1415–1417.

Greenberg, H. B., Pollard, R. B., Lutwick, L. I., Gregory, P. B., Robinson, W. S., and Merigan, T. C., 1976, Effect of human leukocyte interferon on hepatitis B virus infection in patients with chronic active hepatitis, *New Engl. J. Med.* **295**:517–522.

Greene, J. J., Dieffenbach, C. W., and Ts'o, P. O. P., 1978, Inactivation of interferon mRNA in the shut-off of human interferon synthesis, *Nature (London)* **271**:81–83.

Gresser, I., 1961, Production of interferon by suspensions of human leucocytes, *Proc. Soc. Exp. Biol. Med.* **108**:799–803.

Gresser, I., 1977a, Antitumor effects of interferon, in: *Cancer—A Comprehensive Treatise*, Vol. 5: *Chemotherapy* (F. Becker, ed.), pp. 521–571, Plenum Press, New York.

Gresser, I., 1977b, On the varied biologic effect of interferon, *Cell. Immunol.* **34**:406–415.

Gresser, I., and Bourali, C., 1969, Exogenous interferon and inducers of interferon in the treatment of Balb/c mice inoculated with RC$_{19}$ tumor cells, *Nature (London)* **223**:844–845.

Gresser, I., and Bourali, C., 1970, Antitumor effects of interferon preparations in mice, *J. Natl. Cancer Inst.* **45**:365–376.

Gresser, I., and Bourali-Maury, C., 1972, Inhibition by interferon preparations of a solid malignant tumour and pulmonary metastases in mice, *Nature (London) New Biol.* **236**:78–79.

Gresser, I., Coppey, J., Falcoff, E., and Fontaine, D., 1967a, Interferon and murine leukemia. I. Inhibitory effect of interferon preparations on development of Friend leukemia in mice, *Proc. Soc. Exp. Biol. Med.* **124**:84–91.

Gresser, I., Fontaine, D., Coppey, J., Falcoff, R., and Falcoff, E., 1967b, Interferon and murine leukemia. II. Factors related to the inhibitory effect of interferon preparations on development of Friend leukemia in mice, *Proc. Soc. Exp. Biol. Med.* **124**:91–94.

Gresser, I., Falcoff, R., Fontaine-Brouty-Boye, D., Zajdela, F., Coppey, J., and Falcoff, E., 1967c, Interferon and murine leukemia. IV. Further studies on the efficacy of interferon preparations administered after inoculation of Friend virus, *Proc. Soc. Exp. Biol. Med.* **126**:791–797.

Gresser, I., Berman, L., De Thé, G., Brouty-Boye, D., Coppey, J., and Falcoff, E., 1968, Interferon and murine leukemia. V. Effect of interferon preparations on the evolution of Rauscher disease in mice. *J. Natl. Cancer Inst.* **41**:505–522.

Gresser, I., Coppey, J., and Bourali, C., 1969a, Interferon and murine leukemia. IV. Effect of interferon preparations on the lymphoid leukemia of AKR mice, *J. Natl. Cancer Inst.* **43**:1083–1089.

Gresser, I., Bourali, C., Levy, J. P., Fontaine-Brouty-Boye, D., and Thomas, M. T., 1969b, Prolongation de la survie des souris inoculées avec des cellules tumorales et traitées avec des préparations d'interférons, *C. R. Acad. Sci.* **268**:994–997.

Gresser, I., Brouty-Boye, D., Thomas, M. T., and Macieira-Coelho, A., 1970a, Interferon and cell division. I. Inhibition of the multiplication of mouse leukemia

L 1210 cells *in vitro* by interferon preparations, *Proc. Natl. Acad. Sci. USA* **66**:1052–1058.

Gresser, I., Bourali, C., Chouroulinkov, I., Brouty-Boye, D., and Thomas, M. T., 1970*b*, Treatment of neoplasia in mice with interferon preparations, *Ann. N.Y. Acad. Sci.* **173**:694–707.

Gresser, I., Maury, C., and Brouty-Boye, D., 1972, Mechanism of the antitumor effect of interferon in mice, *Nature (London)* **239**:167–168.

Gresser, I., Bandu, M. T., and Brouty-Boye, D., 1974*a*, Interferon and cell division. IX. Interferon-resistant L 1210 cells characteristics and origin, *J. Natl. Cancer Inst.* **52**:553–559.

Gresser, I., Bandu, M. T., Brouty-Boye, D., and Tovey, M., 1974*b*, Pronounced antiviral activity of human interferon on bovine and porcine cells, *Nature (London)* **251**:543–545.

Gresser, I., Maury, C., and Tovey, M., 1976*a*, Interferon and murine leukemia. VII. Therapeutic effect of interferon preparations after diagnosis of lymphoma in AKR mice, *Int. J. Cancer* **17**:647–651.

Gresser, I., Tovey, M. G., Bandu, M. T., Maury, C., and Brouty-Boye, D., 1976*b*, Role of interferon in the pathogenesis of virus diseases in mice as demonstrated by the use of anti-interferon serum. I. Rapid evolution of encephalomyocarditis virus infection, *J. Exp. Med.* **144**:1305–1315.

Gresser, I., Tovey, M. G., Maury, C., and Bandu, M. T., 1976*c*, Role of interferon in the pathogenesis of virus diseases in mice as demonstrated by the use of anti-interferon serum. II. Studies with Herpes simplex, Moloney sarcoma, vesicular stomatitis, Newcastle disease and influenza viruses, *J. Exp. Med.* **144**:1316–1323.

Gresser, I., De Maeyer-Guignard, J., Tovey, M. G., and De Maeyer, E., 1979, Electrophoretically pure mouse interferon exerts multiple biologic effects, *Proc. Natl. Acad. Sci. USA* (in press).

Grossberg, S. E., 1977, Nonviral interferon inducers: Natural and synthetic products, *Tex. Rep. Biol. Med.* **35**:111–116.

Gupta, S. L., Sopori, M. L., and Lengyel, P., 1973, Inhibition of protein synthesis directed by added viral and cellular messenger RNAs in extracts of interferon-treated Ehrlich ascites tumor cells. Location and dominance of the inhibitor(s), *Biochem. Biophys. Res. Commun.* **54**:777–783.

Gupta, S. L., Sopori, M. L., and Lengyel, P., 1974, Release of the inhibition of messenger RNA translation in extracts of interferon-treated Ehrlich ascites tumor cells by added transfer RNA, *Biochem. Biophys. Res. Commun.* **57**:763–770.

Haahr, S., Rasmussen, L., and Merigan, T. C., 1976, Lymphocyte transformation and interferon production in human mononuclear cell microcultures for assay of cellular immunity to Herpes simplex virus, *Infect. Immun.* **14**:47–54.

Haase, A. T., Johnson, J. S., Kasel, J. A., Margolis, S., and Levy, H. B., 1970, Induction of interferon in lymphoblastoid cell lines, *Proc. Soc. Exp. Biol. Med.* **133**:1076–1083.

Hajnicka, V., Fuchsberger, N., and Borecky, L., 1976, Affinity chromatography of mouse interferon: A modified purification procedure utilizing specifically purified antibodies, *Acta Virol.* **20**:326–333.

Havell, E. A., and Vilček, J., 1972, Production of high-titered interferon in cultures of human diploid cells, *Antimicrob. Agents Chemother.* **2**:476–484.

Havell, E. A., Berman, B., Ogburn, C. A., Berg, K., Paucker, K., and Vilček, J., 1975,

Two antigenically distinct species of human interferon, *Proc. Natl. Acad. Sci. USA* **72**:2185–2187.

Havell, E. A., Yip, Y. K., and Vilček, J., 1977a, Correlation of physicochemical and antigenic properties of human leukocyte interferon subspecies, *Arch. Virol.* **55**:121–129.

Havell, E. A., Yamazaki, S., and Vilček, J., 1977b, Altered molecular species of human interferon produced in the presence of inhibitors of glycosylation, *J. Biol. Chem.* **252**:4425–4427.

Havell, E. A., Yip, Y. K., and Vilček, J., 1978a, Characteristics of human lymphoblastoid (Namalva) interferon, *J. Gen. Virol.* **38**:51–59.

Havell, E. A., Hayes, T. G., and Vilček, J., 1978b, Synthesis of two distinct interferons by human fibroblasts, *Virology* **89**:330–334.

Heineberg, H., Gold, E., and Robbins, F. C., 1964, Differences in interferon content in tissues of mice of various ages infected with Coxsackie B1 virus, *Proc. Soc. Exp. Biol. Med.* **115**:947–953.

Heller, E., 1963, Enhancement of Chikungunya virus replication and inhibition of interferon production by actinomycin D, *Virology* **21**:652–656.

Hirsch, M. S., Ellis, D. A., Black, P. H., Monaco, A. P., and Wood, M. L., 1974, Immunosuppressive effects of an interferon preparation *in vivo*, *Transplantation* **17**:234–236.

Ho, M., and Breinig, M. K., 1965, Metabolic determinants of interferon formation, *Virology*, **25**:331–339.

Ho, M., and Ke, Y. H., 1970, The mechanism of stimulation of interferon production by a complexed polyribonucleotide, *Virology* **40**:693–702.

Ho, M., and Kono, Y., 1965, Tolerance to the induction of interferons by endotoxin and virus, *J. Clin. Invest.* **44**:1059.

Ho, M., Kono, Y., and Breinig, M. K., 1965, Tolerance to the induction of interferons by endotoxin and virus. Role of a humoral factor, *Proc. Soc. Exp. Biol. Med.* **119**:1227–1232.

Holtermann, O. A., and Havell, E. A., 1970, Reduced interferon response in mice congenitally infected with lymphocytic choriomeningitis virus, *J. Gen. Virol.* **9**:101–103.

Hovanessian, A. G., and Kerr, I. M., 1978, Synthesis of an oligonucleotide inhibitor of protein synthesis in rabbit reticulocyte lysates analogous to that formed in extracts from interferon-treated cells, *Eur. J. Biochem.* **84**:149–159.

Hovanessian, A. G., Brown, R. E., and Kerr, I. M., 1977, Synthesis of low molecular weight inhibitor of protein synthesis with enzyme from interferon-treated cells, *Nature (London)* **268**:537–540.

Huang, J. W., Davey, M. W., Hejna, C. J., Von Muenchhausen, W., Sulkowski, E., and Carter, W. A., 1974, Selective binding of human interferon to albumin immobilized on agarose, *J. Biol. Chem.* **249**:2665–2667.

Huang, K. Y., Donahoe, R. M., Gordon, F. B., and Dressler, H. R., 1971, Enhancement of phagocytosis by interferon-containing preparations, *Infect. Immun.* **4**:581–588.

Imanishi, J., Yokota, Y., Kishida, T., Mukainaka, T., and Matsuo, A., 1975, Phagocytosis enhancing effect of human leukocyte interferon preparation on human peripheral monocytes *in vitro*, *Acta Virol.* **19**:52–58.

Imanishi, J., Oishi, K., Kishida, T., Negoro, Y., and Izuka, M., 1977, Effects of interferon preparations on rabbit corneal xenograft, *Arch. Virol.* **53**:157–161.

Inglot, A. D., Albin, M., and Chudzio, T., 1973, Persistent infection of mouse cells with Sindbis virus: Role of virulence of strains, auto-interfering particles and interferon, *J. Gen. Virol.* **20**:105–110.

Isaacs, A., 1961, Mechanisms of virus infections, *Nature (London)* **192**:1247–1248.

Isaacs, A., 1963, Interferon, *Adv. Virus Res.* **10**:1–38.

Isaacs, A., and Burke, D. C., 1958, Mode of action of interferon, *Nature (London)* **182**:1073–1074.

Isaacs, A., and Lindenmann, J., 1957a, Virus interference. I. The interferon, *Proc. Roy. Soc. London Ser. B* **147**:258–267.

Isaacs, A., and Lindenmann, J., 1957b, Virus interference. II. Some properties of interferon, *Proc. Roy. Soc. London Ser. B* **147**:268.

Iwakura, Y., Yonehara, S., and Kawade, Y., 1978, Purification of mouse L cell interferon. Essentially pure preparations with associated cell growth inhibitory activity, *J. Biol. Chem.* **253**:5074–5079.

Jankowski, W. J., Davey, M. W., O'Malley, J. A., Sulkowski, E., and Carter, W. A., 1975, Molecular structure of human fibroblast and leukocyte interferons: Probe by lectin and hydrophobic chromatography, *J. Virol.* **16**:1124–1130.

Jankowski, W. J., Von Muenchhausen, W., Sulkowski, E., and Carter, W. A., 1976, Binding of human interferons to immobilized cibacron blue F3GA: The nature of molecular interaction, *Biochemistry* **15**:5182–5187.

Johnson, H. M., and Baron, S., 1976, The nature of the suppressive effect of interferon and interferon inducers on the *in vitro* immune response, *Cell. Immunol.* **25**:106–115.

Johnson, H. M., Smith, B. G., and Baron, S., 1974, Inhibition of the primary *in vitro* antibody response of mouse spleen cells by interferon preparations, *IRCS* **2**:1616.

Joklik, W. K., and Merigan, T. C., 1966, Concerning the mechanisms of action of interferon, *Proc. Natl. Acad. Sci. USA* **56**:558–565.

Jullien, P., De Maeyer-Guignard, J., and De Maeyer, E., 1974, Interferon synthesis in X-irradiated animals. V. Origin of mouse serum interferon induced by polyinosinic-polycytidylic acid and encephalomyocarditis virus, *Infect. Immun.* **10**:1023–1028.

Kawakita, M., Cabrer, B., Taira, H., Rebello, M., Slattery, E., Weideli, H., and Lengyel, P., 1978, Purification of interferon from mouse Ehrlich ascites tumor cells, *J. Biol. Chem.* **253**:598–602.

Kerr, I. M., 1971, Protein synthesis in cell-free systems: An effect of interferon, *J. Virol.* **7**:448–459.

Kerr, I. M., and Brown, R. E., 1978, pppA2'p5'A2'p5'A: An inhibitor of protein synthesis synthesized with an enzyme fraction from interferon-treated cells, *Proc. Natl. Acad. Sci. USA* **75**:256–260.

Kerr, I. M., Friedman, R. M., Brown, R. E., Ball, L. A., and Brown, J. C., 1974a, Inhibition of protein synthesis in cell-free systems from interferon-treated, infected cells. Further characterization and effect of formylmethionyl-tRNA$_F$, *J. Virol.* **13**:9–21.

Kerr, I. M., Brown, R. E., and Ball, L. A., 1974b, Increased sensitivity of cell-free protein synthesis to double-stranded RNA after interferon treatment, *Nature (London)* **250**:57–59.

Kerr, I. M., Brown, R. E., Clemens, M. J., and Gilbert, C. S., 1976, Interferon-mediated inhibition of cell-free-protein synthesis in response to double-stranded RNA, *Eur. J. Biochem.* **69**:551–561.

Kerr, I. M., Brown, R. E., and Hovanessian, A. G., 1977, Nature of inhibitor of cell-free protein synthesis formed in response to interferon and double-stranded RNA, *Nature* (*London*) **268**:540–542.

Kilbourne, E. D., Smart, K. M., and Pokorny, B. A., 1961, Inhibition by cortisone of the synthesis and action of interferon, *Nature* (*London*) **190**:650–651.

Kimball, P. C., and Duesberg, P. H., 1971, Virus interference by cellular double-stranded RNA, *J. Virol.* **7**:697–706.

Kishida, T., Morikawa, K., Ito, H., and Yokota, Y., 1973, Influence de l'interféron sur l'inhibition par les macrophages, de la multiplication *in vitro* de la cellule maligne murine (FM₃A), *C. R. Soc. Biol.* **167**:1502.

Kleinschmidt, W. J., Ellis, L. F., Van Frank, R. M., and Murphy, E. B., 1968, Interferon stimulation by a double-stranded RNA of a mycophage in statolon preparations, *Nature* (*London*) **220**:167–168.

Knight, E., Jr., 1974, Interferon-sepharose: Induction of the antiviral state, *Biochem. Biophys. Res. Commun.* **56**:860–864.

Knight, E., Jr., 1975, Heterogeneity of purified mouse interferons, *J. Biol. Chem.* **250**:4139–4144.

Knight, E., Jr., 1976a, Interferon: Purification and initial characterization from human diploid cells, *Proc. Natl. Acad. Sci. USA* **73**:520–523.

Knight, E., Jr., 1976b, Antiviral and cell growth inhibitory activities reside in the same glycoprotein of human fibroblast interferon, *Nature* (*London*) **262**:302–303.

Knight, E., Jr., 1978, Preparation of ¹²⁵iodine-labeled human fibroblast interferon, *J. Gen. Virol.* **40**:681–684.

Knight, E., Jr., and Korant, B. D., 1977, A cell surface alteration in mouse L cells induced by interferon, *Biochem. Biophys. Res. Commun.* **74**:707–713.

Kohase, M., and Vilček, J., 1977, Regulation of human interferon production stimulated with poly(I·C): Correlation between shutoff and hyporesponsiveness to reinduction, *Virology* **76**:47–54.

Kohn, L. D., Friedman, R. M., Holmes, J. M., and Lee, G., 1976, Use of thyrotropin and cholera toxin to probe the mechanism by which interferon initiates its antiviral activity, *Proc. Natl. Acad. Sci. USA* **73**:3695–3699.

Kono, Y., and Ho, M., 1965, The role of the reticuloendothelial system in interferon formation in the rabbit, *Virology* **25**:162–166.

Kroath, H., Gross, H. J., Jungwirth, C., and Bodo, G., 1978, RNA methylation in vaccinia virus-infected chick embryo fibroblasts treated with homologous interferon, *Nucleic Acids Res.* **5**:2441–2454.

Kronenberg, L. H., 1977, Interferon production by individual cells in culture, *Virology* **76**:634–642.

Kronenberg, L. H., and Friedmann, T., 1975, Relative quantitative assay of the biological activity of interferon messenger ribonucleic acid, *J. Gen. Virol.* **27**:225–238.

Lai, M. H. T., and Joklik, W. K., 1973, The induction of interferon by temperature-sensitive mutants of reovirus, UV-irradiated reovirus, and subviral reovirus particles, *Virology* **51**:191–204.

Lampson, G. P., Tytell, A. A., Nemes, M. M., and Hilleman, M. R., 1963, Purification and characterization of chick embryo interferon, *Proc. Soc. Exp. Biol. Med.* **112**:468–478.

Lampson, G. P., Tytell, A. A., Field, A. K., Nemes, M. M., and Hilleman, M. R., 1967, Inducers of interferon and host resistance. I. Double-stranded RNA from extracts of penicillium funiculosum, *Proc. Natl. Acad. Sci. USA* **58**:782–789.

Lebleu, B., Sen, G. C., Shaila, S., Cabrer, B., and Lengyel, P., 1976, Interferon, double-stranded RNA, and protein phosphorylation, *Proc. Natl. Acad. Sci. USA* **73**:3107–3111.

Lebleu, B., Hubert, E., Content, J., De Wit, L., Braude, I. A., and De Clercq, E., 1978, Translation of mouse interferon mRNA in *Xenopus laevis* oocytes and in rabbit reticulocytes lysates, *Biochem. Biophys. Res. Commun.* **82**:665–673.

Levy, H. B., and Carter, W. A., 1968, Molecular basis of the action of interferon, *J. Mol. Biol.* **31**:561–577.

Levy, H. B., and Wheelock, E. F., 1975, Impaired macrophage function in Friend virus leukemia: Restoration by statolon, *J. Immunol.* **114**:962–965.

Lin, L. S., Wiranowska-Stewart, M., Chudzio, T., and Stewart, W. E., II., 1978, Characterization of the heterogeneous molecules of human interferons: Differences in the cross-species antiviral activities of various molecular populations in human leukocyte interferons, *J. Gen. Virol.* **39**:125–130.

Lindahl, P., Leary, P., and Gresser, I., 1972, Enhancement by interferon of the specific toxicity of sensitized lymphocytes, *Proc. Natl. Acad. Sci. USA* **69**:721–725.

Lindahl, P., Leary, P., and Gresser, I., 1974, Enhancement of the expression of histocompatibility antigens of mouse lymphoid cells by interferon *in vitro*, *Eur. J. Immunol.* **4**:779–784.

Lindahl, P., Gresser, I., Leary, P., and Tovey, M., 1976, Interferon treatment of mice: Enhanced expression of histocompatibility antigens on lymphoid cells, *Proc. Natl. Acad. Sci. USA* **73**:1284–1287.

Lindahl-Magnusson, P., Leary, P., and Gresser, I., 1972, Interferon inhibits RNA synthesis induced in mouse lymphocyte suspensions by phytohaemagglutinin or by allogeneic cells, *Nature (London) New Biol.* **237**:120–121.

Lindenmann, J., Burke, D. C., and Isaacs, A., 1957, Studies on the production, mode of action and properties of interferon, *Br. J. Exp. Pathol.* **38**:551–562.

Lockart, R. Z., Jr., 1963, Production of an interferon by L cells infected with western equine encephalomyelitis virus, *J. Bacteriol.* **85**:556–566.

Lockart, R. Z., Bayliss, N. L., Toy, S. T., and Yin, F. H., 1968, Viral events necessary for the induction of interferon in chick embryo cells, *J. Virol.* **2**:962–965.

Lodmell, D. L., and Notkins, A. L., 1974, Cellular immunity to herpes simplex virus mediated by interferon, *J. Exp. Med.* **140**:764–778.

Lomniczi, B., 1970*a*, Systemic induction of interferon in chicks with various NDV strains. I. Relationship between virulence of the virus and the mechanism of interferon production, *Arch. Gesamte Virusforsch.* **30**:159–166.

Lomniczi, B., 1970*b*, Systemic induction of interferon in chicks with various NDV strains. II. Nature of the interferon inducing agent, *Arch. Gesamte Virusforsch.* **30**:167–172.

Lomniczi, B., 1973, Studies on interferon production and interferon sensitivity of different strains of Newcastle disease virus, *J. Gen. Virol.* **21**:305–316.

Lomniczi, B., and Burke, D. C., 1970, Interferon production by temperature-sensitive mutants of Semliki forest virus, *J. Gen. Virol.* **8**:55–68.

Lonai, P., and Steinman, L., 1977, Physiological regulation of antigen binding to T cells: Role of a soluble macrophage factor and of interferon, *Proc. Natl. Acad. Sci. USA* **74**:5662–5666.

Long, W. F., and Burke, D. C., 1971, Interferon production by double-stranded RNA: A comparison of induction by reovirus to that by a synthetic double-stranded polynucleotide, *J. Gen. Virol.* **12**:1–11.

Manejias, R. E., Hamburg, S. I., and Rabinovitch, M., 1978, Serum interferon and phagocytic activity of macrophages in recombinant inbred mice inoculated with Newcastle disease virus, *Cell. Immunol.* **38**:209–213.

Marcus, P. I., and Sekellick, M. J., 1977, Defective interfering particles with covalently linked ($\pm$) RNA induced interferon, *Nature* **266**:815–819.

Marcus, P. I., and Sekellick, M. J., 1978, Interferon action. III. The rate of primary transcription of vesicular stomatitis virus is inhibited by interferon action, *J. Gen. Virol.* **38**:391–408.

Marcus, P. I., Engelhardt, D. L., Hunt, J. M., and Sekellick, M. J., 1971, Interferon action: Inhibition of vesicular stomatitis virus RNA synthesis induced by virion-bound polymerase, *Science* **174**:593–598.

Margolis, S. A., Oie, H., and Levy, H. B., 1972, The effect of interferon, interferon inducers or interferon induced virus resistance on subsequent interferon production, *J. Gen. Virol.* **15**:119–128.

Mayr, U., Bermayer, H. P., Weidinger, G., Jungwirth, C., Gross, H. J., and Bodo, G., 1977, Release of interferon-induced translation inhibition by tRNA in cell-free extracts from mouse erythro-leukemia cells, *Eur. J. Biochem.* **76**:541–551.

McLaren, C., and Potter, C. W., 1973, The relationship between interferon and virus virulence in influenza virus infections of the mouse, *J. Med. Microbiol.* **6**:21–32.

Meager, A., Graves, H., Walker, R., Burke, D. C., Swallow, D., and Westerwald, A., 1979, Somatic cell genetics of human interferon production in human–rodent cell hybrids, *J. Gen. Virol.* (in press).

Mendelson, J., and Glasgow, L. A., 1966, The *in vitro* and *in vivo* effects of cortisol on interferon production and action, *J. Immunol.* **96**:345–352.

Merigan, T. C., Rand, K. H., Pollard, R. B., Abdallah, P. S., Jordon, G. W., and Fried, R. P., 1978, Human leukocyte interferon for the treatment of herpes zoster in patients with cancer, *New Engl. J. Med.* **298**:981–987.

Metz, D. H., and Douglas, A. R., 1977, Viral resistance to interferon, *Tex. Rep. Biol. Med.* **35**:260–263.

Metz, D. H., Esteban, M., and Danielescu, G., 1975, The effect of interferon on the formation of virus polyribosomes in L cells infected with Vaccinia virus, *J. Gen. Virol.* **27**:197–209.

Metz, D. H., Levin, M. J., and Oxman, M. N., 1976, Mechanism of interferon action: Further evidence for transcription as the primary site of action in Simian virus 40 infection, *J. Gen. Virol.* **32**:227–240.

Metz, D. H., Oxman, M. N., and Levin, M. J., 1977, Interferon inhibits the *in vitro* accumulation of virus specific RNA in nuclei isolated from SV40 infected cells, *Biochem. Biophys. Res. Commun.* **75**:172–178.

Metz, M., and Esteban, D. H., 1972, Interferon inhibits viral protein synthesis in L cells infected with Vaccinia virus, *Nature (London)* **238**:385–388.

Mirchamsy, H., and Rapp, F., 1969, Role of interferon in replication of virulent and attenuated strains of measles virus, *J. Gen. Virol.* **4**:513–522.

Mishell, R. I., and Dutton, R. W., 1967, Immunization of dissociated spleen cultures from normal mice, *J. Exp. Med.* **126**:423–442.

Mobraaten, L., De Maeyer, E., and De Maeyer-Guignard, J., 1973, Prolongation of allograft survival in mice by inducers of interferon, *Transplantation* **16**:415–420.

Mogensen, K. E., and Cantell, K., 1974, Human leukocyte interferon: A role for disulphide bonds, *J. Gen. Virol.* **22**:95–103.

Mogensen, K. E., Pyhala, L., Torma, E., and Cantell, K., 1974, No evidence for a carbohydrate moiety affecting the clearance of circulating human leukocyte interferon in rabbits, *Acta Pathol. Microbiol. Scand.* **82B**:305–310.

Mozes, L. W., and Vilček, J., 1974, Interferon induction in rabbit cells irradiated with UV light, *J. Virol.* **13**:646–651.

Mozes, L. W., and Vilček, J., 1975, Distinguishing characteristics of interferon induction with poly(I·C) and Newcastle disease virus in human cells, *Virology* **65**:100–111.

Nemes, N. M., Tytell, A. A., Lampson, G. P., Field, A. K., and Hilleman, M. R., 1969*a*, Inducers of interferon and host resistance. VI. Antiviral efficacy of poly(I·C) in animal models, *Proc. Soc. Exp. Biol. Med.* **132**:776–783.

Nemes, N. M., Tytell, A. A., Lampson, G. P., Field, A. K., and Hilleman, M. R., 1969*b*, Inducers of interferon and host resistance. VII. Antiviral efficacy of double-stranded RNA of natural origin, *Proc. Soc. Exp. Biol. Med.* **132**:784–789.

Neumann, C., and Sorg, C., 1977, Immune interferon. I. Production by lymphokine-activated murine macrophages, *Eur. J. Immunol.* **7**:719–725.

Northrop, R. L., and Deinhardt, F., 1967, Production of interferon-like substances by human bone marrow tissues *in vitro*, *J. Natl. Cancer Inst.* **39**:685–689.

Notkins, A. L., Mergenhagen, S. E., and Howard, R. J., 1970, Effect of virus infections on the function of the immune systems, *Annu. Rev. Microbiol.* **24**:525–538.

Ogburn, C. A., Berg, K., and Paucker, K., 1973, Purification of mouse interferon by affinity chromatography on anti-interferon globulin-sepharose, *J. Immunol.* **111**:1206–1218.

Oie, H. K., Gazdar, A. F., Buckler, C. E., and Baron, S., 1972, High interferon producing line of transformed murine cells, *J. Gen. Virol.* **17**:107–109.

Orlova, T. G., Georgadze, I. I., Kognovitskaya, A. I., and Solovyov, V. D., 1974, Interferon-inducing and interferon-translating functions of RNA isolated from Newcastle disease virus-infected cells, *Acta Virol.* **18**:210–216.

Osborn, J. E., and Medearis, D. N., Jr., 1967, Suppression of interferon and antibody and multiplication of Newcastle disease virus in cytomegalovirus infected mice, *Proc. Soc. Exp. Biol. Med.* **124**:347–353.

Overall, J. C., Jr., and Glasgow, L. A., 1970, Fetal response to viral infection: Interferon production in sheep, *Science* **167**:1139–1141.

Oxman, M. N., and Levin, M. J., 1971, Interferon and transcription of early virus-specific RNA in cells infected with Simian virus 40, *Proc. Natl. Acad. Sci. USA* **68**:299–302.

Pantelouris, E. M., and Pringle, C. R., 1976, Interferon production in athymic nude mice, *J. Gen. Virol.* **32**:149–152.

Paucker, K., and Boxaca, M., 1967, Cellular resistance to induction of interferon, *Bacteriol. Rev.* **31**:145–156.

Paucker, K., Cantell, K., and Henle, W., 1962, Quantitative studies on viral interferences in suspended L cells. III. Effect of interfering viruses and interferon on the growth rate of cells, *Virology* **17**:324–334.

Paucker, K., Dalton, B. J., Ogburn, C. A., and Torma, E., 1975, Multiple active sites on human interferons, *Proc. Natl. Acad. Sci. USA* **72**:4587–4591.

Peries, J., Levy, J. P., Boiron, M., and Bernard, J., 1964, Multiplication of Rauscher virus in cultures of mouse kidney cells, *Nature (London)* **203**:672–673.

Peries, J., Boiron, M., and Canivet, M., 1965, Recherche d'une production d'interféron et d'une interférence virale hétérologue dans une lignée cellulaire chroniquement infectée par le virus de Rauscher, *Ann. Inst. Pasteur* **109**:595–600.

Peries, J., Canivet, M., Guillemain, B., and Boiron, M., 1968, Inhibitory effect of interferon preparations on the development of foci of altered cells induced *in vitro* by mouse sarcoma virus, *J. Gen. Virol.* **3**:465–468.

Pestka, S., McInnes, J., Havell, E. A., and Vilček, J., 1975, Cell-free synthesis of human interferon, *Proc. Natl. Acad. Sci. USA* **72**:3898–3901.

Pitha, P. M., and Pitha, J., 1974, Interferon induction by single-stranded polynucleotides modified with polybases, *J. Gen. Virol.* **24**:385–390.

Pitha, P. M., Vengris, V. E., and Reynolds, F. H., Jr., 1976*a*, The role of cell membrane in the antiviral effect of interferon, *J. Supramol. Struct.* **4**:467–473.

Pitha, P. M., Rowe, W. P., and Oxman, M. N., 1976*b*, Effect of interferon on exogenous, endogenous, and chronic murine leukemia virus infection, *Virology* **70**:324–338.

Pitha, P. M., Staal, S. P., Bolognesi, D. P., Denny, T. P., and Rowe, W. P., 1977, Effect of interferon on murine leukemia virus infection. II. Synthesis of viral components in exogenous infection, *Virology* **79**:1–13.

Polezhaev, F. I., Makariev, G. S., and Aleksandrova, G. I., 1974, Interferon-inducing ability in human leukocyte cultures of influenza viruses of different virulence, *Acta Virol.* **18**:362.

Radke, K. L., Colby, C., Kates, J. R., Krider, H. M., and Prescott, D. M., 1974, Establishment and maintenance of the interferon-induced antiviral state: Studies in enucleated cells, *J. Virol.* **13**:623–630.

Raj, N. B. K., and Pitha, P. M., 1977, Relationship between interferon production and interferon messenger RNA synthesis in human fibroblasts, *Proc. Natl. Acad. Sci. USA* **74**:1483–1487.

Rasmussen, L. E., Jordan, G. W., Stevens, D. A., and Merigan, T. C., 1974, Lymphocyte interferon production and transformation after herpes simplex infections in humans, *J. Immunol.* **112**:728–735.

Ratner, L., Sen, G. C., Brown, G. E., Lebleu, B., Kawakita, M., Cabrer, B., Slattery, E., and Lengyel, P., 1977, Interferon, double-stranded RNA and RNA degradation. Characteristics of an endonuclease activity, *Eur. J. Biochem.* **79**:565–577.

Repik, P., Flamand, A., and Bishop, D. H. L., 1974, Effect of interferon upon the primary and secondary transcription of vesicular stomatitis and influenza viruses, *J. Virol.* **14**:1169–1178.

Revel, M., 1977, Interferon-induced translational regulation, *Tex. Rep. Biol. Med.* **35**:212–220.

Revel, M., Bash, D., and Ruddle, F. H., 1976, Antibodies to a cell-surface component coded by human chromosome 21 inhibit action of interferon, *Nature (London)* **260**:139–141.

Revel, M., Kimchi, A., Schmidt, A., Shulman, L., and Zilberstein, A., 1978, The interferon system: Studies on the molecular mechanisms of interferon action, in: *Proceedings of the 12th FEBS meeting*, Pergamon Press, Oxford, England.

Reynolds, F. H., and Pitha, P. M., 1974, The induction of interferon and its messenger RNA in human fibroblasts, *Biochem. Biophys. Res. Commun.* **59**:1023–1030.

Reynolds, F. H., Jr., Premkumar, E., and Pitha, P. M., 1975, Interferon activity produced by translation of human interferon messenger RNA in cell-free ribosomal systems and in *Xenopus* oocytes, *Proc. Natl. Acad. Sci. USA* **72**:4881–4885.

Roberts, W. K., Clemens, M. J., and Kerr, I. M., 1976*a*, Interferon-induced inhibition of protein synthesis in L-cell extracts: An ATP-dependent step in the activation of an inhibitor by double-stranded RNA, *Proc. Natl. Acad. Sci. USA* **73**:3136–3140.

Roberts, W. K., Hovanessian, A., Brown, R. E., Clemens, M. J., and Kerr, I. M.,

1976*b*, Interferon-mediated protein kinase and low-molecular weight inhibitor of protein synthesis, *Nature (London)* **264**:477–480.

Rossi, G. B., Marchegiani, M., Matarese, G. P., and Gresser, I., 1975, Brief communication: Inhibitory effect of interferon on multiplication of Friend leukemia cells in vivo, *J. Natl. Cancer Inst.* **54**:993–996.

Rubinstein, M., Rubinstein, D., Familletti, P. C., Miller, R. S., Waldmann, A. A., and Pestka, S., 1979, Human leucocyte interferon: Production, purification to homogeneity, and initial characterization, *Proc. Natl. Acad. Sci. USA* **76**:640–644.

Rytel, M. W., and Hooks, J. J., 1977, Induction of immune interferon by murine cytomegalovirus, *Proc. Soc. Exp. Biol. Med.* **155**:611–614.

Rytel, M. W., and Kilbourne, E. D., 1966, The influence of cortisone on experimental viral infection. VIII. Suppression by cortisone of interferon formation in mice injected with Newcastle disease virus, *J. Exp. Med.* **123**:767–776.

Saito, S., Matsuno, T., Furuya, E., and Kohno, S., 1976, Priming activity of mouse interferon: Effect on interferon messenger RNA synthesis, *Arch. Virol.* **52**:159–163.

Salvin, S. B., Youngner, J. S., and Lederer, W. H., 1973, Migration inhibitory factor and interferon in the circulation of mice with delayed hypersensitivity, *Infect. Immun.* **7**:68–75.

Salvin, S. B., Ribi, E., Granger, D. L., and Youngner, J. S., 1975, Migration inhibitory factor and type II interferon in the circulation of mice sensitized with mycobacterial components, *J. Immunol.* **114**:354–359.

Samuel, C. E., and Farris, D. A., 1977, Mechanism of interferon action. Species specificity of interferon and of the interferon-mediated inhibitor of translation from mouse, monkey, and human cells, *Virology* **77**:556–565.

Samuel, C. E., Farris, D. A., and Eppstein, D. A., 1977, Mechanism of interferon action. Kinetics of interferon action in mouse L 929 cells: Translation inhibition protein phosphorylation and messenger RNA methylation and degradation, *Virology* **83**:56–71.

Sarma, P. S., Baron, S., Huebner, R. J., and Shiu, G., 1969, Inhibitory effect of a synthetic interferon inducer on murine sarcoma and leukaemia virus infection *in vitro*, *Nature (London)* **224**:604–605.

Schultz, R. M., Papamatheakis, J. D., Stylos, W. A., and Chirigos, M. A., 1976, Augmentation of specific macrophage mediated cytotoxicity: Correlation with agents which enhance antitumor resistance, *Cell. Immunol.* **25**:309–316.

Schultz, R. M., Papamatheakis, J. D., and Chirigos, M. A., 1977, Interferon: An inducer of macrophage activation by polyanions, *Science* **197**:674–676.

Schultz, R. M., Chirigos, M. A., and Heine, U. I., 1978, Functional and morphologic characteristics of interferon-treated macrophages, *Cell. Immunol.* **35**:84–91.

Sehgal, P. B., and Tamm, I., 1976, An evaluation of messenger RNA competition in the shutoff of human interferon production, *Proc. Natl. Acad. Sci. USA* **73**:1621–1625.

Sehgal, P. B., Tamm, I., and Vilček, J., 1975, Human interferon production: Superinduction by 5,6-dichloro-1-β-D-ribofuranosylbenzimidazole, *Science* **190**:282–284.

Sehgal, P. B., Dobberstein, B., and Tamm, I., 1977, Interferon messenger RNA content of human fibroblasts during induction, shutoff, and superinduction of interferon production, *Proc. Natl. Acad. Sci. USA* **74**:3409–3413.

Sehgal, P. B., Lyles, D. S., and Tamm, I., 1978, Superinduction of human fibroblast interferon production: Further evidence for increased stability of interferon mRNA, *Virology* **89**:186–198.

Sen, G. C., Lebleu, B., Brown, G. E., Kawakita, M., Slattery, E., and Lengyel, P., 1976, Interferon, double-stranded RNA and mRNA degradation, *Nature (London)* **264**:370–373.

Sen, G. C., Shaila, S., Brown, G. E., Desrosiers, R. C., and Lengyel, P., 1977, Impairment of reovirus mRNA methylation in extracts of interferon-treated Ehrlich ascites tumor cells: Further characteristics of the phenomenon, *J. Virol.* **21**:69–83.

Shaila, S., Lebleu, B., Brown, G. E., Sen, G. C., and Lengyel, P., 1977, Characteristics of extracts from interferon-treated Hela cells: Presence of a protein kinase and endoribonuclease activated by double-stranded RNA and of an inhibitor of mRNA methylation, *J. Gen. Virol.* **37**:535–546.

Shapiro, S. Z., Strand, M., and Billiau, A., 1977, Synthesis and cleavage processing of oncornavirus proteins during interferon inhibition of virus particle release, *Infect. Immun.* **16**:742–747.

Sheaff, E. T., Meager, A., and Burke, D. C., 1972, Factors involved in the production of interferon by inactivated Newcastle disease virus, *J. Gen. Virol.* **17**:163–175.

Simon, E. H., Kung, S., Koh, T. T., and Brandman, P., 1976, Interferon-sensitive mutants of mengovirus. I. Isolation and biological characterization, *Virology* **69**:727–736.

Sipe, J. D., De Maeyer-Guignard, J., Fauconnier, B., and De Maeyer, E., 1973, Purification of mouse interferon by affinity chromatography on a solid-phase immunoadsorbent, *Proc. Natl. Acad. Sci. USA* **70**:1037–1040.

Slate, D. L., and Ruddle, F. H., 1979, Fibroblast interferon in man is coded by two loci on separate chromosomes, *Cell* **16**:171–180.

Slate, D. L., Shulman, L., Lawrence, J. B., Revel, M., and Ruddle, F. H., 1978, Presence of human chromosome 21 alone is sufficient for hybrid cell sensitivity to human interferon, *J. Virol.* **25**:319–325.

Smith, T. J., and Wagner, R. R., 1967, Rabbit macrophages interferons. I. Conditions for biosynthesis by virus-infected and uninfected cells, *J. Exp. Med.* **125**:559–577.

Sonnenfeld, G., Salvin, S. B., and Youngner, J. S., 1977a, Cellular source of interferons in the circulation of mice with delayed hypersensitivity, *Infect. Immun.* **18**:283–290.

Sonnenfeld, G., Mandel, A. D., and Merigan, T. C., 1977b, The immunosuppressive effect of type II mouse interferon preparations on antibody production, *Cell. Immunol.* **34**:193–206.

Sonnenfeld, G., Mandel, A. D., and Merigan, T. C., 1978, Time and dosage dependence of immunoenhancement by murine type II interferon preparations, *Cell. Immunol.* **40**:285–293.

Sonnenfeld, G., Mandel, A. D., and Merigan, T. C., 1979, *In vitro* production and cellular origin of murine type II interferon, *Immunology* **36**:883–890.

Stebbing, N., Dawson, K. M., and Lindley, I. J. D., 1978, Requirement for macrophages for interferon to be effective against encephalomyocarditis virus infection of mice, *Infect. Immun.* **19**:5–11.

Stern, R., and Friedman, R. M., 1971, Ribonucleic acid synthesis in animal cells in the presence of actinomycin, *Biochemistry* **10**:3635–3645.

Stewart, W. E., II, 1974, Distinct molecular species of interferons, *Virology* **61**:80–86.

Stewart, W. E., II, and Desmyter, J., 1975, Molecular heterogeneity of human leukocyte interferon: Two populations differing in molecular weights, requirements for renaturation and cross-species antiviral activity, *Virology* **67**:68–73.

Stewart, W. E., II, Gosser, L. B., and Lockart, R. Z., Jr., 1971, Priming: A non antiviral function of interferon, *J. Virol.* **7**:792–801.

Stewart, W. E., II, De Clercq, E., and De Somer, P., 1972, Recovery of cell-bound interferon, *J. Virol.* **10**:707–712.

Stewart, W. E., II, De Clercq, E., and De Somer, P., 1974a, Stabilisation of interferons by defensive reversible denaturation, *Nature (London)* **249**:460–461.

Stewart, W. E., II, De Somer, P., and De Clercq, E., 1974b, Protective effects of anionic detergents on interferons: Reversible denaturation, *Biochim. Biophys. Acta* **359**:364–368.

Stewart, W. E., II, De Somer, P., Edy, V. G., Paucker, K., Berg, K., and Ogburn, C. A., 1975, Distinct molecular species of human interferons: Requirements for stabilization and reactivation of human leukocyte and fibroblast interferons, *J. Gen. Virol.* **26**:327–331.

Stewart, W. E., II, Gresser, I., Tovey, M. G., Bandu, M. T., and Le Goff, S., 1976, Identification of the cell multiplication inhibitory factors in interferon preparations as interferons, *Nature (London)* **262**:300–302.

Stewart, W. E., II, Lin, L. S., Wiranowska-Stewart, M., and Cantell, K., 1977a, Elimination of size and charge heterogeneities of human leukocyte interferons by chemical cleavage, *Proc. Natl. Acad. Sci. USA* **74**:4200–4204.

Stewart, W. E., II, Le Goff, S., and Wiranowska-Stewart, M., 1977b, Characterization of two distinct molecular populations of type I mouse interferons, *J. Gen. Virol.* **37**:277–284.

Stewart, W. E., II, Chudzio, T., Lin, L. S., and Wiranowska-Stewart, M., 1978, Interferoids: *In vitro* and *in vivo* conversion of native interferons to lower molecular weight forms, *Proc. Natl. Acad. Sci. USA* **75**:4814–4818.

Stinebring, W. R., and Absher, P. M., 1970, Production of interferon following an immune response, *Ann. N.Y. Acad. Sci.* **173**:713–714.

Stobo, J., Green, I., Jackson, L., and Baron, S., 1974, Identification of a subpopulation of mouse lymphoid cells required for interferon production after stimulation with mitogens, *J. Immunol.* **112**:1589–1593.

Strander, H., Mogensen, K. E., and Cantell, K., 1975, Production of human lymphoblastoid interferon, *J. Clin. Microbiol.* **1**:116–117.

Stringfellow, D. A., 1975, Hyporeactivity to interferon induction: Characterization of a hyporeactive factor in the serum of encephalomyocarditis virus-infected mice, *Infect. Immun.* **11**:294–302.

Stringfellow, D. A., 1976, Murine leukemia: Depressed response to interferon induction correlated with a serum hyporeactive factor, *Infect. Immun.* **13**:392–398.

Stringfellow, D. A., Kern, E. R., Kelsey, D. K., and Glasgow, L. A., 1977, Suppressed response to interferon induction in mice infected with encephalomyocarditis virus, Semliki forest virus, influenza A2 virus, herpes virus hominis type 2, or murine cytomegalovirus, *J. Infect. Dis.* **135**:540–551.

Sulkowski, E., Davey, M. W., and Carter, W. A., 1976, Interaction of human interferons with immobilized hydrophobic amino acids and dipeptides, *J. Biol. Chem.* **251**:5381–5385.

Sutton, R. N. P., and Tyrrell, D. A. J., 1961, Some observations on interferon prepared in tissue cultures, *Br. J. Exp. Pathol.* **42**:99–105.

Swart, B. E., and Young, B. G., 1969, Inverse relationship of interferon production and virus content in cell lines from Burkitt's lymphoma and acute leukemias, *J. Natl. Cancer Inst.* **42**:941–944.

Takemoto, K. K., and Baron, S., 1966, Nonheritable interferon resistance in a fraction of virus populations, *Proc. Soc. Exp. Biol. Med.* **121**:286–287.

Talas, M., Szolgay, E., and Rozsa, K., 1972, Further study of spontaneous interferon produced by hamster peritoneal cells, *Arch. Gesamte Virusforsch.* **38**:149–158.

Tan, Y. H., 1975, Chromosome-21-dosage effect on inducibility of antiviral gene(s), *Nature (London)* **253**:280–282.

Tan, Y. H., and Berthold, W., 1977, A mechanism for the induction and regulation of human fibroblastoid interferon genetic expression, *J. Gen. Virol.* **34**:401–411.

Tan, Y. H., and Greene, A. E., 1976, Subregional localization of the gene(s) governing the human interferon induced antiviral state in man, *J. Gen. Virol.* **32**:153–155.

Tan, Y. H., Armstrong, J. A., Ke, Y. H., and Ho, M., 1970, Regulation of cellular interferon production: Enhancement by antimetabolites, *Proc. Natl. Acad. Sci. USA* **67**:464–471.

Tan, Y. H., Armstrong, J. A., and Ho, M., 1971a, Accentuation of interferon production by metabolic inhibitors and its dependence on protein synthesis, *Virology* **3**:503–509.

Tan, Y. H., Armstrong, J. A., and Ho, M., 1971b, Intracellular interferon: Kinetics of formation and release, *Virology* **45**:837–840.

Tan, Y. H., Jeng, D. K., and Ho, M., 1972, The release of interferon: An active process inhibited by p-hydroxymercuribenzoate, *Virology* **48**:41–48.

Tan, Y. H., Tischfield, J. and Ruddle, F. H., 1973, The linkage of genes for the human interferon-induced antiviral protein and indophenol oxidase-B traits to chromosome G-21, *J. Exp. Med.* **137**:317–330.

Tan, Y. H., Creagan, R. P., and Ruddle, F. H., 1974a, The somatic cell genetics of human interferon: Assignment of human interferon loci to chromosomes 2 and 5, *Proc. Natl. Acad. Sci. USA* **71**:2251–2255.

Tan, Y. H., Schneider, E. L., Tischfield, J., Epstein, C. J., and Ruddle, F. H., 1974b, Human chromosome 21 dosage: Effect on the expression of the interferon induced antiviral state, *Science* **186**:61–63.

Tan, Y. H., Tan, C., and Berthold, W., 1977, Genetic control of the interferon system, *Tex. Rep. Biol. Med.* **35**:63–68.

Tarr, G. C., Armstrong, J. A., and Ho, M., 1978, Production of interferon and serum hyporeactivity factor in mice infected with murine cytomegalovirus, *Infect. Immun.* **19**:903–907.

Taylor, J., 1964, Inhibition of interferon action by actinomycin, *Biochem. Biophys. Res. Commun.* **14**:447–451.

Thang, M. N., Thang, D. C., De Maeyer, E., and Montagnier, L., 1975, Biosynthesis of mouse interferon by translation of its messenger RNA in a cell-free system, *Proc. Natl. Acad. Sci. USA* **72**:3975–3977.

Thang, M. N., Bachner, L., De Clercq, E., and Stollar, B. D., 1977a, A continuous high molecular weight base-paired structure is not an absolute requirement for a potential polynucleotide inducer of interferon, *FEBS Lett.* **76**:159–165.

Thang, M. N., De Maeyer-Guignard, J., and De Maeyer, E., 1977b, Interaction of interferon with tRNA, *FEBS Lett.* **80**:365–370.

Törma, E. T., and Paucker, K., 1976, Purification and characterization of human leukocyte interferon components, *J. Biol. Chem.* **251**:4810–4816.

Torrence, P. F., and De Clercq, E., 1977, Inducers and induction of interferons, *Pharmacol. Ther.* **A2**:1–88.

Tovey, M., Brouty-Boye, D., and Gresser, I., 1975, Early effect of interferon on mouse

leukemia cells cultivated in a chemostat, *Proc. Natl. Acad. Sci. USA*
72:2265–2269.

Trinchieri, G., Santoli, D., Dee, R. R., and Knowles, B. B., 1978, Antiviral activity
induced by culturing lymphocytes with tumor-derived or virus-transformed cells.
Identification of the antiviral activity as interferon and characterization of the
human effector lymphocyte subpopulation, *J. Exp. Med.* **147**:1299–1313.

Tsukui, K., 1977, Influenza virus-induced interferon production in mouse spleen cell
culture: T cells as the main producer, *Cell. Immunol.* **32**:243–251.

Tytell, A. A., Lampson, G. P., Field, A. K., and Hilleman, M. R., 1967, Inducers of
interferon and host resistance. III. Double-stranded RNA from reovirus type 3
virions (REO 3-RNA), *Proc. Natl. Acad. Sci. USA* **58**:1719–1722.

Tytell, A. A., Lampson, G. P., Field, A. K., Nemes, M. M., and Hilleman, M. R.,
1970, Influence of size of individual homopolynucleotides on the physical and biological properties of complexed $rI_n:rI_c$ (poly I·C), *Proc. Soc. Exp. Biol. Med.*
135:917–921.

Ustacelebi, S., and Williams, J. F., 1972, Temperature-sensitive mutants of adenovirus
defective in interferon induction at non-permissive temperature, *Nature (London):*
235:52–53.

Valle, M. J., Jordan, G. W., Haahr, S., and Merigan, T. C., 1975a, Characteristics of
immune interferon produced by human lymphocyte cultures compared to other
human interferons, *J. Immunol.* **115**:230–233.

Valle, M. J., Bodrove, A. M., Strober, S., and Merigan, T. C., 1975b, Immune specific
production of interferon by human T cells in combined macrophage-lymphocyte
cultures in response to herpes simplex antigen, *J. Immunol.* **114**:435–441.

Vengris, V. E., Stollar, B. D., and Pitha, P. M., 1975, Interferon externalization by
producing cell before induction of antiviral state, *Virology* **65**:410–417.

Vengris, V. E., Reynolds, F. H., Jr., Hollenberg, M. D., and Pitha, P. M., 1976,
Interferon action: Role of membrane gangliosides, *Virology* **72**:486–493.

Vilček, J., 1963, Production of interferon by newborn and adult mice infected with
Sindbis virus, *Virology* **22**:651–652.

Vilček, J., and Kohase, M., 1977, Regulation of interferon production: Cell culture
studies, *Tex. Rep. Biol. Med.* **35**:57–62.

Vilček, J., and Ng, M. H., 1971, Post-transcriptional control of interferon synthesis, *J.
Virol.* **7**:588–594.

Vilček, J., and Rada, B., 1962, Studies on an interferon from Tick-borne encephalitis
virus-infected cells (IF) III. Antiviral action of interferon, *Acta Virol.* **6**:9–16.

Vilček, J., and Stancek, D., 1963, Formation and properties of interferon in the brain
of tick-borne encephalitis virus-infected mice, *Acta Virol.* **7**:331–338.

Vilček, J., Rossman, T. G., and Varacalli, F., 1969, Differential effects of actinomycin
D and puromycin on the release of interferon induced by double stranded RNA,
Nature (London) **222**:682–683.

Vilček, J., Havell, E. A., and Kohase, M., 1976, Superinduction of interferon with
metabolic inhibitors: Possible mechanisms and practical applications, *J. Infect.
Dis.* **133**:A22–A29.

Vilček, J., Havell, E. A., and Yamazaki, S., 1977, Antigenic, physicochemical and biologic characterization of human interferons, *Ann. N.Y. Acad. Sci.* **284**:703–710.

Virelizier, J. L., and Gresser, I., 1978, Role of interferon in the pathogenesis of viral
diseases of mice as demonstrated by the use of anti-interferon serum. V. Protective
role in mouse hepatitis virus type 3 infection of susceptible and resistant strains of
mice, *J. Immunol.* **120**:1616–1619.

Virelizier, J. L., Virelizier, A. M., and Allison, A. C., 1976, The role of circulating interferon in the modifications of immune responsiveness by mouse hepatitis virus (MHV 3), *J. Immunol.* **117**:748–753.

Virelizier, J. L., Allison, A. C., and De Maeyer, E., 1977*a*, Production by mixed lymphocyte cultures of a type II interferon able to protect macrophages against virus infections, *Infect. Immun.* **17**:282–285.

Virelizier, J. L., Chan, E. L., and Allison, A. C., 1977*b*, Immunosuppressive effects of lymphocyte (type II) and leucocyte (type I) interferon on primary antibody response *in vivo* and *in vitro*, *Clin. Exp. Immunol.* **30**:299–304.

Volckaert-Vervliet, G., and Billiau, A., 1977, Induction of interferon in human lymphoblastoid cells by Sendal and Measles viruses, *J. Gen. Virol.* **37**:199–203.

Von Pirquet, C., 1908, Das Verhalten der kutanen tuberkulin-reaktion während der masern, *Dtsch. Med. Wochenschr.* **34**:1297–1300.

Wagner, R. R., 1963, The interferons: Cellular inhibitors of viral infection, *Annu. Rev. Microbiol.* **17**:285–296.

Wagner, R. R., 1964, Inhibition of interferon biosynthesis by actinomycin D, *Nature (London)* **204**:49–51.

Wagner, R. R., and Huang, A. S., 1965, Reversible inhibition of interferon synthesis by puromycin: Evidence for an interferon specific messenger RNA, *Proc. Natl. Acad. Sci. USA* **54**:1112–1118.

Wallen, W. C., Dean, J. H., and Lucas, D. O., 1973, Interferon and the cellular immune response: Separation of interferon-producing cells from DNA-synthetic cells, *Cell. Immunol.* **6**:110–122.

Wheelock, E. F., 1965, Interferon-like virus-inhibitor induced in human leukocytes by phytohemagglutinin, *Science* **149**:310–311.

Wheelock, E. F., 1966, Virus replication and high-titered interferon production in human leukocyte cultures inoculated with Newcastle disease virus, *J. Bacteriol.* **92**:1415–1421.

Wiebe, M. E., and Joklik, W. K., 1975, The mechanism of inhibition of reovirus replication by interferon, *Virology* **66**:229–240.

Wietzerbin, J., Falcoff, R., Catinot, L., and Falcoff, E., 1977, Affinity chromatographic analysis of murine interferons induced by viruses and by T and B cell stimulants, *Ann. Immunol.* **128C**:699–708.

Wietzerbin, J., Stefanos, S., Falcoff, R., Lucero, M., Catinot, L., and Falcoff, E., 1978, Immune interferon induced by phytohemagglutinin in nude mouse spleen cells, *Infect. Immun.* **21**:966–972.

Williams, B. R. G., and Kerr, I. M., 1978, Inhibition of protein synthesis by 2′-5′ linked adenine oligonucleotides in intact cells, *Nature (London)* **276**:88–89.

Wiranoswaks-Stewart, M., and Stewart, W. E., 1977, The role of human chromosome 21 in sensitivity to interferons, *J. Gen. Virol.* **37**:629–633.

Yakobson, E., Revel, M., and Winocour, E., 1977*a*, Inhibition of simian virus 40 replication by interferon treatment late in the lytic cycle, *Virology* **80**:225–228.

Yakobson, E., Prives, C., Hartman, J. R., Winocour, E., and Revel, M., 1977*b*, Inhibition of viral protein synthesis in monkey cells treated with interferon late in simian virus 40 lytic cycle, *Cell* **12**:73–81.

Yamamoto, K., Yamaguchi, N., and Oda, K., 1975, Mechanism of interferon-induced inhibition of early simian virus 40 (SV40) functions, *Virology* **68**:58–70.

Yamamoto, Y., and Kawade, Y., 1976, Purification of two components of mouse L cell interferon: Electrophoretic demonstration of interferon proteins, *J. Gen. Virol.* **33**:225–236.

Young, C. S. H., Pringle, C. R., and Follett, E. A. C., 1975, Action of interferon in enucleated cells, *J. Virol.* **15**:428–429.

Youngner, J. S., and Hallum, J. V., 1969, Inhibition of induction of interferon synthesis in L-cells pretreated with interferon, *Virology* **37**:473–475.

Youngner, J. S., and Salvin, S. B., 1973, Production and properties of migration inhibitory factor and interferon in the circulation of mice with delayed hypersensitivity, *J. Immunol.* **111**:1914–1922.

Youngner, J. S., and Stinebring, W. R., 1965, Interferon appearance stimulated by endotoxin, bacteria, or viruses in mice pre-treated with *Escherichia coli* endotoxin or infected with mycobacterium tuberculosis, *Nature (London)* **208**:456–458.

Youngner, J. S., Stinebring, W. R., and Taube, S. E., 1965, Influence of inhibitors of protein synthesis on interferon formation in mice, *Virology* **27**:541–550.

Youngner, J. S., Scott, A. W., Hallum, J. V., and Stinebring, W. R., 1966, Interferon production by inactivated Newcastle disease virus in cell cultures and in mice, *J. Bacteriol.* **92**:862–868.

Zajac, B. A., Henle, W., and Henle, G., 1969, Autogenous and virus-induced interferons from lines of lymphoblastoid cells, *Cancer Res.* **29**:1467–1475.

Zilberstein, A., Dudock, B., Berissi, H., and Revel, M., 1976a, Control of messenger RNA translation by minor species of leucyl-transfer RNA in extracts from interferon-treated L cells, *J. Mol. Biol.* **108**:43–54.

Zilberstein, A., Federman, P., Shulman, L., and Revel, M., 1976b, Specific phosphorylation *in vitro* of a protein associated with ribosomes of interferon-treated mouse L cells, *FEBS Lett.* **68**:119–124.

Zilberstein, A., Kimchi, A., Schmidt, A., and Revel, M., 1978, Isolation of two interferon-induced translational inhibitors: A protein kinase and an oligo-isoadenylate synthetase, *Proc. Natl. Acad. Sci. USA* **75**:4734–4738.

Zoon, K. C., and Buckler, C. E., 1977, Large-scale production of human interferon in lymphoblastoid cells, *Tex. Rep. Biol. Med.* **35**:145–149.

Index